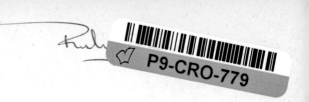

FEARS AND PHOBIAS

PERSONALITY AND PSYCHOPATHOLOGY:
A Series of Monographs, Texts, and Treatises

1. The Anatomy of Achievement Motivation, *Heinz Heckhausen.* 1966
2. Cues, Decisions, and Diagnoses: A Systems-Analytic Approach to the Diagnosis of Psychopathology, *Peter E. Nathan.* 1967
3. Human Adaptation and Its Failures, *Leslie Phillips.* 1968
4. Schizophrenia: Research and Theory, *William E. Broen, Jr.* 1968
5. Fears and Phobias, *I. M. Marks.* 1969

FEARS AND PHOBIAS

by

ISAAC M. MARKS

Senior Lecturer at the Institute of Psychiatry and Honorary Consultant Psychiatrist at Bethlem Royal and Maudsley Hospitals, London, S.E.5

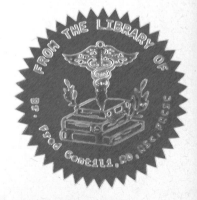

ACADEMIC PRESS · NEW YORK AND LONDON

Printed in Great Britain by R. J. Acford, Ltd., Industrial Estate, Chichester, Sussex.

Preface

Phobias are an important and fashionable topic today as a result of advances in the behavioural sciences. Hundreds of articles about phobias have appeared in recent years, but these are scattered widely in journals and books across many areas. It is therefore difficult for the interested doctor, psychologist or research worker to appraise the subject. This book is a pilot attempt by a psychiatrist to review the field and to synthesise the different viewpoints of learning theory, psychoanalysis, ethology and clinical psychiatry. Present insights into such a growing field are necessarily provisional and will have to be modified repeatedly as knowledge increases.

Much dispute has arisen about the causes and treatment of phobias because psychologists and psychiatrists see rather different populations of phobics and are arguing from different clinical material. Only when the differing populations are compared does it become obvious that generalisations which are true for one population are not true for another, and that more complex formulations are necessary to account for the whole range of populations. In fact, many phobias do behave like simple learned habits, and these are the ones usually seen by psychologists rather than psychiatrists. Equally, however, many other phobias are part of a complex disorder which is more the province of psychiatrists. Proper understanding of phobic disorders can only come eventually from survey of the area as a whole, with due regard for biological and psychological developments which are relevant to the subject. This book was written as a small step in that direction.

I.M.M.

London, January 1969

Acknowledgements

The ideas in this book have crystallised during several years' research into the treatment of phobias at the Maudsley Hospital and Institute of Psychiatry. They reflect discussions with many psychiatrists and psychologists on both sides of the Atlantic. Of particular help in shaping the concepts were Dr. Michael Gelder, now professor of psychiatry at Oxford, with whom I have enjoyed many years of fruitful collaboration, and Dr. Malcolm Lader and Mr. Andrew Mathews, who also read the manuscript and made many valuable suggestions in the final stages. Dr. Alwyn Lishman, Mr. David Milner and Mr. Richard Passingham kindly read and commented on Chapter 2. Many other seminal ideas arose from discussions with Professors Albert Bandura, Jerome Frank, Sir Denis Hill, Fred Kanfer, and Martin Roth and Drs. Stewart Agras, David Malan, Desmond Morris, Jack Rachman, Cyril Rashbass, Henry Rey, Joseph Sandler and Heinz Wolff. The sections on children's phobias were written together with Dr. Gelder. The clinical research into treatment of phobias was generously supported by the Medical Research Council. I am also very grateful to Mrs. Eileen Wade and Mr. Claude Inniss for their sterling secretarial aid.

Acknowledgements for permission to reproduce material in the book: Table 2.1: Mrs. T. C. Schneirla for kind permission in the name of her late husband Dr. Theodore C. Schneirla, and Academic Press Inc., who hold the copyright. Figs. 2.1 and 2.2: Dr. G. P. Sackett and Science, Copyright 1966 by the American Association for the Advancement of Science. Fig. 2.3: Professor Stanley Schachter and Stanford University Press. Fig. 2.4: Dr. Albert F. Ax and Hoeber Medical Journals. Figs. 2.5 and 2.6: Dr. Glenn D. Wilson, and to Perceptual and Motor Skills and the New Zealand Medical Journal. Fig. 2.7: Dr. Michael Gelder and Mr. Andrew Mathews. Fig 2.8: Dr. Denis Williams and Brain. Fig. 2.9: Mrs. Berry Weil for kind permission in the name of her late husband Dr. André A. Weil and Archives of Neurology. Fig. 4.1: Professor Peter J. Lang and McGraw-Hill Book Co. Figs. 4.5, 4.6, 4.7, 4.9, 4.11: British Journal of Psychiatry. Fig. 4.10: Pergamon Press Ltd., copyright 1967. Fig. 4.13: Professor Albert Bandura. Fig. 4.14: Dr. W. Stewart Agras and American Medical Association. The Appendix: Professor Arnold A. Lazarus and Pergamon Press Ltd., copyright 1966.

Contents

CHAPTER   PAGE

PREFACE

ACKNOWLEDGEMENTS

1. INTRODUCTION   1
   Historical aspects of phobias   7

2. AETIOLOGY OF FEAR   13
   Section   I. The origins of fear   13
                 A. Innateness maturation and learning   13
                 B. Innate and maturational elements
                     in fear   16
                     I. Genetic aspects of timidity   16
                     II. The kinds of situations which are
                         feared   18
                 Summary   34

   Section   II. Physiology and learning of fear   36
                 A. Physiological mechanisms for
                     expressing and learning fear   36
                 B. Psychological mechanisms for learning
                     fear   55
                 Summary   69

   Section III. Aetiology of phobias   72
                 A. Background features   72
                 B. Direct influences   85
                 Summary   100

3. THE CLINICAL SYNDROMES   102
   Section   I.   Classification of phobic disorders   102
      ,,   II.   The agoraphobic syndrome   119
      ,,   III.   Specific animal phobias   147
      ,,   IV.   Social phobias   152
      ,,   V.   Miscellaneous other phobias   157
      ,,   VI.   Illness phobias   159
      ,,   VII.   Obsessive phobias   163
      ,,   VIII.   Autonomic equivalents to phobic disorders   165
      ,,   IX.   Children's fears and phobias   166

PAGE

4. TREATMENT OF PHOBIAS 178
   Section   I. Introduction 179
   ,,   II. Desensitisation 182
   ,,   III. Techniques other than desensitisation which improve phobias 234
           A. Experimental methods 234
           B. Clinical methods 245
   ,,   IV. Treatment of phobias in children 255
   ,,   V. The psychiatric management of phobic patients 260
          Summary 267

Bibliography 271

Appendix 289

Author index 292

Subject index 297

Chapter 1

INTRODUCTION

"Many lamentable effects this fear causeth in men, as to be red, pale, tremble, sweat; it makes sudden cold and heat to come all over the body, palpitation of the heart, syncope.... Many men are so amazed and astonished with fear, they know not where they are, what they do; and (that which is worst) it tortures them, many dayes before, with continual affrights and suspicion. It hinders most honourable attempts, and makes their hearts ake, sad and heavy. They that live in fear, are never free, resolute, secure, never merry, but in continual pain; ... no greater misery, no rack, no torture, like unto it; ever suspicious, anxious solicitous, they are childishly drooping without reason, without judgement . . ." (Burton, 1621, p. 143–144).

Every man has experienced the emotion of fear. The word 'fear' comes from the Old English 'faer' for sudden calamity or danger, and was later used to describe the emotion of uneasiness caused by the sense of impending danger (OED). In Middle English it continued to denote a state of alarm or dread, and does so still today. Fear is a normal response to active or imagined threat in higher animals, and comprises an outer behavioural expression, an inner feeling, and accompanying physiological changes (Landis, 1964).

Two of the most obvious behavioural effects of fear present a striking contrast (Miller, 1951). One is the tendency to remain motionless and mute, which reaches its extreme form in the deathfeigning of certain animals. The other is the pattern of startle, withdrawal, running and vocalisation. Both of these incompatible patterns seem to be activated by fear, and behaviour may shift rapidly from one to the other, as when a frightened animal first freezes, then suddenly scurries for shelter.

Strong fear causes unpleasant subjective feelings of terror, a pounding heart, muscular tenseness, trembling, exaggerated startle, dryness of the throat and mouth, a sinking feeling in the stomach, nausea, perspiration, an urge to urinate and maybe to defaecate, irritability, aggresssion, a great urge to cry, run or hide, difficulty in breathing, paraesthesiae of the extremities, feelings of unreality, paralysing weakness of the limbs and a sensation of faintness and falling. Common chronic

1

effects of fear in healthy people are fatigue, a feeling of depression, slowing down of movements and mental processes, restlessness, aggression, loss of appetite, trembling, being easily startled, avoidance of further frightening situations, insomnia and nightmares (Wickert, 1947).

Many physiological changes accompany fearful behaviour and feelings. Among these are pallor, sweating, pilomotor erection, pupillary dilatation, tachycardia, hypertension, increased blood flow through the muscles, rapid breathing, fluctuations in the skin conductance, failure of habituation of the galvanic skin response, and contractions of the bladder and rectum leading to desires to urinate and defaecate. Biochemical changes include secretion of adrenaline by the adrenals, noradrenaline at the peripheral nerve endings, and an increase in the plasma free fatty acids. These physiological changes are not unique for fear alone, and may be found in other forms of intense emotional arousal.

The usefulness of fear: Fear is obviously useful since it often leads to rapid action in the face of threat. Fear can also motivate the learning and performance of socially useful responses such as driving carefully or writing an examination. Of men in aerial combat 50% reported that mild fear had a beneficial effect, and 37% thought they performed their duties better even when very afraid (Wickert, 1947, p. 131). Fear normally accompanies activities like parachuting, and fluctuates with other feelings at different phases of the activity. During preparation for the parachute jump both fear and enthusiasm increase. At the start of the jump run fear decreases and enthusiasm increases, reaching a nadir and zenith respectively when the parachute is opened. Near landing, fear again increases and enthusiasm decreases, while upon touching the ground fear drops to a new nadir and enthusiasm rises to a zenith above the first. Fear and enthusiasm are negatively correlated at successive points during parachute jumps (Klausner, 1966).

During frightening activities like parachuting the timing and amount of fear which is felt changes with experience. Walk (1956) showed that subjective fear diminished with experience in parachute jumping. Fenz and Epstein (1966) examined the timing of this change. Continuous recordings of the skin conductance, heart rate and respiration rate were measured in parachutists before and during a jump. Novice jumpers showed increasing reactivity right to the moment of the jump, whereas in experienced parachutists reactivity showed an initial rise but then a sharp drop shortly before the jump. It appeared that after repeated exposure to threat an adaptive mechanism developed. This provided for an initial increase in activation which gave an early signal of danger; this was then inhibited from becoming disruptive at the crucial moment of the jump.

Excessive fear can become disruptive, even though lesser amounts may be useful in activities like parachuting. High fear is correlated with poor performance in trainee parachutists (Walk, 1956) and even trained paratroopers become so afraid that they 'lose their nerve' and become unable to jump (The Times, 2nd and 3rd June, 1966).

Phobias

Phobias are a special kind of fear. The term 'phobia' derives from the Greek word *phobos* meaning flight, panic-fear, terror, and from the deity of the same name who could provoke fear and panic in one's enemies. The Greeks made fear masks by depicting the likeness of Phobos on weapons such as shields, and examples of these appear on vase paintings (Errera, 1962).

Although morbid fears were described by doctors from Hippocrates onwards, its sole medical usage before the 19th century was in Celsus's term hydrophobia for a prominent symptom of rabies (Errera, 1962). Only in 1801 was 'phobia' used on its own (OED), and during the next 70 years it slowly gained acceptance in the same sense as today, viz., a persistent excessive fear attached to an object or situation which objectively is not a significant source of danger. Definitions in the literature are remarkably alike:

Jaspers (1923): "an irresistible and terrifying fear of perfectly natural situations and performances".

Ross (1937): "a specific fear which the patient himself knows is ridiculous but which he cannot overcome".

Terhune (1949): "a strong unreasonable fear of specific situations inhibiting the person from entering or remaining in them".

Laughlin (1956): "a morbid fear out of proportion to the apparent stimulus . . . fear which is inappropriate and unreasoning. It is beyond voluntary control, and cannot adequately or logically be explained by the patient".

Errera (1962): "a persisting fear of an object or of an idea which does not ordinarily justify fear".

A *phobia* can thus be defined as a special form of fear which 1. *is out of proportion to demands of the situation*, 2. *cannot be explained or reasoned away*, 3. *is beyond voluntary control*, and 4. *leads to avoidance of the feared situation*.

Phobic patients usually recognise that their fear is excessive and unrealistic as most other people would not be unduly afraid of the same situation. Because they are unable to quell their phobia it is considered irrational and involuntary though rationalisations may be offered for it. The disproportion between a phobia and its stimulus is obvious in phobias of simpler situations such as feathers or minor heights, but such disproportion is also found in more complex phobias such as those of cancer or venereal disease, where the object or situation can only be avoided when it is external to the patient's own person. Phobic stimuli arising within themselves naturally cannot be avoided—such are phobias of disease or death, or of one's own harmful impulses. Phobias of this variety thus differ from phobias of external situations.

Patients experience overwhelming anxiety when confronted with their phobic situation. They manifest physiological signs of sweating, tremor, pallor, tachycardia, rapid breathing, diarrhoea, urinary frequency, nausea and vomiting and tightness of the chest. Phobic patients often rehearse their frightening experiences in their minds until they are in an agony of fearful anticipation about the next time they will meet their phobic object. The fear of fear is now a fresh source of dread. To escape such anxiety patients avoid their phobic situations and may greatly constrict their activities and daily function. Such avoidance reduces the phobia to more manageable proportions. Phobic patients develop selective attention to anything resembling the phobic object in their environment. As Rangell (1952) noted, the phobic patient becomes "married to the (phobic) object. In order to avoid it his eyes seek it out, he finds it in obscure places, he sees it with his peripheral vision". Conversely, one sign of improvement in a phobic patient during treatment is decreased awareness of the phobic object in his surroundings.

Many phobic objects are common and cannot easily be avoided. The life of a patient with phobias of cats, of crossing streets or bridges, of being in a crowd, or of travelling on a bus or train can be seriously disrupted. Kraupl Taylor (1966) has described the difficulties which beset phobic patients. The more common and familiar the phobic objects are the greater is the incomprehension and lack of compassion which the plight of the phobic arouses in normal people. It surpasses the intuitive understanding of normal people how anybody can be scared of a playful puppy, a fluttering bird or of going outside his home. It is often thought that the patient pretends or exaggerates, and should pull himself together or be forced to do so.

Concealment in an unsympathetic environment

Phobic patients are often sensitive to the lack of understanding among normal people. They are ashamed of their fears, and of ridicule by others for having these fears, so they often suffer in silence and hide their symptoms from an unsympathetic environment as long as they can. Even when the fears can no longer be hidden they may try to complain only of symptoms which are secondarily caused by their anxiety, such as headaches, palpitations, diarrhoea or fatigue. Phobic patients who keep their fears to themselves may develop the additional fear that they are mentally disturbed, and can obtain great comfort by meeting other patients with the same phobias and problems as themselves.

Because of the secretiveness of phobic patients the casual observer may not become aware of their fears. Agoraphobic housewives can be housebound for years without acquaintances or relatives realizing there is any problem. Many new cases of agoraphobia, for example, were discovered by accident in the course of a rehousing scheme in New York (Perman, 1966). Negro and Puerto Rican families who had been living in single rooms were rehoused and followed up by welfare workers. In many women phobic symptoms became apparent as soon as they moved into new homes in a new neighbourhood. Some mothers who could not sleep without close contact with their children or another adult tried to restore this sleeping arrangement, and might invite a sister or previous paramour to come and stay with them. Although the new apartments had several rooms only a single room would be used. Travel phobias became obvious, and clients were found to be fearful of doing anything alone.

As Kraupl Taylor (1966, p. 158) pointed out, phobic symptoms cannot be shed as easily as normal superstitions, but are less resistant to psychological pressure than psychotic delusions. In extreme adversity when survival is hard and dependent on constant vigilance and exertion, psychotic patients perish because they cannot compromise but phobic patients do not show their phobias. In the concentration camp of Theresienstadt in Nazi-occupied Europe in which 120,000 people (86%) died or were sent east to extermination camps, phobic symptoms either disappeared completely or improved to such a degree that patients could work. No new cases of phobia occurred, though schizophrenia and manic-depression developed in some people: several months after liberation and return home some of the old neurotics who had been free of complaints during their stay in the camp again developed their former symptoms (Kral, 1952).

The components of phobias

Fears and phobias involve at least 3 distinct components: a subjective inner state felt by patients, outer aspects visible to observers, and the physiological changes so far known to accompany these. Usually these 3 components are congruent and what a patient says he is feeling corresponds to what the clinician infers from the patient's visible behaviour. Difficulties of recognition do arise occasionally where fear appears present but is denied, where fear seems absent to the observer while the patient claims it is present, or where there is subtle disproportion between these two aspects, as, for example, in histrionic patients or in those states which we call stoicism and belle indifference.

Though the different components of fear are congruent, they are related imperfectly to one another. Subjective and behavioural aspects of fear are sometimes separable, as Lang showed (1966). About 20% of students reported fears of snakes on a questionnaire he gave them, yet only 1-2% actually avoided snakes when tested, and during the avoidance test subjective reports of fear correlated only $\cdot 40$ (n=23, p < $\cdot 05$)

with ability to approach the snake. Agras (1967) showed that physiological and behavioural aspects of fear do not always vary together. In five agoraphobic subjects the galvanic skin response to imagined phobic scenes only partly reflected subjects' ability to enter the phobic situations concerned. Thus the subjective, behavioural and physiological ingredients of fear together form a complex but not necessarily unitary response.

Anxiety is an emotion closely allied to fear and phobias. Derived from the Latin *anxius*, the term dates back at least to 1661, (OED), when it suggested a condition of agitation and depression with a sensation of tightness and distress in the praecordial region, but was also used to indicate solicitude, concern or disturbing suspense. Today it continues to describe apprehension or uneasiness without apparent cause; the assumption is sometimes made that this must be a response to an unknown internal stimulus. Many patients cannot recognise even an internal stimulus to their anxiety, and some writers speak here of an object 'completely obscure to conscious awareness' (Laughlin, 1956, p. 1).

Though the distinction between fear, anxiety and phobia must be arbitrary at some point, the three terms are best kept separate for most purposes since they describe rather different ranges of phenomena. Within this area of emotional experience varying nuances of feeling are implied by other terms such as misgiving, perturbation, haunt, apprehension, trepidation, dread, alarm, peril, horror and terror. Phobic patients commonly use such terms to express their experiences.

Panic denotes a sudden surge of acute terror. The term was in use by 1603 (OED) and derives from the Greek rural deity Pan. Not only was Pan supposed to preside over shepherds and flocks, and to delight in rural music, but he was also regarded as the author of abrupt and inexplicable terror. In later times he became an impersonation of Nature.

Certain phenomena shade into the phobias, yet it is possible and important to separate them as they generally have rather distinct correlates. Such phenomena include *superstitious fears and taboos*—the collective beliefs about dangerous situations which are shared by other members of the same cultural group; *obsessions*—the insistent recurrence of unwanted thoughts despite the patient's active resistance against their intrusion; *preoccupations*—the repetitive rumination of ideas without a subjective feeling of resistance; *sensitive ideas of reference*—the fear that actions and words of other people refer to oneself when they don't; and finally, some *paranoid delusions*, where the patient is convinced for no good reason that other persons or forces are threatening him.

Counterphobic behaviour: This is the attraction some patients have to their phobic situation or object so that they seek it out repeatedly. Such behaviour may occur when the phobia is relatively mild or when the patient attempts to master it. An example of this is a woman who was originally so afraid of heights that she would not ride on elevators, but who mastered her fear by subsequently becoming an air hostess (Frazier and Carr, 1967). Counterphobic behaviour may thus help the patient overcome his fear by gradually familiarising him with the phobic situation until it loses its frightening aspect. The phobic situation may then become an overvalued and highly attractive object for a while (Kraupl Taylor, 1966, p. 172). The patient with a phobia of the sea then turns into an enthusiastic swimmer and sailor, or a person with former stage fright then seizes every opportunity for public speaking.

Counterphobic behaviour is similar to that observed in children who enjoy playing frightening games, or in adults who derive pleasure from risky endeavours like high speed racing or dangerous mountaineering.

A *soteria* is the converse of a phobia. The term was coined by Laughlin (1956) to describe the disproportionate comfort some people get from certain objects or situations. The word derives from the Greek *soteria* denoting a festive entertainment given on a person's recovery from illness or escape from danger.

Examples of soterias are the toys and stuffed animals which young children carry around with them, and the talismans and charms which many adults wear. Phobic patients may develop a soterial attachment to an object which reduces their fear, e.g. some get comfort from carrying round a bottle of smelling salts in case they feel in danger of fainting, while others are comforted by the knowledge that they have a supply of sedative drugs in their pocket, and this reassures them without their having to take the drug. Further descriptions of soterial behaviour appear in Laughlin (1967).

HISTORICAL ASPECTS OF PHOBIAS

The main point of this historical review is that clinical pictures of phobic disorders have not changed significantly since their earliest descriptions. This section is only intended for those who savour historical anecdotes. Other readers might prefer to skip these and proceed directly to the next chapter. As we have seen, the word 'phobia' was first used in a medical context by Celsus, the Roman encyclopaedist, in the first century, when he coined the term hydro-phobia. However, the term only appeared on its own in the psychiatric literature in the 19th century.

Clinical descriptions of morbid fears long antedate the appearance of the word phobia. As one might expect, Hippocrates gave good accounts of two phobic subjects (Ep. VII, 86 and 87). He referred to

"... the morbid condition of Nicanor. When he used to begin drinking, the girl flute-player would frighten him; as soon as he heard the first note of the flute at a banquet, he would be beset by

terror. He used to say he could scarcely contain himself when
night fell; but during the day he would hear this instrument
without feeling any emotion. This lasted a long time with him.

Damocles, who was with him, appeared to have dim vision and
to be quite slack in body; he could not go near a precipice, or over
a bridge, or beside even the shallowest ditch; and yet he could
walk in the ditch itself. This came upon him over a period of
time".

From Elizabethan times onwards" many references were made
to phobic behaviour. Shakespeare wrote of "some, that are mad if
they behold a cat" (Merchant of Venice) while Descartes (1650) alluded
to "the strange aversions of some, who cannot endure the smell of
roses, the sight of a cat, or the like . . .". Pascal, a contemporary of
Descartes, was said to have suffered from what we now call agoraphobia
(Weiss, 1964, p. 101). Sir Kenelm Digby (1644) described the discrimination of psychological aversion from physical allergy by a patch-test:

"Lady Heneage (who was of the bedchamber to the late Queen
Elizabeth) that had her cheeke blistered by laying a rose upon it
whiles she was asleepe, to try if her antipathy against that flower,
were so great as she used to pretend".

Digby also noted that "the antipathy of beasts towards one another
may be taken away by assuefaction", a treatment akin to modern
methods of desensitisation in which pleasant stimuli are administered
simultaneously with phobic ones.

The first comprehensive description of phobias appeared in 1621,
when Robert Burton published his monumental "Anatomy of Melancholy". In it he distinguished carefully between the emotions of
depression and of fear (p. 269), and gave an excellent account of normal
fear. Several historical figures were mentioned who had normal
fears. Tully and Demosthenes had stage fright, while Augustus Caesar could
not sit in the dark (p. 143–4).

Burton was also a keen observer of morbid fears, including agoraphobia and obsessive phenomena, and of the stratagems patient
adopted to obtain relief (p. 170–1).

"Montanus speaks of one that durst not walk alone from home,
for fear he should swoon, or die. A second fears every man he meets
will rob him, quarrel with him, or kill him. A third dares not venture to walk alone, for fear he should meet the devil, a thief, be
sick; fears all old women as witches; and every black dog or cat
he sees, he suspecteth to be a devil; . . . another dares not go over
a bridge, come near a pool, rock, steep hill, lye in a chamber where
cross beams are, for fear he be tempted to hang, drown or precipitate himself. If he be in a silent auditory, as at a sermon, he is
afraid he shall speak aloud, at unawares, something indecent, unfit
to be said. If he be locked in a close room, he is afraid of being

stifled for want of air, and still carries bisket, aquavitae, or some strong waters about him, for fear of deliquiums, or being sick; or if he be in a throng, middle of a church, multitude, where he may not well get out, though he sit at ease, he is so misaffected".

Burton made shrewd comments on the role of willpower in overcoming phobias, and his advice could well be heeded by relatives and physicians of phobic patients today. He observed (p. 306) that phobias were not the result of insufficient willpower but were due to causes outside the control of the patient, "take away the cause; and otherwise counsel can do little good: you may as well bid him that sick of an ague, not to be adry; or him that is wounded, not to feel pain".

Finally, Burton noted the role of the therapeutic relationship and the placebo effect on the relief of melancholy (p. 347):

". . . to be required in a patient, is confidence to be of good chear, and have sure hope that his physician can help him. . . . as Galen holds, 'confidence and hope do more than physick'; he cures most, in whom most are confident".

The learning of fear is a fashionable subject today. That innate and learned elements both play a part in the origin of fears was already clearly enunciated by Locke in 1700, when he wrote "Of the Association of Ideas":

". . . most of the antipathies, I do not say all, for some of them are truly natural, depend upon our original constitution and are born with us; but a great part of those which are counted natural, would have been known to be from unheeded, though perhaps early, impressions, or wanton fancies at first, which would have been acknowledged the original of them, if they had been warily observed . . . . The ideas of goblins and spirits have really no more to do with darkness than light; yet let but a foolish maid inculcate these often on the mind of a child, and raise them there together, possibly he shall never be able to separate them again so long as he lives; but darkness shall ever afterwards bring with it those frightful ideas, and they shall be so joined, that he can no more bear the one than the other".

A comprehensive study of phobias was made by the French surgeon Le Camus in his book "Des Aversions" (1769). He classified the aversions according to the five senses which might be affected—sight, hearing, touch, taste and smell. Le Camus listed many clinical cases, such as that of James I of England, who would be terrified at the sight of an unsheathed sword, and noted the contemporary comment on his personality—"Elizabeth was King, James 1st was Queen". Another sovereign, Germanicus, couldn't stand the sight or sound of cocks, and Montaigne, the French moralist, reported people who "flee from the smell of apples more than from the dangers of gunfire. Others have become frightened by the sight of a mouse or cream". Le Camus also described a doctor who had such an aversion for milk and cheese that he couldn't even smell or see it without falling in a faint. During this period typical features of phobic syndromes were described. Sauvages (1770) described the giddiness of phobic anxious patients and labelled their condition *vertigo hysterique* or *vertigo hypocondriaque*, since he thought vertigo was the dominant aspect of the disorder. He reported a woman who was afraid of falling and had attacks of vertigo whenever she entered an empty church. A century later Benedikt (1870) was to regard the same feature of giddiness as the hallmark of the agoraphobic syndrome (phobic anxiety state) to the extent that he labelled the disorder *platzschwindel*. The dizziness was ascribed to dysfunction of the eye muscles. A few years earlier Simon (1858) cited Sauvages' interest in vertigo and fear, and described phobic patients with *vertige nerveux idiopathique ou primitif*. Not long after Sauvages' observations Beauchêne (1783) noted how the presence of a companion often resulted in relief of the symptoms of a phobic patient.

Bru (1789) recounted cases of syphilophobia at this time, which he named *manie verolique*—syphilitic mania. The history of syphilophobia was outlined by MacAlpine (1957) who cited many works not generally available. Syphilophobia was well described already in the 17th century medical and surgical literature, and by 1721 Freind wrote about a salient feature of syphilophobia that still applies:

> "if but a pimple appears or any slight ache is felt, they distract themselves with terrible apprehensions: by which means they make life uneasy to themselves and run for help ... And so strongly are they for the most part possessed with this notion that an honest practitioner generally finds it more difficult to cure the imaginary evil than the real one".

An autobiographical account of syphilophobia appeared in John Hunter's 'Treatise on the Venereal Disease' in 1810. The term "syphilophobia" itself appeared first in a dictionary of medical science published in 1848 in Philadelphia by Dunglison, and was defined as "a morbid dread of syphilis giving rise to fancied symptoms of the disease". Throughout the 19th century many French and English writings appeared on the condition.

Until 1870 sporadic references to other phobias continued. Connolly's textbook in 1830 made brief comments on morbid fears. He cited examples of historical figures with phobias, instancing fears of cats in Henry III of France and in the Duke of Schonberg, and a famous Russian general who "entertained a singular antipathy to mirrors, and the Empress Catherine always took care to give him audience in a room without any "(p. 97–8). A contemporary of Connolly's who suffered from agoraphobia was the Italian writer Manzoni who was afraid of leaving home alone, had fears of fainting when he left home, and would carry a small bottle of concentrated vinegar wherever he went (Weiss, 1964, pp. 86 and 104).

Other writings at this time were reviewed by Errera (1962), whose article is a useful introduction to many historical aspects of phobic disorders. Etiological theories in the early 19th century concerned poor upbringing, stomach ailments and autonomic dysfunction. Hereditary factors were regarded as important, and a family was described where the grandmother, mother and daughter experienced an identical fear of water. The well-known neuro-psychiatrist Morel described his own fear of heights in 1866. However, many authors still failed to separate the phobic disorders from other conditions which gave rise to delusional fears.

Full clinical description of phobic disorders in their own right began with Westphal's (1871) classic description of three male patients who feared going into streets and public places, like the 'agora' of ancient Greece, and he coined the term agoraphobia to describe this condition. He pointed out that the thought of a feared situation was as distressing as the situation itself, and noted the relief afforded by companionship, alcohol, a vehicle or use of a cane.

At the time that Westphal described morbid fears so accurately, Charles Darwin (1872) turned his attention to the features of normal fear, and suggested that past selection processes had shaped present-day expressions of fear, even though those past pressures operated no longer. This foreshadowed Stanley Hall's observation in 1897 that the "relative intensity (of different fear elements) fits past conditions better than it does present ones". Darwin wrote (pp. 307–9):

"Men, during numberless generations, have endeavoured to escape from their enemies or danger by headlong flight, or by violently struggling with them; and such great exertions will have caused the heart to beat rapidly, the breathing to be hurried, the chest to heave, and the nostrils to be dilated. As these exertions have often been prolonged to the last extremity, the final result will have been utter prostration, pallor, perspiration, trembling of all the muscles, or their complete relaxation. And now, whenever the emotion of fear is strongly felt, though it may not lead to any exertion, the same results tend to reappear, through the force of inheritance and association.

With respect to the involuntary bristling of the hair, we have good reason to believe that in the case of animals this action, however it may have originated, serves, together with certain involuntary movements, to make them appear terrible to their enemies; and as the same involuntary and voluntary actions are performed by animals nearly related to man, we are led to believe that man has retained through inheritance a relic of them, now become useless. It is certainly a remarkable fact, that the minute unstriped muscles, by which the hairs thinly scattered over man's almost naked body are erected, should have been preserved to the present day; and that they should still contract under the same emotions, namely, terror and rage, which cause the hairs to stand on end in the lower members of the Order to which man belongs".

The period of Westphal and after was a seminal one for clinical psychiatry, and excellent accounts of different psychiatric syndromes began appearing from this time onwards. Phobic disorders were not clearly distinguished from delusional fears and many other disorders. Westphal himself also gave the earliest full description of obsessive-compulsive neurosis in 1878, while Kraepelin's observations on schizophrenia were made a few years later.

Many observers now gave good detailed case histories of phobic disorders. In 1894 Freud wrote an illuminating description of anxiety neurosis, which also included agoraphobic symptoms. In the following year Henry Maudsley wrote a memorable account of agoraphobia and related symptoms in his well-known textbook "The Pathology of Mind" (pp. 409–411). Further good clinical descriptions of the agoraphobic syndrome were published by du Saulle (1878), Clevenger (1890), Prince (1912) and Kraepelin (1913), while Freud gave a vivid portrayal of animal phobias in 1913.

Among prominent figures of this period who showed phobic symptoms were Freud himself, who had fears of travel and anxiety symptoms for a number of years (Jones, 1953), and Feydeau, the French dramatist, who practically never went out during the day because of a morbid fear of daylight (Charon, 1967).

After this period we reach modern times, and publications of this century form the substance of this book.

Chapter 2

AETIOLOGY OF FEAR

Section I. THE ORIGINS OF FEAR

A. Innateness, maturation and learning
B. Innate and maturational elements in fear
   I. Genetic aspects of timidity
  II. The kinds of situations which are feared
     1. The hawk effect
     2. Fears of heights—the "visual cliff"
     3. Social approach—avoidance behaviour
     4. Fear of novelty
     5. Fear of snakes
     6. Fears of being looked at
     7. Other fears with an innate origin
     8. The earliest fears of childhood
Summary

A. INNATENESS, MATURATION AND LEARNING

Phobias are persistent fears in an abnormal context. We therefore need to discuss what is known about the origin of normal fear before reviewing clinical evidence on the genesis of abnormal phobias.

In general fear, like other behaviour, develops through the interaction of three kinds of phenomena, those which are innate, those dependent on maturation and those developed through learning from individual and social experience. The contribution of these three sources to a particular response varies roughly according to the degree of evolution of the cerebral cortex. The more primitive the species, the more it depends on innate mechanisms of response, the shorter is the time it takes to mature, and the less is its capacity for learning. In snakes the newborn animal closely resembles the adult in form and behaviour and learns little beyond its innate repertoire of responses (Morris and Morris, 1965). In birds the newly hatched chick matures quite rapidly; its innate responses are modified slightly by subsequent experience, and there is even room for embryo traditions to develop, as Thorpe (1961a) has shown in chaffinches, which learn different song dialects in different geographical areas. In higher primates the infant matures quite slowly and innate responses show appreciable change after learning by individual and social experience; already in primates tradition (imitative learning) is an important mode of transmitting behaviour, including that of fear. The human infant takes a long time to mature, and its limited repertoire of innate responses is soon altered beyond recognition as the infant matures and learns by his own experience and by modelling.

It is difficult to separate out the contribution of innate, maturational and learned elements to the fears of higher animals, and much that was thought to be innate in the past has turned out to be the result of learning. Man is not a species rich in inborn reactions and has evolved more as a learning machine. It has accordingly become unfashionable to talk about innate responses in man, but the pendulum has perhaps swung too far in this regard. As Valentine (1930) noted, we cannot assume that because learning has begun by the second month of life maturing of the innate has therefore been completed by then, though undoubtedly the fact that learning has begun imposes on us the utmost caution in inquiring how far the various supposed instinctive responses are genuinely innate. Fantz (1961) has lucidly discussed the problem in the special instance of visual form perception, and his remarks apply equally to fear responses:

If the perception of visual forms (and fear responses to them) depended wholly upon innate mechanisms, it would be evident without experience at any age, and deprivation of visual experience would have no effect. If maturation were the controlling factor, younger infant animals would be less responsive than older ones, regardless of visual experience. If form perception were entirely learned, some visual experience would be required regardless of age and length of deprivation.

Fantz's scheme should also include two other factors. First, visual deprivation itself can cause irreversible optic damage (Walk, 1965) and so obscure the mechanisms at work. Second, from conception onwards no firm line divides innate from acquired characteristics, since the expression of innate features depends upon their interplay with a normal environment in the uterus and the world outside. In the words of Piaget (1966), the phenotype constitutes the reply of the genotype to the pressures of the environment. Even the innate tendency of a human embryo to develop two hands depends upon its chemical environment, as the thalidomide tragedies have shown. That more than 10 years elapse between birth and the onset of puberty in man does not argue against its innate basis, even though its emergence depends upon the maturation of complex neuroendocrinal factors. Maturation in a normal environment allows the gradual emergence of different characteristics at successive phases of development.

We will examine experimental work on fear with this framework in mind: innate elements are those which appear early in life before there has been significant experience; maturational phenomena are those innate elements which require growth of the animal to a particular stage of development before they are finally expressed; finally, elements due to learning appear mainly as a function of particular experiences, although maturation is necessary before learning can begin. It is not always possible to separate maturational from learning phenomena. On the one hand what appears to be maturation may in fact be learning since every species requires certain conditions in its environment in order to survive, and experience of these constant conditions may be the determinant of a particular fear rather than maturational changes within the animal itself. On the other hand, learning may obscure maturation in two ways. First, very early experience of an object may subsequently inhibit fear to it at the later age when fear to that object usually appears. Second, at the critical age at which a response matures very brief experiences can greatly enhance the maturational response although at an earlier or later age such experiences would have had little effect.

Fears need not be either completely innate or completely learned since another possibility exists. Certain stimuli that do not spontaneously arouse fear may have a latent tendency to elicit it, with the result that the subject will learn to fear these stimuli much more quickly than others, and if the subject is already mildly afraid these stimuli can intensify the fear. In other words, fear can be high in the innate hierarchy of responses to a stimulus without being the dominant response (Miller, 1951). Such latent fears may manifest as pseudoconditioning. A stimulus may seem neutral at first, but after the subject has received a few electric shocks he shows strong fear of the stimulus in spite of the fact that it has never been paired with the shock.

In the pages which follow the reader may wonder why so much space is devoted to innate and maturational aspects of fear when undoubtedly in man learning plays the more important part. The reason is simple. Many principles behind the learning of fear have been mapped out from sound experimental evidence over the last 50 years—these are now freely accepted, but innate factors have been neglected and the subject is in disfavour, so that correspondingly more space is needed to correct the current distorted perspective. Of course, acceptance that there are innate elements in fear responses does not imply that they are immutable since environmental factors can modify the expression of inborn elements.

B. INNATE AND MATURATIONAL ELEMENTS IN FEAR

Fear is an innate emotional response in higher animals which has obvious survival value. This emotional response varies in strength in two ways. First, regardless of situation, the overall fearfulness of an animal varies from one individual to another. This is true for variation both between and within species. Without experimental evidence to the contrary few people would doubt that rabbits are more timid than tigers, and that these differences are largely genetically determined. In addition, some rabbits are more timid than other rabbits. This enduring characteristic we call a trait, which is one aspect of temperament. Second, regardless of individuals, some situations are more feared than others and this variation may also be species specific. To take three contrasting situations, as soon as young birds and mammals are mobile they avoid obvious heights, but only a few species of birds fear the shadow of a passing hawk, and hardly any animals are afraid of trees.

In the following pages we will briefly discuss the trait of fearfulness which characterises certain species and individuals, and then pass on to the kinds of situation feared in animals and man.

I.   GENETIC ASPECTS OF TIMIDITY

From Hippocrates to Pavlov it has been recognised that people and animals vary in temperament according to their hereditary endowment. Timidity (fearfulness) is one aspect of temperament, and it is reasonable to expect that this trait depends in part upon genetic makeup. Several workers support this expectation.   In rats Broadhurst and Bignami (1965) have described two strains of rats bred selectively for slow and for rapid acquisition of escape-avoidance conditioned responses in a shuttlebox. The parent stock came from two strains of rats preselected for high and low avoidance. Progressive divergence of the mean scores for these high and low avoidance strains indicated a strong genetic control over the development of the conditioned avoidance response, especially that to shock. Autonomic reactivity as measured by emotional elimination was not important in differentiating the strains, but they differed in ambulatory activity and in aversion to alcohol in their drinking water. The selection also affected body weight.

In pointer dogs, Murphree and co-workers (Murphree et al, 1966, Peters et al. 1966) succeeded in selectively breeding two separate strains of dogs, one of which was excessively fearful, the other reasonably stable. They began with two contrasting pairs of pointers preselected by dog breeders, one pair being fearful, the other stable.   By the F–2 generation excessively fearful behaviour was shown by 90% of the offspring of the originally timid pair, and stable behaviour by 80% of the offspring of the originally healthy pair. Since the environments were constant for all dogs these differences were best accounted for by hereditary factors, and the mode of inheritance was most probably polygenic. Fearful behaviour was measured by the duration of immobility after a loud noise, the amount of exploratory activity in an empty room, several conditioning measures and standardised field trials with live birds. Repetitive measures showed that maturation was important, since the freezing time to noise and activity scores became characteristic of the nervous dogs near the age of 3–4 months, though some differences between the strains were seen earlier. In both strains of dog, independently of fearfulness, there was a wide variation in friendliness to man.

Yerkes' (1948, p. 120) observations in chimpanzees are worth noting. Two dizygotic chimpanzee twins born in captivity showed marked differences in timidity from early infancy to adult life. Yerkes inferred tentatively that the trait called timidity is probably hereditary in chimpanzees though we now know that environmental factors are also of importance in primates (Harlow, 1965).

Genetic variation between species is so striking that it hardly needs discussion—contrast the timidity of deer and aggression of wolves. In island species long free of predators the trait of fearfulness is almost lost, e.g. birds on the Galapagos Islands are in danger of extinction since they allow themselves and their eggs to be taken without alarm or attempt at protection or cover. Furthermore, decades of contact with men have not led to significant variation in this behaviour—learning does not occur since this behaviour results mainly from genetic makeup.

Of course, fearfulness in higher animals depends upon both heredity and experience, and hunted animals soon learn to avoid man. In dogs, Krushinskii (1962) showed that passive-defensive behaviour (fearfulness) depends upon both breed and manner of rearing. A deprived "kennel" rearing produced more passive-defensive behaviour than home rearing. But regardless of manner of rearing, German shepherds showed more passive-defensive behaviour than Airedales.

Genetic aspects of timidity in man are not well known. Freedman (1965) studied the development of smiling and fear of strangers in a series of twins over the first year of life. He found greater concordance for monozygotic twins than for dizygotic twins. In a series of adult twins Shields (1962) gave a neuroticism questionnaire which included questions on emotionality, nervousness and shyness. Evidence suggested a genetic contribution to neuroticism. Neuroticism scores were closer for monozygotic than for dizygotic twins. Furthermore, the discordance between dizygotic twins was greater than the discordance between monozygotic twins reared apart; the difference between these two groups was much greater than that between monozygotic twins reared apart and together. However, further work is needed on this point. Certainly siblings differ from birth onwards in the intensity of their startling and fears, as Valentine (1930) noted, so it is highly likely that genes affect timidity, but systematic work is needed to delimit the extent of this influence.

II. THE KINDS OF SITUATIONS WHICH ARE FEARED

In 1897 Stanley Hall suggested (p. 246–7) that the best evidence for phylogenetic influences on human fear rests

"on the proportional strength of different fear elements and tendencies. Their relative intensity fits past conditions far better than it does present ones . . . serpents are no longer among our most fatal foes and most of the animal fears do not fit the present conditions of civilized life; strangers are not usually dangerous, nor are big eyes and teeth . . . . Yet again, the intensity of many fears, especially in youth, is out of all proportion to the exciting cause. The first experiences with water, the moderate noise of the wind, or distant thunder, etc., might excite faint fear, but why does it sometimes make children on the instant frantic with panic? Must we not conclude that . . . the human instinct feelings . . . have been felted and macerated into their present form very gradually by social, telluric and cosmic influences, some of which still persist unchanged, but more of which have been either modified or are now extinct?"

Subsequent work has confirmed that although animals and humans may show fear of any situation at some time or other, in general certain situations are much more feared than others. Furthermore, these fears may follow little or no experience of such situations. The situations which are feared vary according to species, age and experience of the animal. Schneirla (1965) examined this variation in early approach—withdrawal behaviour in vertebrates. He suggested that approach and withdrawal are elicited by different classes of stimuli which form a biphasic functional system from embryonic stages onwards; low stimulus intensities tend to elicit approach responses, whilst high stimulus intensities tend to arouse withdrawal behaviour. Schneirla thought that in evolution and ontogenesis these functional conditions are related to the fact that low-intensity stimuli are more likely to be followed by beneficial results and high intensity stimulation by noxious consequences. Stimuli producing withdrawal are generally abrupt, of high magnitude, and irregular in timing; they are summarised in Table 2. 1.

The idea has often been expressed that the escape reactions of birds to certain stimuli depend upon the inheritance of "innate schemata" of dangerous objects. In contrast, Schneirla thought that the distinction between stimuli for approach and withdrawal lay rather in the qualities described in Table 2. 1. From these elements the animal gradually differentiates the kinds of objects which are feared on the basis of contiguity conditioning and selective learning.

Table 2.1: Types of stimuli which produce approach or withdrawal in vertebral neonates (adapted from Schneirla, 1965).

Type of stimulus	Effect	
	Approach	Withdrawal
Proximal Tactile, proprioceptive and chemoceptive patterns of—	low magnitude, regular timing.	high magnitude, irregular timing.
Distance *Visual* Succession	gradual changes, regular intervals, low motion parallax	abrupt changes, irregular intervals, high motion parallax.
Intensity	low, low-medium, or decreasing	high, high-medium, sharply or irregularly increasing.
Contour	rounded	angular, abrupt corners.
Movement	regular, low to medium speed away from subject	irregular, high speed, toward subject.
Size	small, medium-small	large.
Auditory Succession	regular	irregular
Intensity	low to low-medium	high
Frequency	medium-low, low; regular	medium to high, irregular
Pattern	simple	complex, irregular ("noisy")

Schneirla's view simplifies the elements which need to be inherited, and takes little account of the role of maturation (e.g. Harlow, 1961). This does not dispel the basic observation that certain stimuli trigger avoidance more readily than others in neonatal animals. Schneirla summarises evidence that newly hatched chicks are disturbed by harsh sounds such as sneezing and chair scraping. When neonatal chicks hear such sounds they become disturbed, cease uttering pleasure notes, give frequent distress calls and, later, escape reactions. The same occurs to bright light or sudden movement. For example, eight species of gallinaceous birds and waterfowl were disturbed when a black rectangle was advanced rapidly towards the chicks. Distress calls were produced at the age of 5 hours, and avoidance after 2 to 35 days. This phenomenon is akin to the famous hawk effect, which we will now examine in more detail.

1. The hawk effect

As we have seen, very young birds and mammals have a nucleus of simple sensory percepts to which fear is shown, and from these the animal develops more complex fears. Lorenz (see Tinbergen, 1951, p. 31) made the now classic observation that newly hatched ducks and geese showed fear when a hawk/goose model (looking rather like the silhouette of a monoplane) was moved about their heads. This innate response was thought to be of biological advantage because the silhouette of the plane resembled the shape of a short necked bird of prey in flight. When the monoplane was moved in the opposite direction it resembled a harmless long-necked waterfowl in flight and produced no escape reaction. To use Lorenz's term current among some ethologists (Thorpe, 1961 b), the short neck was thought to be an innate releasing mechanism for the innate fear response. It is clear that an innate releasing mechanism is one form of unconditioned stimulus and that an innate fear response is one form of unconditioned response.

Schneirla (1965) suggested that the necessary factor for the hawk effect is a sudden, massive increase in retinal stimulation. In support of this idea are observations that the hawk/goose model produced escape reactions in chicks far more when it swooped than when it sailed toward them. The condition of swooping ensures, much better than does sailing, that the subject will receive quickly an intensive increase in the visual input adequate to arouse withdrawal. The same effect was produced in newly hatched gallinaceous birds when objects as different as a stuffed bird, tea-tray, black rectangle, green box and a large black disc were swooped rapidly towards the chick.

Even the earliest fears of birds are modified by embryonic experience. Dimond (1966) found differences between chicks hatched from eggs incubated in darkness compared with those hatched from eggs incubated in light. Chicks of the same age hatched from dark- or light-incubated eggs were placed at one side of a large square enclosure while a balloon was moved backwards and forwards at the other side. When chicks were placed in the enclosure, light-incubated broods exhibited more freezing responses, spent less time in the section of the enclosure containing the moving object, and showed frequent gross avoidance responses which were absent in the dark-incubated brood. In contrast, imprinting at the age of 36 hours occurred much more readily in dark- than in light-incubated broods. We can thus see that from conception onwards the interaction begins between genetically programmed and environmentally influenced behaviour.

2. Fears of heights—the "visual cliff"

An innate fear of heights is present in chickens and goats which depends upon the innate ability to perceive depth. Gibson and Walk (1960) showed this by an experimental "visual cliff" simulated by a board laid across the centre of a large sheet of heavy glass supported a foot or more above the floor. On one side of the board a sheet of patterned material was placed flush against the undersurface of the glass, giving the glass the appearance as well as the substance of solidity. On the other side a sheet of the same patterned material was laid upon the floor a foot or more below the glass—this side of the board became the "visual cliff" when seen from above. If an experimental animal is placed on the centre board, it has the choice of descending onto the "shallow" or the "deep" side. This choice is the critical feature of the apparatus. If the animal consistently chooses the shallow side it must have the ability to discriminate visual depth and avoid receding edges. Gibson and Walk found that newborn kids froze reflexly if they were placed on the "deep" side of the glass, and only relaxed again to move freely when they were removed to the "shallow" side of the glass. The same was shown for day-old chickens. It is thought that motion parallax is the main element producing this response, without visual experience as a necessary factor (Schneirla, 1965).

For some species light stimulation is not necessary for development of the visual cliff effect. Most species which avoid or show distress on the visual cliff from birth onwards (chicks, ungulates and monkeys) have adequate locomotion within 24 hours of birth. However, rats may be reared in the dark for at least 3 months without affecting visual depth discrimination (Walk, 1965). Other species such as the cat and the rabbit may need light stimulation to develop normal visual depth discrimination. These animals are adversely affected rather quickly if raised in the dark, but after short periods of light deprivation (4 weeks) little visual stimulation is needed to develop avoidance of a visual cliff (Walk, 1965).

Human infants aged 6–14 months avoided the "deep" cliff side but crawled readily on the "shallow" side of the board. Most human infants discriminate and avoid depth as soon as they can crawl. Fantz (1961) has shown that even infants aged 1–6 months can discriminate spheres from flat circles, which again demonstrates the infant's ability to perceive depth. Fear of a receding edge remains amongst adults on the edge of a precipice, with a feeling of being drawn down and a protective reflex to withdraw from the edge. A similar frightening effect is produced in passengers when a low-flying helicopter skims the edge of a plateau or of a high building.

3. Maturation and social approach-avoidance behaviour

The role of maturation is seen in the phasic emergence of fear and avoidance of the unfamiliar in various species after an initial period during which the very young animal approached most objects fearlessly. At the end of a brief period of imprinting certain species of birds avoid strange stimuli (Sluckin, 1964, p. 85). This is not evident during the first 24 hours but thereafter avoidance behaviour increases up to 4–6 days after hatching. The innate following response in ducks usually results in the duckling imprinting on its mother, and the subsequent avoidance of strange stimuli checks that the duckling does not stray away from its mother. Knowledge of what is strange must be acquired before the bird can show a tendency to flee from strange objects. Sluckin also reviewed studies of 2 other forms of fear in domestic chicks. The first was distress calls, which are in evidence at any time from hatching onwards. The second was the immobility reaction to handling, which is absent before the 7th day of handling.

Sackett (1966) reported excellent evidence that maturation influences the development of avoidance behaviour in primates, and that certain stimuli were prepotent in eliciting such avoidance. Sackett experimented with rhesus monkeys who were socially naive. Four male and 4 female monkeys were reared in isolation without ever seeing a monkey or a human after the first 9 days of life. In a daily test session slides were projected onto a screen on one side of the cage. In some of these tests the monkey could control the showing of the slides. The slides showed monkeys in poses of threat, play, fear, withdrawal, exploration, sex, and inactivity, and there were also slides of infants and of mother and infant.

Little disturbance occurred throughout the 9 months of testing to any of the pictures except those of threat. However, beginning at 2 to $2\frac{1}{2}$ months and peaking at $2\frac{1}{2}$ to 3 months, markedly disturbed behaviour occurred whenever pictures of threatening monkeys appeared on the screen (fig. 2. 1). The disturbed behaviour consisted of fear, withdrawal, rocking and huddling. Each of the different animals behaved similarly toward the threat pictures. Lever-touching by the monkeys to turn on the threat pictures was very low during this period from the age of $2\frac{1}{2}$ to 4 months (fig. 2.2).

Pictures of infants aroused more vocalisation and play than any of the other picutres but did not produce the disturbance evoked by pictures of threat.

Sackett concluded that at least two kinds of socially meaningful visual stimuli—pictures of monkeys threatening and pictures of infants —appear to have unlearned prepotent activating properties for socially naive infant monkeys. From the second month of life these two stimuli produced higher levels of all behaviours in all monkeys. Sackett further concluded that "the visual stimulation involved in threat behaviour appears to function as an 'innate releasing stimulus' for fearful behaviour. This innate mechanism appears maturational in nature. Thus, at 60–80 days threat pictures release disturbance behaviour, although they fail to do so before this age. These fear responses waned about 110 days after birth. This could be due to habituation occurring because no consequences follow the fear behaviour released by threat pictures—consequences that would certainly appear in a situation with a real threatening monkey."

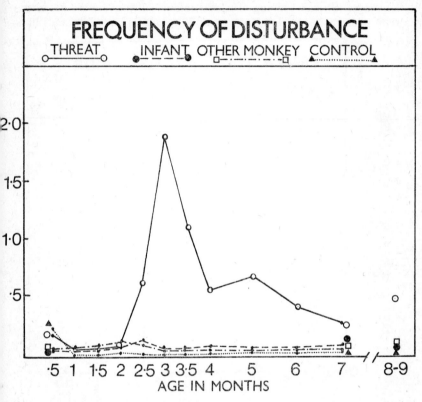

Fig. 2.1: Reactions of monkeys to experimenter controlled slides (Sackett, 1966): the development of disturbed behaviour in response to pictures of threatening monkeys, infants, all other monkey pictures pooled, and control pictures.

This experiment has important implications for the development of complex social interaction in primates and man. It suggests that at least certain aspects begin with innate recognition mechanisms which lead to social interaction and learning which then modifies the behaviour concerned. This is probably true for fear, for the smiling response, and for language.

The smiling response develops first as an innate recognition process which is subsequently changed through social learning. This will be described presently. The development of language may have similar beginnings. Congenitally deaf infants spontaneously babble in the first year of life, but cease to do so in their second year, presumably because they cannot hear the response of adults to this babbling. Their sounds are not reinforced, whereas in a normal child the adults' responses to the infant's sounds gradually shape the child's sounds into language. Special training of a deaf infant will provide the necessary reinforcement to develop language and prevent its lapse into mutism.

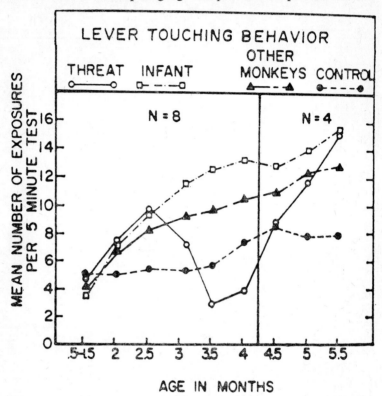

Fig. 2.2: Frequency of self exposures to threat, infant, other monkey and control pictures for the first 6 months of animal controlled tests. (Sackett, 1966).

In Sackett's monkeys the waning of fear responses to threat after the age of about 4 months, possibly due to lack of social reinforcement, is reminiscent of the waning of the babblings of deaf infants who are left without special training. When these isolated monkeys were later brought into contact with other monkeys they did not show fear or withdrawal when attacked. The appropriate response had atrophied and did not develop, not having been reinforced at the time it first appeared.

Harlow (1961, p. 76) noted that in rhesus monkeys avoidance behaviour appeared after a period of approach behaviour. Very young rhesus monkeys approach almost all stimuli, and the larger, stronger, brighter and more mobile the stimuli, the stronger the approach responses. Such a system would undoubtedly be lethal if it were not held in early abeyance by the mother monkey in the wild and by the experimenter in the laboratory. However, at about the age of 20–40 days a check and balance system gradually develops—the fear-response system. Stimuli, particularly large, mobile, strange stimuli, cease to call forth approach responses and come to elicit avoidance responses, and the same is true for new, strange environments even though they are devoid of any specific fear-arousing stimulus objects.

Homologous periods are seen in human infants who progress first through the stage of the smiling response to that of the fear of strangers. The smiling response is phasic. It is readily elicited by any human face by approximately 2 months of age, reaches a maximum at 3–4 months and declines in response to unfamiliar faces after 6 months of age (Morgan and Ricciuti, 1966). Only one study, that of Gewirtz (1965) has found that smiling to strangers continued unchanged through to 18 months of age. Smiling appeared in 98% of a sample of infants aged 2 to 6 months in response to the face of any individual, friend or stranger, regardless of sex or colour (Spitz and Wolff, 1946; Spitz, 1965). Before the age of 2 months only 2% of the infants smiled in response to the presentation of any stimulus. After the age of 6 months indiscriminate smiling at any face ceased in 95% of the infants. The smiling response is first elicited by a specific configuration of forehead, eyes and nose (Ahrens, 1954, cited by Ambrose, 1961). Two eyes have been regarded as the key stimulus of an innate releasing mechanism which produces a smiling response (Spitz, 1965, p. 94). Smiling has obvious survival value in humans as it elicits parental care, and it is the first evidence of social interaction in humans which forms the basis for subsequent social learning.

In the second half of the first year of life human infants gradually develop a fear of strangers (Freedman, 1965) which Gewirtz (1961) regarded as homologous to that occurring in animals of certain species at the end of the imprinting period; in lower mammals and birds the flight response to strangers often follows a period in which indiscriminate attachments are possible (Freedman, 1965). The fear is especially pronounced when the stranger is seen next to the mother, that is, when an unfamiliar stimulus is combined with a familiar one, Spitz (1965) termed this fear "eight month anxiety" but Morgan and Ricciuti (1966) lucidly reviewed studies of this phenomenon which indicated that fear of strangers begins to appear between 6 and 8 months, increases to its maximum by 12 months and continues through the second year of life. The universality of this fear at a particular age, regardless of experience though modifiable by it, suggests a blending of innate, maturational and learned factors in its production. This fear response marks a further stage in social interaction where intimates are discriminated from strangers.

Morgan and Ricciuti (1966) carefully tested 80 infants for fear of strangers in the presence of their mothers. The behaviour of the infants in the experimental session correlated highly with the mothers' reports of the infants' usual reactions to strangers. Almost all $4\frac{1}{2}$ and $6\frac{1}{2}$ months old infants reacted positively to 2 different strangers, especially when the stranger approached and touched them. At $8\frac{1}{2}$ and $10\frac{1}{2}$ months the infants became less positive, and by $12\frac{1}{2}$ months the reactions were predominantly negative. At these ages negative reactions were greater when the infant was separated from mother by 4 feet than when the infant was on the mother's lap. The fear was also greater in older infants when the stranger approached and touched them, though this same approach elicited positive responses in younger infants. However, when the stranger did not touch the infant but smiled, talked and moved his head as if playing peek-a-boo, even the 10 and 12 month infants reacted mildly positively. Thus even when these older infants were separated from their mothers the stranger's behaviour was an important factor in eliciting fear from the infant. In summary, the major determinants of fear of strangers in infancy included the age of the infant, the degree of its proximity to mother and finally, the particular identity, behaviour and proximity of the stranger. Morgan and Ricciuti's meticulous study did not discuss fear of strangers in the absence of the mother.

4. Fear of novelty

Fear of strangers is a special instance of the well known phenomenon that the novel, the strange and the unfamiliar is apt to provoke fear in many species (Bronson, 1968). Hebb and Thompson (1954) reported that chimpanzees manifest a phasic emergence of fear to the model of a chimpanzee's head; none of the 1 to 2-year old chimpanzees paid any attention to the model head, looking only at the experimenter; the 5–6 year group were fascinated by it, coming close to stare persistently and excitedly at it; and the older animals, 9 years and up, showed strong avoidance with screaming, erection of hair and in about a third of the animals, outright terror. None of the older animals would approach, even with cage wire between them and the fear-producing object, which was a reasonably faithful clay model of a chimpanzee head, about half life size. Kohler (1925) noted similar behaviour in a young chimpanzee which went into paroxysms of terror when Kohler tried to give him some stuffed toys which faintly resembled animals and had black buttons for eyes. The uncanny quality of the objects may have resided in their combination of strangeness with the very familiar.

Strong fear of novelty was noted in monkeys by Harlow and Zimmermann (cited by Berlyne, 1960). When an infant monkey is reared away from its natural mother but in the presence of a cloth-covered model, the model becomes a mother substitute. When such an animal is placed in a room full of novel objects but without the model, it will freeze in a crouched position or run rapidly from object to object screaming and crying. If the model is present it will cling to it. After a few trials with the model, fear will diminish sufficiently for exploration to begin. The monkey will use the mother substitute as a "base of operations" and "will explore and manipulate a stimulus and then return to the mother before adventuring again into the strange new world".

Human children also show an admixture of curiosity and fear to uncanny stimuli; fears of the uncanny nearly all occurred after the age of 1 year in the children described by Valentine (1930).

Though novelty is apt to provoke fear, those same novel stimuli can on other occasions cause pleasure and be eagerly sought out. Novel stimulus patterns can attract and repel in turn, and so cause a conflict between approach and avoidance responses.

Berlyne (1960) cites an excellent description by Lorenz of this approach-avoidance conflict in the raven:

> A young raven, confronted with a new object, which may be a camera, an old bottle, a stuffed polecat, or anything else, first reacts with escape responses. He will fly up to an elevated perch and from this point of vantage, stare at the object . . . maintaining all the while a maximum of caution and the expressive attitude of intense fear. He will cover the last distance from the object hopping sideways with half-raised wings, in the utmost readiness to flee. At last, he will deliver a single fearful blow with his powerful beak at the object and forthwith fly back to his safe perch. If nothing happens he will repeat the same procedure in much quicker sequence and with more confidence. If the object is an animal that flees, the raven loses all fear in the fraction of a second and will start in pursuit instantly. If it is an animal that charges, he will either try to get behind it or, if the charge is sufficiently unimpressive, lose interest in a very short time. With an inanimate object, the raven will proceed to apply a number of further instinctive movements. He will grab it with one foot, peck at it, try to tear off pieces, insert his bill into any existing cleft and then pry apart his mandibles with considerable force. Finally, if the object is not too big the raven will carry it away, push it into a convenient hole and cover it with some inconspicuous material.

Monkeys and apes show the same mixture of fear and curiosity in the presence of strange objects. Berlyne cites Russian experimenters who observed this. The primates were watched from behind a one-way screen while objects such as tin boxes, toys, geometric figures and smaller animals were placed in their cages. The first reaction was inhibitory—the subject remained frozen in one posture and stared at the object from a distance. After a while the animals would explore by approaching the object, looking at it, sniffing, touching and finally handling it. This exploration might last an hour, during some of which time the animals would return to staring fixedly at the object.

Inhibition was more prominent in certain individuals, with living stimulus objects, and on the first day the object was encountered.

Whether a novel situation will elicit fear or exploration depends upon many factors. Individuals differ greatly in their traits of timidity and curiosity. What is novel will of course depend upon the previous experience of an individual. The degree of novelty is also important, as Berlyne noted. Extreme novelty tends to induce avoidance, while moderate novelty induces approach. But a lot also depends upon whether an animal is plunged into a totally unfamiliar environment or whether novel and familiar aspects are combined. A totally unfamiliar environment elicits rapid intense exploration which soon dies down. A mixture of old and new elements produces greater initial caution with increasing exploration as time goes on. Finally, fears of novelty are attenuated by the presence of the mother animal (Bronson, 1968).

5. Fear of snakes

Fear of snakes is fairly universal in primates and in man, but it is difficult to exclude the role of tradition in the origins of this fear. The obvious experiment to settle this issue is extremely difficult to arrange in primates or in humans, since their infants require prolonged contact with a mother or mother substitute to develop normally, and endless precautions would be needed to ensure that the mother and child never saw snake-like objects over several years. However tradition alone would be unlikely to be responsible for this fear if one encountered multiple instances of fears of snakes in cases where previous exposure to such objects was highly improbable. Morris and Morris (1965), after surveying relevant researches in this field, commented: "We would not dare to offer them as proof of an inborn fear of snake-like objects. But we trust that they will make you as sceptical as we are, concerning the evidence collected to date by psychologists, supposedly disproving an inborn fear of snakes".

Morris and Morris cited some interesting observations made by Chalmers Mitchell in the London Zoo in the early part of the present century. When snakes were carried into the monkey-house "the monkeys at once fled back shrieking whilst the lemurs crowded to the front of the cage". The lemurs are a species confined to Madagascar, which is one of the few parts of the world which has no poisonous snakes. There are thus sound evolutionary reasons for the absence of fear of snakes in lemurs despite its presence in other primates. However, this difference between lemurs and other primates could be the result of primate tradition rather than of inborn characters. Chalmers Mitchell also recorded the intriguing fact that once, when a chimpanzee passed particularly large nematode worms in its faeces, the other chimpanzees who shared its cage were terrified of them. Chalmers Mitchell went on to exhibit snakes to animals all over the London

Zoo and found that only Passerine birds, Parrots and Primates, excluding the lemurs, were afraid of them.

At the Harvard Primate Laboratory Robert and Ada Yerkes tested which objects triggered fear in young and adult chimpanzees (1936, p. 64). To be really frightening, objects had to be endowed with the properties of "visual movement, intensity, abruptness, suddenness and rapidity of change in stimulus". A writhing snake would naturally provide all these stimuli, and an inborn fear of such stimuli would automatically lead a chimpanzee towards a fear of a snake, without the apes being born with a small portrait of a snake, labelled "danger", inside their brain. Haslerud (1938) confirmed the results of the Yerkses. Dogs too, show more fear of harmless strange moving objects than of similar stationary objects (Melzack, 1952).

Like Kohler 30 years earlier, Morris and Morris found from experiments in a chimpanzee that there were certain powerful fear-producing stimuli which had a quite different impact from all other novel objects. These stimuli included model snakes, and the more life-like the model the greater the fear evoked. The chimpanzee had been reared in captivity from the time it was a tiny nursling. They also noted that two orang-utans accidentally saw a tame python in a television studio and leapt away up into the studio rigging, though the orang-utans had been 6 years in captivity since they were tiny babies. "If, by some extraordinary process, the young suckling ape does have snake hate drummed into its tiny mind by its mother, then its persistence in such an intense form, without reinforcement of any kind for 3 and even 6 years, is a truly remarkable feat".

In human infants two American psychologists, (Jones and Jones, 1928) reported that there was no fear of snakes up to 2 years of age. By the age of $3\frac{1}{2}$ some caution had appeared and the snake might be tentatively touched. Definite fear was often present after the age of 4. Morris and Morris found that dislike of snakes increases from age 4 to 6, at which stage it is present in one-third of British children, and then declines to the age of 14. This prevalence is striking when one considers how small the actual danger is from snakes in the British Isles.

6. Fears of being looked at

Fear of two staring eyes is ubiquitous throughout the animal kingdom including man. Naturally in man most aspects of such social fears depend upon the individual's experience. However, there is some evidence to suggest that the recognition of the look in another is instinctive, and that to see a pair of eyes looking at one acts as a releaser for specifically social action (Kendon, 1965; Argyle and Kendon, 1967). Kendon adduced 3 kinds of evidence for an innate basis for the response to looking. First, Ambrose (1963) suggested that the eyes of another are one of the first figural entities perceived by the infant; of all the features of the face the eyes possess the greatest combination of those qualities which attract an infant's fixation: figure, small enough to be perceived with a minimum of multiple fixation, colour, movements and light reflection. It has been shown in human infants that two eyes are the minimal visual stimulus required to elicit the first social response in man, viz., the smiling response (Spitz and Wolff, 1946; Ahrens, quoted by Ambrose, 1961). The infant's smile and his fixation of the eyes of the person looking at him may be seen as component instinctual responses of the infant which themselves elicit further approach and caring behaviour in the mother.

The eye spots are part of the first figural entity expressed in the paintings of young children from all over the world (Jameson, personal communication). Out of the earliest scribbles the "big head figure" is the first to emerge between the ages of 3–4 (Kellogg, 1959). This figure is the outline of a circle containing eye spots inside it and sometimes outside it as well. Legs are then added to the circle, followed by other parts of the body.

Kendon's second point is that belief in the power of the look seems quite universal and independent of culture, as is the use of large staring eyes in defensive magic (Tomkins, 1963). Finally, the effect of gaze is also seen in animals. When they see a human face observing them in the laboratory Rhesus monkeys show a change in behaviour and in electrical activity in the brain stem (Wada, 1961). Many species of mammals use their eyes and eye markings to intimidate intruders (Hingston, 1933; p. 56) and eyes and conspicuous eye-like markings are used in birds and insects as threat displays and defence against attack (Cott, 1957; p. 387–9).

It is thus not surprising how important looking is to someone with social fears. Starting with innate mechanisms we learn that being looked at means being the object of another's attention and intention, so naturally the gaze of others triggers acute discomfort in self-conscious persons.

7. Other fears with an innate origin

Certain species of animals constantly show avoidance behaviour which parallels some aspects of human phobias. As a species hamsters avoid bright light, yet they will stay on the "solid" side of a "visual cliff" even if it is illuminated while the "cliff" side is rather dim (Lawlor, personal communication). Their fear of heights is thus prepotent over their fear of bright light, which makes sense in terms of the survival value of each response. Hamsters, rats and mice are "agoraphobic" in their behaviour in that they generally cling to the boundaries of an open space; however, if the light is dimmed to a level just above the human threshold the hamsters make much more use of the unbounded space in an open field. In other words, most of the hamster's "agoraphobic" behaviour is a response to illumination above the level which is optimal for the animal, rather than a response to the openness of the situation. Confinement of hamsters or rats in a transparent cylinder in the middle of a lighted field will increase their stress by blocking the searching behaviour which would normally dissipate the avoidance response aroused by bright light.

In this connection in humans it is interesting that agoraphobics tend to feel easier in the dark rather than in the light, and feel less anxious if they skirt the edge when crossing an open space. They also become far more anxious if they feel confined and unable to escape immediately from a frightening situation.

Other stimulus configurations can also elicit fear reflexly in children and adults; we will see later that these shape the forms of various phobias. Though evidence in man is anecdotal, it agrees with the experimental results obtained in chimpanzees by the Yerkses (1936) and by Haslerud (1938). Such stimuli concern movement; young children at the toddler stage may handle live or toy animals with impunity until they see the animal stalking or rushing towards them—this is likely to cause immediate fear. The fear dissipates as soon as the same animal changes to another posture. The fear is thus triggered by a particular configuration of movement rather than by the animal itself. This was well described by Valentine (1930). For example, a 14 month old girl showed great fear of a teddy bear when it was moved toward her; she turned away, trembling in every limb, yet when the teddy bear was still she would pick it up and kiss it.

Other observations concern space and light perception. In expensive skyscraper apartments with exterior walls of glass from floor to ceiling, many inhabitants feel uncomfortable. This is partly because they feel they lack privacy, partly because they feel dizzy looking down outside through windows which extend from floor to ceiling, and partly because they feel their apartments are too brightly lit. These discomforts are alleviated to some extent by curtaining the window, which darkens the room and makes it feel smaller. This however, defeats the original purpose of the window, and instead makes the tenant feel uncomfortable about the high rental he pays for an amenity he doesn't enjoy. At daytime parties in apartments of this kind it is observed that many guests retreat from the well-lit side of the room to throng the darker interior in preference.

What applies to luxury apartments in New York applies with equal force to working class flats in London. A housewife who lived in a flat 22 floors above London described the discomfort produced by a sense of space and light:

(The Observer, 18th Feb, 1968, p. 21) . . . "When my husband first saw the view he was lyrical. He said at night it was like fairyland. When we've company, they often spend the first half-hour looking out of the window. Some get dizzy, though. We'd a fellow here, like a wrestler he is, short but muscly, and he wouldn't go near the windows at all. Just stood by the cooker all evening. I felt like that at first. Now I only notice it when I'm cleaning the windows. The windows run right over for cleaning, but I have to get my husband to do it. My stomach just leaves me.

To begin with, we put the children's bunks in the little bedroom. It's such a tiny room we had to put them up against the window, and my elder daughter just refused to go to bed in the top bunk: she got in with the little one down below. I didn't know what was wrong, so one day I got up myself to see what put her off. It was terrifying! Like lying on the edge of a cliff, just the glass between you and all that space."

Another highliving tenant commented:

"There's something about it which makes it feel unlike home. If you draw the curtains, you're cosy, but you're cut off from the world till next morning."

Further evidence emphasises how certain conditions of space and light can produce discomfort and fear. Many everyday incidents suggest the importance of space and light perception in the production of fear, but we lack experimental evidence for the mechanisms involved. A man went for a stroll on a vast expanse of mud flats exposed by the sea at low tide. These were so extensive that at one point the walker was surrounded by an unbroken featureless surface of mud stretching from one horizon to the other. All visual reference points were thus lost, and definite fear overcame the subject until, as he continued walking, the sea-line finally broke the horizon again to provide a visual reference point, and the fear then abated. Another man at a theatre performance sat high up at the side of the stage above the orchestra pit. As the performance began the lights in the auditorium dimmed, the curtain rose on a dark stage, and only the orchestra pit remained lit between the two dark expanses on either side of the subject. Immediately he felt drawn down into the orchestra pit below, had a sudden fear of the height and withdrew from the edge of the balcony. As soon as the lights came on again in the auditorium the sensation disappeared. The experience was repeated under the same conditions in another theatre.

8. The earliest fears of childhood

At birth human infants already have an innate startle reflex to noise. Extension of this reflex is seen in the regular fear of sudden noise found in young infants, who show innate fear of "any intense, sudden, unexpected or novel stimulus for which the organism appears to be unprepared" (Jersild, 1950). We have already seen that infants avoid perceived heights as soon as they can crawl, and that they develop a fear of strangers in the second-half of the first year of life which reaches its peak at about 12 months. A fear of weird, uncanny stimuli develops later.

We can further understand the contribution of innate elements to the earliest fears of children by considering an important but neglected paper by Valentine (1930), who described the conditions which elicited fear in his own five young children. Although his was a small sample, the observations deserve detailed comment since they are based on careful study and experiments over a decade. Valentine found that loud sounds usually caused reactions suggesting fear in infants from the age of 2 weeks to a few months. Novelty was at times a factor in determining whether a sound caused a fear reaction, but not all novel sounds caused fear. Qualitative differences between sounds, e.g. the high or low pitch of piano notes, influenced the occurrence of fear.

Fears of uncanny objects, especially if the unfamiliar object was combined with a familiar one, were found after about the age of 1 year. Valentine also described fears of the sea in his children between age 1 and 3. These were not explicable in terms of experience or suggestion, as he was with 4 of his 5 children on the occasion of their first sight of the sea, and every encouragement was given to the children to like and go into the sea. Their only previous experience of water was in their baths, which were always a delight to them. He thought there must be something in the great expanse of water which strikes awe into the child.

Valentine also found fear of animals in several of his children after the age of 1 year, despite their previous familiarity and ease with animals, and the absence of any unpleasant experiences to account for the fear. He noted that fear of the dark only appeared in 2 of his children at the age of 5 years, but thought suggestion played an important part in this. These fears contrasted sharply with the fearlessness noted after painful experinces such as falling over obstacles.

There was great individual variability in the tendencies of different children to show fear, since one of them rarely showed fears to anything from infancy to adult life, whereas the other children often showed fear. Valentine did not draw any conclusion from this, but the evidence suggested a genetic constitutional basis for timidity.

A given stimulus did not produce fear in any inevitable and invariable manner. "If it is true of some reflexes that their recurrence is dependent upon conditions other than the mere stimulus, it is still more true of fear". For example the presence of a companion could banish fear and appear comforting from early infancy. The precise nature of the stimulus itself also affected whether fear would result, for example a teddy bear would cause fear when it was moving towards the child, but not when it was still. The children could also enjoy playing at fear, even to an extent which eventually caused screams of fear.

Much of Valentine's paper tilts against the extreme behaviourist position espoused at the time by Watson, viz., that all fears are learned.

Valentine subtly traces the delicate interaction between innate and learned elements in the development of children's fears: "while suggestion is undoubtedly very effective in stimulating fears, the power of suggestion seems to be so much greater in certain ways, as in stimulating the fear of animals or of the dark, than it is in others of the many occasions that a parent uses it (as in suggesting that foods are (nasty), or that children will fall if they climb), that we can more reasonably believe that in the former cases suggestion is appealing to a latent impulse in the same direction, whereas in the latter cases there is no such innate tendency".　He suggested not that there is a specific fixed innate fear of definite objects such as furry animals.　Rather the facts suggest that there is a general tendency to fear the very strange, especially when closely associated with the familiar, which varies greatly with the temperament and condition of the individual.　He thought "we must assume a further tendency to especially fear live, moving things, a faint tendency, so that it can easily be modified by repeated experience or even suggested away; yet sensitive, so that it can easily be stimulated by suggestion or by a supplementary stimulus causing a general disturbance".　Some of Watson's own observations on infants were used to support this position:

> "Vincent showed no fear of the rabbit, even when it was pushed against his hands or face. His only response was to laugh and reach for the rabbit's fur.　On the same day he was taken into the pen with Rosey, who cried at the sight of the rabbit.　Vincent immediately developed a fear response; in the ordinary playroom situation he would pay no attention to her crying, but in connection with the rabbit, her distress had a marked suggestion value.　The fear transferred in this way persisted for over two weeks".

Valentine pointed out that, ordinarily, Vincent took no notice of Rosey's crying.　But the rabbit, previously unfeared, combined with the suggestion due to Rosey crying, at once set up a fear.　This might be explained on the assumption that there was latent in Vincent an innate tendency to fear things like the rabbit.　To say that it was entirely due to suggestion is to leave unexplained the complete absence of response to Rosey's crying previously.

Valentine's argument is similar to that of Morris and Morris about fear of snakes: that children are not born with a picture of furry animals labelled "danger" inside their cortex, rather they have a low threshold for showing fear to a few stimulus configurations which automatically lead to fear of animals under certain conditions.

Summary

Fear is an innate emotional response in animals. This response occurs in differing situations as the animal matures and learns.　Regardless of situation, the overall fearfulness (timidity) of an animal varies both between and within species; this enduring trait of timidity has an important genetic component in animals and probably in man. Regardless of individuals, certain situations are more feared than others. This is the result of innate tendencies to fear particular stimulus configurations rather than particular objects; some of these fears require maturation before they are expressed.

From birth certain species of birds show fear of stimuli resembling birds of prey. Birds and mammals avoid perceived depth as soon as they can walk. Photophobia leads rats and guinea-pigs to avoid wide open spaces while confinement increases their fear by blocking searching behaviour. Young primates, after an initial period of approach to large, mobile stimuli, develop fear of these same stimuli, especially if the stimuli are of threat displays or are strange and combined with familiar cues; fear of the uncanny develops later. Most primates show fears of snakes which are based in part on fears of sudden or writhing movement.

In man, fears of similar kinds of stimuli occur regularly independent of experience, and thus are probably the result of inborn mechanisms which take time to mature. At birth human infants already have an innate startle reflex to sudden noise. Young infants show innate fear of any intense, sudden, unexpected or novel stimulus for which the organism is unprepared. As soon as infants crawl they avoid perceived heights, and at about 12 months show a fear of strangers. Later they show fear of other unusual stimuli. After the age of 1 year children show fear of animals, arising partly out of fears of certain types of movement. Some children, on their first encounter, fear expanses of water like the sea.

None of these fears occur invariably each time a particular stimulus is presented. The degree of fear varies with the overall timidity of the child, the presence of a companion, the details of the stimulus and the condition of the child at the time.

As the child grows, subsequent experience greatly modifies the expression of those few innate mechanisms which originally triggered fear, so that in adults the traces of these inborn mechanisms are largely obscured by learned behaviour. Nevertheless, such mechanisms influence the form which phobias take in adult life.

Section II. PHYSIOLOGY AND LEARNING OF FEAR

A. **Physiological mechanisms for expressing and learning fear**
    1.   Peripheral mechanisms
          Measures of skin conductance
          Forearm blood flow
          Biochemical changes during fear
    2.   Central mechanisms
    3.   Epilepsy and fear

B. **Psychological mechanisms for learning fear**
    1.   Experimental paradigms of fear
    2.   Unity of the learning process
    3.   Acquisition of fear
          Maintenance of fear after acquisition
          Effect of drugs and alcohol
    4.   Extinction of fear
          Factors influencing resistance to extinction
          Responses antagonistic to fear
    5.   The notion of conditionability
    6.   Vicarious learning (modelling)
    7.   Symbolic aspects of fear
    8.   Experimental fear in children

Summary

A. PHYSIOLOGICAL MECHANISMS FOR EXPRESSING AND LEARNING FEAR

It is necessary at this point to examine the physiological mechanisms which are known so far to subserve the expression and learning of fear. It is not proposed to enter the experimental literature in any detail, but simply to sketch the main outlines which are apparent.

James and Lange long ago suggested that emotion consisted solely in the perception of peripheral concomitants of affect, while others maintained that the experience was purely central in origin. In an excellent review of the problem Schachter (1964) described evidence that peripheral components play some part in reinforcing emotional feelings although central mechanisms have an important role. Experiments of Schachter and Singer (1962) indicate that an emotional state can begin as a non-specific increase in arousal to which cognitive cues are secondarily attached which help the subject to label the affect as fear, anger, sexual excitement, etc., depending upon the context of the emotional arousal.

A purely visceral formulation of emotion was criticised most lucidly by Cannon (1929). One objection was that artificial induction of the visceral changes typical of strong emotions does not produce them, e.g. the injection of adrenaline by itself produces apparently genuine emotional states in only a tiny minority of subjects. However, humans who have been injected with adrenaline can be readily manipulated into different emotional states by placing them in an appropriate environmental setting. "With the addition of cognitive propositions we are able to specify and manipulate the conditions under which such an injection will or will not lead to an emotional state" (Schachter, 1964).

Another objection to the equating of emotion with visceral changes alone was that similar visceral changes occur in very different emotional states.

Since we are aware of a great variety of emotional feelings, it must follow from a purely visceral formulation that the variety of emotions will have a corresponding variety of different bodily states. However, although there is no clearcut pattern of physical changes for each emotion, certain differences have been claimed, for example between fear and anger (Ax, 1953; Schachter, 1957).

A third objection raised by Cannon was that emotions may occur without any visceral activity, as in sympathectomized animals and men. Wynne and Solomon (1955) showed that sympathectomized dogs acquired an avoidance response far more slowly than control dogs, and were quick to extinguish such responses. However, when deprived of visceral innervation only after acquisition, the animals behaved like normal dogs and failed to extinguish. These animals had learned to act as if they were emotional. Nevertheless, one might still ask "But did they *feel* emotional?"

This problem was studied by Hohmann (cited by Schachter, 1964) in 25 paraplegics and tetraplegics. The patients were divided into 5 groups according to the level of their lesions in the spinal cord. These groups fell along a continuum of visceral innervation and sensation from minimal impairment at the sacral level to maximal disruption at the level of the cervical cord. If visceral activity was important for the experience of emotion, then the higher the lesion, the less the emotion which the subjects should feel. Hohmann interviewed each subject about specific feelings in situations of fear, anger, grief, sexual excitement and sentimentality. He asked them to recall an emotional incident prior to their injury and a comparable event following the injury. The subjects were then asked to compare the intensity of their emotional experiences before and after injury.

Changes reported by Hohmann's patients for fear and anger were plotted by Schachter (1964) and can be seen in figure 2.3. It is obvious that the higher the lesion and the less the visceral sensation, the greater the loss of emotionality. The same applied to states of sexual excitement and grief. The only exception to this consistent trend was sentimentality, which Schachter suggested was a cognitive rather than a feeling state.

Hohmann's subjects who had cervical lesions repeatedly described themselves as acting emotionally but not feeling emotional e.g. "I say I am afraid, like when I'm going into a real stiff exam. at school, but I don't really feel afraid, not all tense and shaky, with that hollow feeling in my stomach, like I used to".

Schachter (1964) pointed out the contrast of these descriptions to the introspections of Maranon's subjects who described their feelings after an injection of adrenaline in an "as if" manner, e.g. "I feel as if

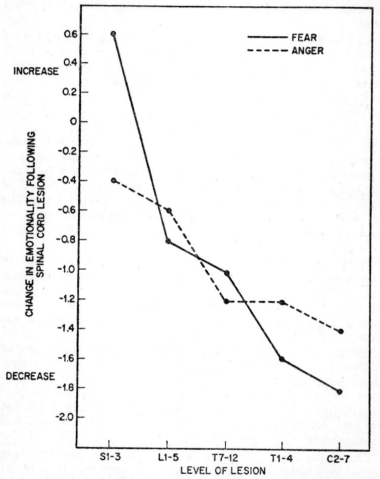

Fig. 2.3: Change in fear and anger following spinal cord lesions at different levels (Hohmann, cited by Schachter, 1964), reproduced with permission from Hohmann, G. W. "The effect of dysfunctions of the autonomic nervous system on experienced feelings and emotions." Paper read at Conference on Emotions and Feelings at New School for Social Research, New York, Oct. 1962 (cited by Schachter, 1964).

I were very frightened; however, I am calm". "The two sets of intro-spections are like opposite sides of the same coin. Maranon's subjects reported the visceral correlates of emotion, but in the absence of veridical cognitions do not describe themselves as feeling emotion. Hohmann's subjects described the appropriate reaction to an emotion-inducing situation, but in the absence of visceral arousal do not seem to describe themselves as emotional. It is as if they were labelling a situation, not describing a feeling. Obviously, this contrasting set of introspections is precisely what should be anticipated from a formula-tion of emotion as a joint function of cognitive and physiological factors".

It appears, therefore, that autonomic activity greatly aids the acquisition of emotional behaviour, but is not necessary for its main-tenance once it has been acquired. In the absence of autonomic arousal during overt emotional behaviour, less emotion is felt subjectively. Finally, given a state of physiological arousal for which an individual has no immediate explanation, he will label this emotion in terms of the cognitions available to him.

1. Peripheral mechanisms

The peripheral pathways for the expression of fear include the sympathetic nervous system. Excitation of this system causes pallor, sweating, pilomotor erection, pupillary dilation, tachycardia and hypertension. Accompanying this during fear there is rapid breathing, trembling, a desire to urinate and defaecate, paraethesiae of the extremities, and a subjective feeling of tension. These signs are not unique for fear alone, and can be found in other forms of intense emotional arousal. To date it has been difficult to differentiate a unique autonomic pattern for fear as opposed, for example, to anxiety or rage.

Wolff and Wolff (1947) studied one patient whose gastric mucosa was visible through a gastric fistula which opened on the surface of the abdominal wall. During periods of fear the patient's mucosa would blanch, whereas during periods of anxiety the gastric mucosa would increase in vascularity and acidity.

The most successful attempt so far to differentiate fear from anger physiologically was made by Ax (1953). He studied 43 volunteers during periods in which they were made to feel alternately frightened or angry by ingenious stratagems. Of 14 physiological measures taken during these periods, 7 discriminated significantly between fear and anger (figure 2.4). Three variables had a greater average reaction for fear—these were increases in skin conductance (SC+), number of muscle tension peaks (MTP), and increases in respiration rate (RR+). Four variables had greater average reactions for anger—rises in diastolic blood pressure (DBP+), falls in heart rate (HR—), number of galvanic skin responses (GSR) and increases in muscle tension (MT+).

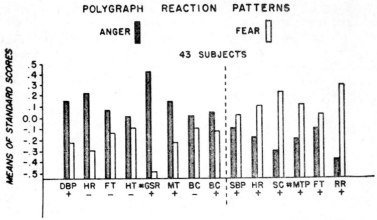

Fig. 2.4: Autonomic response patterns for fear and anger (Ax, 1953).

Variables which did not discriminate significantly were changes in face and hand temperature (FT—, FT+, HT—), ballistocardiogram changes (BC—, BC+), increases in heart rate (HR+) and increases in systolic blood pressure (SBP+). The physiological profile significantly discriminated between fear and anger in all but one subject. Physiological reactions showed very low inter-correlations. The physiological pattern of fear was similar to that produced by the injection of adrenaline alone. The physiological pattern of anger was similar to that of the injection of adrenaline and noradrenaline together.

Since fear involves a complex pattern of physiological responses, no single physiological measure is entirely satisfactory as an index of fear or anxiety though several measures have been of some value in clinical research.

Using a method similar to that of Ax, Schachter (1957) differentiated physiological responses to fear, anger and pain in 48 subjects, 15 of whom had also been included in Ax's report. Schachter studied subjects who were hypertensive and subjects who were normotensive. Regardless of blood pressure level there was a predominantly adrenaline like effect with fear, a predominantly noradrenaline like effect with pain, and in anger either effect or both. Criteria for a noradrenaline like effect were 1. marked rise in peripheral resistance, 2. drop in at least 2 of the 3 variables cardiac output, stroke-volume and heart rate, and 3. marked rise in diastolic pressure. Criteria for an adrenaline like effect were 1. marked drop in peripheral resistance, 2. marked rise in at least 2 of the 3 variables cardiac output, stroke-volume and heart rate and 3. marked rise in systolic pressure.

The work of both Ax and Schachter thus showed that on a large number of variables fear and anger were characterised by a similarly high level of autonomic activation, but on several indices they did differ in the degree of activation.

Measures of skin conductance: Various aspects of skin conductance show significant correlations with overt and subjective anxiety. In a study by Lader et al (1967) the rate of spontaneous fluctuations in palmar skin conductance correlated ·61 (p < ·001) with overt anxiety, while the rate at which the galvanic skin response habituated to successive auditory stimuli correlated —·36 (p < ·05) with overt anxiety. These 2 measures of skin conductance successfully discriminated between groups of phobic patients with high and low overt anxiety, and also discriminated successfully between patients with anxiety states and normals (Lader and Wing, 1966).

A limitation on the value of the habituation rate as an indicator of anxiety is the fact that repetition yields a distorted value, rather as it does in measures of conditioning. However, changes in skin conductance and the rate of spontaneous fluctuations in skin conductance can be determined repeatedly over long periods of time, and so can serve as a useful objective monitor of changes in anxiety in many subjects. Geer (1966) showed that changes in skin conductance were significantly greater and of longer duration in phobic subjects while they watched pictures of their phobic object than while they watched neutral pictures and than the changes in non-phobic subjects who saw similar pictures.

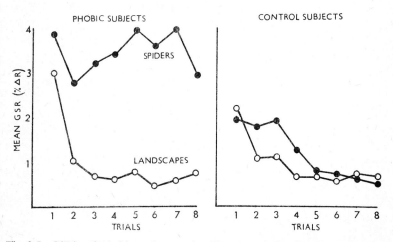

Fig. 2.5: GSR's of phobic and control subjects to phobic and neutral stimuli (Wilson, 1967b).

Using the ratio of change in galvanic skin response Wilson (1967b) obtained even clearer discrimination between phobic and nonphobic students. Twenty undergraduates were chosen—10 who reported intense fears of spiders and 10 who admitted no unreasonable fears. Subjects sat in a dark booth facing a translucent screen onto which coloured slides were projected for 1 second at 15-second intervals.

Eight pictures of spiders and 8 of landscapes in alternating order were presented twice to each subject while bipalmar skin resistance was continuously recorded. The GSR was defined as maximum percentage change in resistance occurring within 10 seconds after stimulus presentation. Response to lansdcapes did not differ for the two groups, but GSR's to spiders were much larger for phobic subjects (figure 2.5). Perfect separation of the two groups could be achieved over trials 5 to 8 using as an index, the *ratio* of response to pictures of spiders over response to landscapes.

The galvanic skin response can also be a useful monitor of changes over time. Wilson (1966) showed how repeated exposure to the same phobic stimulus can be accompanied by extinction of phobic GSR's (figure 2.6). However, the relationship of changes in skin resistance

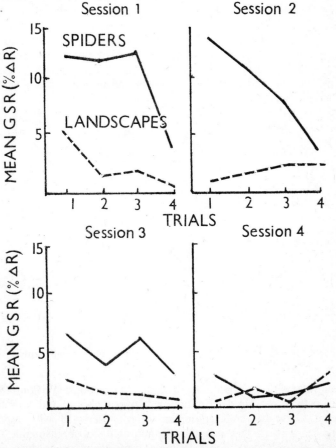

Fig. 2.6: Extinction of GSR's by repeated exposure to the same phobic stimuli (Wilson, 1966).

to changes in subjective fear and overt behaviour is imperfect, as Agras (1967) has demonstrated during treatment of agoraphobic patients.

A drawback to the value of changes in skin conductance in monitoring anxiety is that fluctuations also occur during states of emotional arousal other than fear, so that measures can only be made usefully under limited conditions. Another limitation is the fact that some subjects show no increase despite subjective report of intense fear (Wilson, 1966).

Forearm blood flow. Forearm blood flow has also been used as a measure of anxiety. Kelly (1966) noted that forearm blood flow was more than twice as great in patients with chronic anxiety states than in normals, and showed that forearm blood flow diminished in parallel to decrease in self ratings of anxiety after anxious patients had a modified leucotomy (Kelly et al., 1966). Forearm blood flow differentiated between diagnostic groups more clearly than other measures such as heart rate and blood pressure, and correlated significantly with psychometric measures of neurotic symptoms (Kelly and Walter, 1968).

Unfortunately the forearm blood flow correlates rather lowly, even if significantly, with subjective measures of anxiety. The correlation was only ·24 (p <·001) in the study of Kelly and Walter (1968) and ·28 (p <·01) in a study by Gelder and Mathews (1968). Gelder and Mathews measured the forearm blood flow in 19 phobic patients while they imagined neutral and phobic scenes. The blood flow was significantly higher during scenes concerning intense phobias than during scenes concerning mild phobias or neutral topics. As in the studies by Kelly, however, the forearm blood flow increased most of all while patients did mental arithmetic at speed, whereas subjective anxiety was greatest during visualisation of intensely phobic scenes. Figure 2.7 summarises the changes in forearm blood flow and subjective anxiety during the different conditions.

Drawbacks to use of forearm blood flow as a measure of anxiety are not only its low correlation with subjective ratings of anxiety but also the fact that it increases in many other states of arousal. Furthermore it cannot be used for continuous monitoring of anxiety as technical problems only enable one to obtain intermittent samples over any given period.

Biochemical changes during fear. Visible autonomic effects of fear are also accompanied by biochemical changes at peripheral nerve endings and in the blood stream. There are changes in the levels of adrenaline, noradrenaline, 17-hydroxycorticosteroids, free fatty acids and other chemicals. The pattern of these changes varies to some extent in different emotions such as fear and anger, though no unique pattern for fear is yet discernible, and the changes are not yet clearly understood.

Some of these biochemical patterns were described by Brady (1966). He measured changes in rhesus monkeys during the acquisition of a conditioned emotional response, viz. disruption of instrumental lever-pressing responses for food. During this disruption there were consistent rises in both 17-hydroxycorticosteroids and noradrenaline with no change in adrenaline levels. Adrenaline increase occurred with other emotional behaviour in the monkeys.

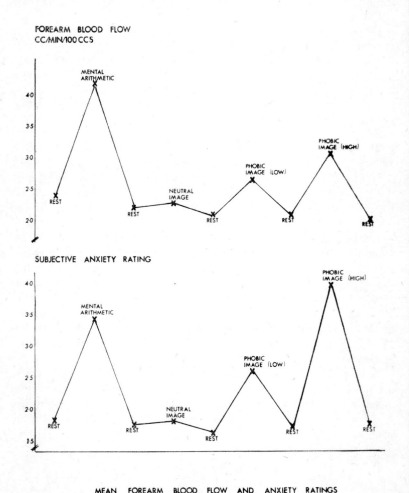

MEAN FOREARM BLOOD FLOW AND ANXIETY RATINGS

OF 19 PHOBIC PATIENTS

Fig. 2.7: Mean forearm blood flow and subjective anxiety ratings of 19 phobic patients (Gelder and Mathews, 1968).

Brady also analysed hormonal patterns in monkeys during conditioned avoidance of shocks. Measures of thyroid, gonadal and adrenal hormone secretion before, during and after 72 hour avoidance sessions suggested that changes may endure for a long time after avoidance behaviour has stopped.

2. Central mechanisms

Peripheral aspects of emotion depend ultimately upon more central mechanisms. These are gradually becoming clearer after recent experimental work. It appears so far that the expression of emotions depends more upon deep brain structures than upon the cerebral cortex (e.g. Smirnov, 1966; Fonberg, 1966). The relevant deep structures include the hypothalamus, amygdala, other parts of the limbic system and the thalamus. For example, Smirnov (1966) studied nine patients suffering from post-encephalitic hyperkinesia who in all had 300 electrodes inserted into different regions of the cortex and deep brain structures for therapeutic reasons. Different points in the brain were stimulated or coagulated. The cortical regions were emotionally neutral to electrical influence, and less than 10% of the regions studied revealed emotional reactions. These were in the ventro-lateral and ventro-posterior thalamic nuclei, the subthalamic region, hippocampus, amygdala and tegmentum. Stimulation of these areas made patients feel sudden emotion unconnected with their current thoughts or environment, yet the emotion was not felt as alien or extraneous. The subjective emotion was accompanied by corresponding motor and autonomic changes.

Miller (1966) has noted that electrical stimulation of certain areas of the brain produces many features usually associated with pain and fear; it can motivate the learning and performance of new instrumental responses, and escape from such central stimulation can serve as a reward to reinforce learning.

Chemical stimulation of certain areas of the brain can also produce behaviour suggestive of fear. In rats Olds (1966) produced escape behaviour by injecting cholinergic and calcium binding compounds into the boundary between the tectum and tegmentum; these were antagonized by the addition of adrenaline or noradrenaline to the active solution.

Subcortical areas of the brain relevant to fear are related to a series of systems for positive and negative reinforcement which integrate complex forms of fearful, defensive, aggressive and alimentary behaviour (Fonberg, 1966). Stimulation of points belonging to a particular system has an effect similar to that of a complex unconditioned stimulus such as noxious stimulation, presence of aggressor or prey, or feeding. Fonberg reviewed evidence that the hypothalamus and parts of the limbic system subserve this effect. She thought it probable that for each behavioural sequence there exist several "centres" with different anatomical locations, possibly organised in hierarchical dependence. For example, in dogs stimulation of the dorsomedial part of the amygdala evokes fear and flight responses which can serve as negative reinforcement in avoidance training. In the basolateral part of the amygdala there are several inhibitory "centres" whose stimulation causes inhibition of some forms of complex behaviour (fear, attack, feeding and conditioned alimentary reactions) while leaving intact other reactions such as general motor ability, walking, playing and instrumental avoidance responses. The same differential excitation and inhibition is also found in the hypothalamus and other parts of the limbic system. Fonberg thought that the systems mediating emotion may be organised in such a way that each excitatory centre is reciprocally connected with the inhibitory one. We do not yet know how all these subcortical centres are controlled by the cortex, thalamus, sensory input and humoral factors. Fonberg (1963) produced evidence that the aversive system is not uniform but is divided into subsystems mediating different forms of defensive-aggressive behaviour, details of which are given in her paper.

In dogs who had hypothalamic stimulation through chronically implanted electrodes Fonberg (1966) observed the following behaviour: fear and flight, fear and defence, rage and attack, appetite and food intake. All these reactions appeared similar or even identical in all their features with the normal behaviour displayed by the same animals in natural situations. Stimulation of the same point regularly gave in every successive trial in different experimental sessions the same form of behaviour, so she concluded that the various forms of behaviour are controlled by different anatomical points. This point to point correlation with behaviour has not always been found by other workers.

After selection of the most suitable electrode points the animals began avoidance training. The CS was an acoustic stimulus, the UCS was brain stimulation and an instrumental response was then trained. Fonberg found that the fastest negative reinforcement in avoidance training occurred when the UCS was stimulation of fear-flight points. Fear-flight and avoidance responses conditioned rapidly to the acoustic stimulus.

In contrast, avoidance training occurred much more slowly when stimulation of fear-defence points was used as the UCS, even though classical conditioning still occurred quickly. The difference between these two groups in avoidance training supported the distinction between fear-flight and fear-defence responses, even though the emotional expression of fear was similar in both cases. Fear-flight and fear-defence are related to one another but depend upon different neurophysiological systems. More than one kind of fear response has also been distinguished in other species. Snowdon et al. (1966)

found in goldfish that removal of the forebrain, which contains precursors of the mammalian limbic system, enhances extinction of conditioned avoidance but not of conditioned escape responses.

Further evidence that different aspects of fear reactions depend upon different parts of the brain comes from Carlson (1966). She found in rats that emotional and cue aspects of an aversive situation can be stored subcortically and influence behaviour regardless of the presence or absence of the cerebral cortex; complex motor response to the same aversive situation, however, only occurred when the cerebral cortex was intact.

Lesions of the mammillothalamic tract affect conditioned avoidance responses. In cats and rats Krieckhaus, (1966) found that such lesions expedite extinction of the conditioned avoidance response. In rats and hamsters Bunnell (1966) noted that such lesions have less effect on conditioned avoidance responses which were learned with low rather than with high emotional arousal.

Many experiments on amygdaloid stimulation were reviewed by Gloor (1960). He noted that the commonest sequence of responses with increasing intensity of stimulation was attention merging into fear and finally rage. Each response was associated with the usual motor and autonomic changes for that response. The sequence of attention, fear and rage corresponds closely to the orienting reflex and its modifications with increasing intensity of the alerting stimulus.

Fonberg (1966) summarised work on emotional reactions as follows: Particular global emotional reactions, including fear, are mediated and integrated by "centres" or "systems" located in various parts of the hypothalamus and limbic systems. Although these systems are connected with work in close relation with each other, they are both anatomically and functionally specific. We may consider them as corresponding to the hypothetical Pavlovian unconditioned centres.

3. Epilepsy and fear

When epileptic discharges evoke emotions such as fear they can illuminate the neurophysiological substrate of those emotions. As early as 1879 Jackson described fear with an epigastric aura which he felt was an integral part of the epileptic attack. Since then fear during epilepsy has often been described, and Williams (1956) wrote an excellent review of the subject. He saw 2,000 epileptics living normal home lives, half of whom were seen in hospital and half in private practice. In all, 165 patients had complex feelings in the epileptic attack, and 100 of these (5% of all cases) felt an emotion as part of the epileptic experience itself and not simply as a response to ictal events. Williams was not concerned with other emotional disturbances surrounding the epileptic fit such as apprehension that an attack may occur, fear evoked by the knowledge of an impending fit, alarm, dismay or distress caused

by the ictal events, and subsequent malaise with depression and distress
in the post-ictal period.

Of the 100 patients who experienced emotion as part of the epileptic
experience, the great majority (61%) felt fear, 21% felt depression,
and the rest experienced pleasure or unpleasure. Location of the focus
causing ictal emotions was made through demonstration of the lesion
at operation by angiography, encephalography, or by inference when
emotion occurred as part of a march of several ictal events. Of the 61
cases who felt fear as part of the ictal experience, 35 patients had an
anterior temporal lesion and 17 patients had a middle temporal disorder
(see fig. 2.8).

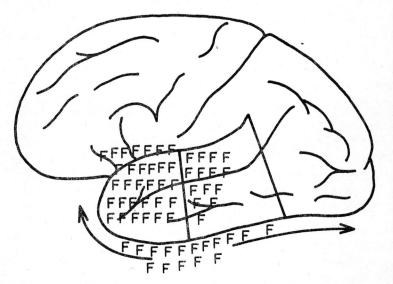

Fig. 2.8: Site of the lesion in 61 cases of epilepsy who felt fear as part of the ictal
experience (Williams, 1956).

Fear was experienced in 70% of patients when the epileptic discharge
involved the anterior half of either temporal lobe, both with disturbance of the outer and of other surfaces of the lobe. In contrast,
when depression was felt lesions were diffusely distributed in the
temporal part of the brain. Pleasure and unpleasure were principally
associated with posterior temporal lesions. When lesions or foci were
above the fissure of Sylvius, ictal emotions were unlikely to arise.
The evidence from Williams' series of patients agrees with Macrae's
account (1954) of 7 instances of epileptic fear arising with organic
lesions of the medial surface of the temporal lobe.

Williams' observations were largely borne out by Weil (1959) who
found temporal lobe epilepsy in 132 patients out of his series of 388

subjects with "symptomatic" epilepsy. Of these, 28 subjects (7% of all cases and 21% of those with temporal lobe epilepsy) experienced ictal emotions, in half of these the emotion being fear and in the other half depression. Like Williams, Weil noted that ictal fear was associated with cortical temporal lobe pathology, while ictal depression was associated with diffuse temporal lobe lesions.

These observations of anterior temporal lobe disturbances being associated with the experience of ictal fear accord with the observations of Fonberg (1966) and Gloor (1960) reviewed earlier that amygdaloid stimulation in animals commonly produces fear. The amygdaloid nucleus is partly situated in the anterior temporal lobe and has links with other parts of the limbic system such as the hypothalamus.

During ictal fear it is possible to distinguish between the emotional experience itself and its somatic, visceral and cognitive accompaniments. The separation between the different components of ictal fear highlights the complex nature of fear, a point also brought out in the work of Lang (1968), Brady et al. (1968) and Fonberg (1966) referred to elsewhere in this book. The following case illustrates the separation of the emotional and cognitive elements of fear.

Ictal fear with Secondary Cognition (Williams, Case 1)

A woman, aged 45, had had brief stereotyped attacks for sixteen years without cause. She suddenly feels "terribly frightened" and "horrible all over". This fear is intense and unnatural and with it she always has the thought "Now I'll know what I am frightened about" but never does. She says she goes stone cold, sweats profusely, has visceral activity—"my inside feels like a washing machine", and her body feels light. She is seen to go very pale. There is no loss of consciousness and the whole attack, which begins and ends abruptly, is over in a few seconds.

Fear during an ictal experience varies from slight unease to stark terror, and may be brief or more prolonged, so that the patient may describe a feeling of anxiety. The patient may say "I feel afraid *as if* something may happen", rather than "I am afraid that (a definite event) will occur". What thought there is is secondary to the emotion whereas normally the emotion arises in response to an evoked thought. This is an interesting contrast to the experiments of Schachter (1964) described elsewhere in which emotions were labelled secondarily to their surrounding cognitions.

Fear may occur anywhere in the march of an epileptic experience, early in the attack, in the middle, at the end, or alone.

Ictal fear can be provoked by natural fear, as in the following case, where the attack began with vertigo and visceral changes (pallor and sighing) accompanying the emotion of fear.

"Unnatural" ictal fear provoked by natural fear (Williams, Case 3)

A girl, aged 11, had had frequent brief attacks for 5 years. They happened in the morning particularly, and were induced by a sudden fright or surprise. Her parents said that she would stare and go pale, then for a few seconds she would go quiet or say a few confused words. Then she would take a big sigh and say "I was so frightened". The patient said she felt as if she were spinning round, then felt fear, "as if someone is going to be knocked over, or as if someone has gone away". Questioned, she said it was unnatural, it was not caused by the attack but "is something inside me". "Then I turn natural and am alright". There was a very sharp spike focus in the left temporal lobe. The girl was physically, intellectually and emotionally normal.

Ictal fear is often felt to be unnatural, unexplainable and contentless, without relation to environmental factors (Williams, 1956; Weil, 1959). Williams suggested that the unnatural quality resulted from epileptic fear being out of context, an hallucination induced by the local epileptic discharge, and having arisen, the affective experience is without previous causal percept or cognition.

Ictal fear often arises during a state of clouded consciousness, and the behavioural accompaniments of fear are then seen in an amnesic state when the experience of fear itself could not be recalled.

Ictal fear is commonly associated with other experiences during the attack, related to the site of the disturbance and its march over the cortex. In 12 cases seen by Williams a visual or auditory hallucination was closely related to the fear state. In other cases ictal fear was linked to disturbances of the body concept, or with other emotions. One case showed a mixture of ictal fear with ictal pleasure. The discharge arose in the anterior half of the left temporal lobe. Williams suggested this pointed to "The emotional anatomy of some complex feelings—the 'sweet agonies', for to be thrilled is compounded of fear and pleasure".

Of patients with ictal fear all of Weil's and half of Williams' series also experienced some visceral changes with the ictal fear, e.g. holding of breath, nausea, retching, belching, flatus, epigastric sensations, palpitations, tachycardia, gooseskin, sweating. Visceral changes immediately preceded or followed the affect as commonly as all other ictal disturbances together. Each of the visceral changes occurring with ictal fear is a fragment of the normally occurring fear syndrome. There is evidence that autonomic and visceral activity is mediated at the cortical level through the inferior part of the frontal cortex, the insular cortex and the adjacent "limbic" temporal cortex. Since the emotion of fear may be subserved in the anterior temporal cortex, Williams suggested that the cortices subserving fear-motor and fear-sensory events are contiguous.

Although the ictal fear does not usually involve all components, sometimes all elements of fear are integrated, as the following case shows. It also demonstrates that operative removal of the abnormal focus abolished the fear attacks.

Total fear response during epilepsy (Williams, Case 19)

A 7-year-old epileptic boy experienced very frequent attacks of pure fear, many of which were witnessed in hospital. When in bed he would often be seen suddenly to show fear in his expression, and would rapidly burrow under the bed-clothes, to emerge in a few seconds, flushed and sweating, saying he had had a terrible fear. If this boy were about the ward he would impulsively rush to the nearest nurse, or failing a nurse, a male patient, clasp them round the legs and bury his face in them, to emerge in a moment flushed with the same explanation. He later became an aggressive delinquent and at the age of 14 had an extensive right temporal lobotomy performed on the basis of electrocorticographic changes, with cessation of the fear attacks.

In some cases a moment to moment correlation can be demonstrated between the experience of emotion and temporal lobe abnormalities, as in the following example, in which, as in the previous case, surgical removal of the lesion abolished both the seizures and the accompanying anxiety.

Ictal fear during abnormal temporal lobe activity (Weil, Case B, see fig. 2.9)

A 29-year-old housewife had seizures from the age of 17. Originally these lasted a few seconds and consisted of a few dyskinetic movements followed by a brief confusional state with automatisms. After age 22 her affect became labile and she experienced episodes of "strangeness and fear". An EEG while on anticonvulsant drugs was normal (fig. 2.9, I). After the drugs were discontinued a second EEG after hyperventilation showed left temporal focal spikes and delta waves (fig. 2.9, II). Coinciding with this focal abnormality the patient experienced inexplicable "anxiety" and "terrible fear". Shortly after this she had a left temporal lobe seizure with masticatory movements, contralateral head turning and confusion. A left carotid arteriogram revealed a large racemose angioma in the entire left temporal lobe and part of the left frontal lobe. After the angioma was removed by surgery the temporal lobe seizures and anxiety episodes ceased.

Selective post-ictal phobias

Very rarely a phobia may manifest in the period shortly after an epileptic attack without it being present in the interictal phase. No

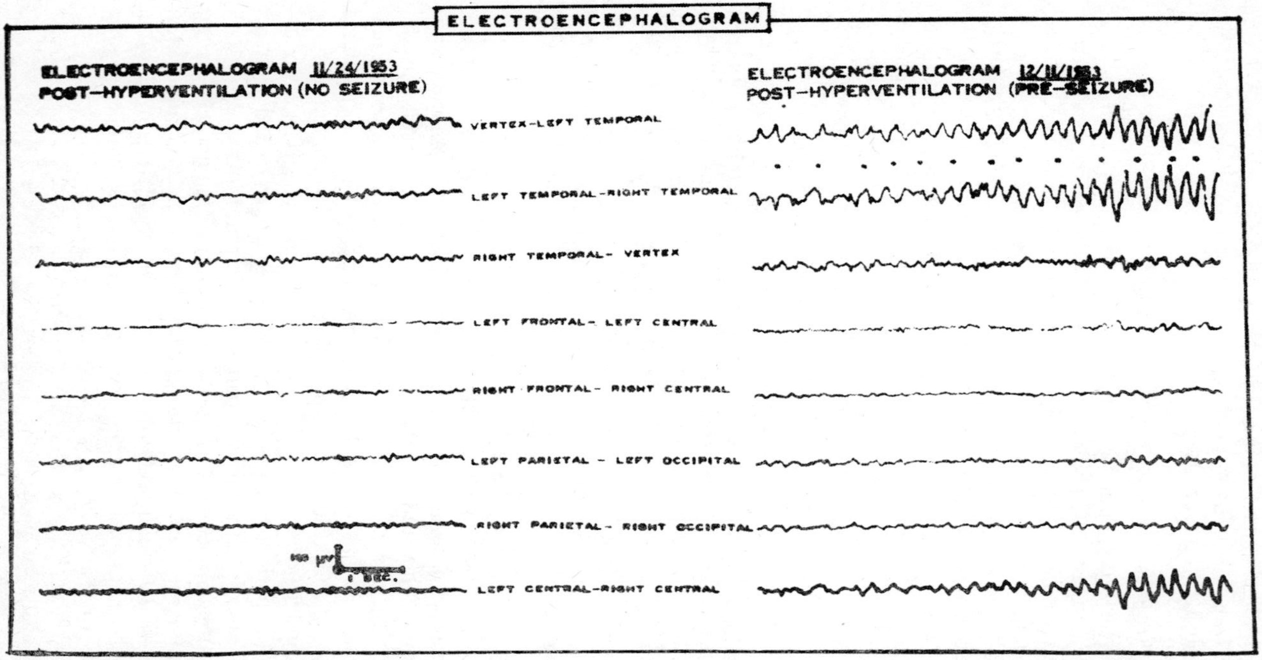

PT. "FEELS FINE" "TERRIBLE FEAR"

Fig. 2.9: Left-sided EEG of a 29-year-old woman with an angioma of the left temporal lobe, temporal lobe seizures and episodes of ictal fear (Weil, 1959).

cases of this kind appear to have been previously described. The author is indebted to Dr. W. A. Lishman for drawing attention to the following case.

Post-ictal phobia absent in inter-ictal phase

The patient was a 51-year-old telephonist who suffered from temporal lobe epilepsy since the age of 29. At the start she had an uncinate olfactory aura. Of late she experienced bilateral numbness of the face before a seizure. During attacks she had brief impairment of consciouness associated with incontinence. Seizures would come in bouts of 5–6 daily at intervals of several months. Until the age of 43 mild depression would ensue postictally for 1–2 days. At that time a few hours after an attack the patient's husband made sexual demands of the patient, who fled in terror from the bedroom. Thereafter each epileptic seizure was followed for 7–10 days by marked depression, retardation and a severe phobia of men and of darkness. In the interictal phase there was no fear at all.

EEG showed spiking in the right anterior temporal region, which continued in serial EEG's during the period of postictal mood change. Polygraph recordings in the postictal phase showed increased fluctuations of skin conductance during the visualisation of phobic fantasies but not during visualisation of neutral fantasies (fig. 2.10, I). During the interictal phase fluctuations of skin conductance did not increase during visualisation of phobic or neutral fantasies (fig. 2.10, II). Physiological measures thus confirmed the patient's report that phobic anxiety was present postically but absent interictally.

As a child the patient had been afraid of the dark until the age of 16. Between the ages of 37 and 43 she had 4 bouts of depression and 3 suicidal attempts related to marital disharmony. The depression cleared after her separation from her husband at the age of 43.

In this patient it seems that psychologically significant events became engrammed in the neurological mechanism of her epilepsy and were reactivated as a phobia whenever seizures occurred.

In summary, epileptic attacks of fear point to both temporal lobes, especially the anterior portions, as part of the neurophysiological substrate for the experience of fear. They also highlight the different components which go to make up fear—experiential, cognitive and autonomic. These components occur separately in some cases. Very rarely a phobia may occur selectively postictally while absent at other times.

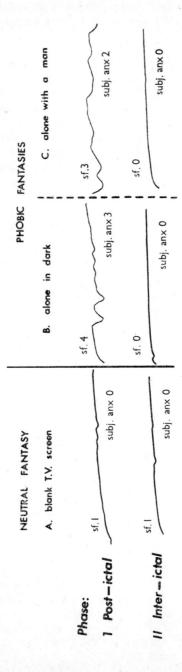

Fig. 2.10: Change from postictal to interictal phase in spontaneous fluctuations of the GSR during phobic and neutral fantasies.

B. PSYCHOLOGICAL MECHANISMS FOR LEARNING FEAR

We have seen earlier that selected stimuli produce innate fear responses in very young animals, as in fears of heights, and that as animals develop the ability to discriminate between different stimuli new fears emerge, for example the fear of strangers in 20–40 day old rhesus and year-old human infants. In adult animals and humans we find fears to many complex situations which cannot possibly be innate and must have been learned. How did fears of these situations develop from the few stimuli which trigger fear very early in life. This development is a complex learning process.

An enormous literature exists on the way fears are learned, yet Kimble (1961) has noted that no single theory covers all the data, and that the mechanism involved differs from one kind of learning situation to another. Useful summaries of the subject are provided by Kimble (1961), Miller (1951; 1966) and Bancroft (1966).

1. Experimental paradigms of fear

Strong fears can be learned easily and become an important drive. Fear is learnable because it can be learned as a response to previously neutral stimuli. It is a drive because it can motivate the learning and performance of new responses in the same way as hunger, thirst, or other drives (Miller, 1951, p. 436).

Evidence for the learning of fear comes chiefly from experiments in animals. In these experiments we do not know for certain what emotion the animal is experiencing and have to infer this indirectly from the animal's overt motor and autonomic responses. Though animal experiments on fear responses are relevant to the problem of fear in man, we must be guarded in translating these experimental results into human terms. In descriptions of such experiments the terms learning and conditioning are often used interchangeably. In general, however, conditioning refers to simpler stimulus-response connections, while learning refers to the acquisition of rather more complex new behaviour.

Most animal experiments about fear involve simple situations of which the following is a paradigm. The animal, say a rat, will be in a cage with a floor through which shocks can be delivered. The cage may contain a lever which will turn off the shocks if the rat happens to press it. The case may also have a door which opens into a second cage. Typically the animal will be trained to fear new stimuli such as a particular tone from a buzzer. This is done by sounding the tone just before a shock is delivered through the floor. After several repetitions the rat will show fear to the tone even if the shock is not delivered. The shock is the original conditioned stimulus (UCS) and the tone is the neutral stimulus of which the animal now becomes afraid (CS). The fear which the rat showed to the shock is the original uncon-ditioned response (UCR), and the fear to the tone is the new conditioned response (CR), also called the conditioned emotional response (CER). This is the *classical conditioning* situation in which a new connection is made by pairing an unconditioned stimulus with a new stimulus (temporal contiguity).

Rats may show fear either by freezing or by increased activity. They can be trained to show either response. When frightened rats become active, further behaviour can be trained. On receipt of a shock the animal may run around its cage until eventually by chance it presses the lever which turns off the shock. After this happens several times the rat will learn to stop the shock by pressing the lever with its paw every time the shock begins. It can also be taught to escape from the shock by jumping through the door leading into a second cage. This is *escape conditioning* in which the rat learns to stop the noxious stimulus after it has begun.

Eventually the rat may learn to avoid the shock by pressing the lever or by jumping into the second cage immediatdely it hears the tone, before the shock is delivered, and so avoiding it. This is *avoidance conditioning*.

Since escape and avoidance conditioning depend upon the rat doing something (operating on its environment), both these situations are forms of instrumental (operant) conditioning, alternative terms for which are trial-and-error learning and law-of-effect learning. They are accompanied by all the signs of fear and correspond to the tendency of human phobic patients to escape from and to avoid those situations of which they are afraid.

In instrumental conditioning situations the animal's responses determine whether he will be reinforced (i.e. rewarded or punished). This is in contrast to classical conditioning situations, where the animal's responses make no difference to the reinforcing events, e.g. whether the animal is shocked or given food does not depend upon lever pressing or any other action of the animal.

Another experimental situation is *temporal pacing*, also known as the Sidman avoidance schedule (Sidman, 1953). Here there is no conditioned stimulus (CS), but the rat learns to delay onset of a shock (the UCS) by pressing a lever. The schedule is arranged so that a shock is given, say, every 20 seconds, unless the rat presses a lever before those 20 seconds have passed. Pressing the lever resets the timing mechanism to start a new 20-second period. The rat soon learns to prevent the occurrence of any shocks by pressing the lever repeatedly for long periods.

Finally there is *punishment training*, in which the animal is punished repeatedly for a particular response, and then appears afraid of making that response.

These experimental situations are not all mutually exclusive. They produce various stimulus-response relationships in the acquisition of

fear responses. With these experimental situations one can systematically study which variables are important in the learning of fear, e.g. the
species, age and sex of the animal, its physiological and psychological
state, the quality of the noxious and neutral stimulus, intensity and
duration of such stimuli, the time interval between the neutral and
noxious stimuli, and the manoeuvres which the animal learns to avoid
or to escape from the feared situation.

2. Unity of the learning process

Most experiments with classical conditioning involve involuntary
autonomic responses such as salivation and heart rate. By contrast,
experiments on instrumental (operant) conditioning generally require
a voluntary motor act to be performed such as bar pressing or jumping.
It was accordingly thought for some time that two different learning
processes were at work. Recently, however, Miller (1966) has shown
in an elegant series of experiments that autonomic responses can also
be acquired by operant conditioning. Autonomic reactions of the
salivary glands, cardiovascular system and large intestine are all
subject to instrumental learning reinforced by a reward such as brain
stimulation. Yet other internal responses, such as those of the brain
waves at different levels of arousal, may also be modified by instrumental training.

Kimble (1966) also concluded from several studies that classical
and instrumental conditioning were the same as regards the basic
associative mechanism involved, and that differences between the two
forms of conditioning are derived from the elaborate feedback associated
with instrumental acts.

There is thus both unity and diversity in the ways fears are learned,
depending on the particular features under consideration. This is just
what we would expect from complex behaviour controlled by an
interacting series of neurophysiological systems of the kind sketched
out by Fonberg (1966).

3. The acquisition of fear

The commonest view holds that fear is first conditioned to new
situations by contiguity learning; fear then serves as a drive to motivate
the instrumental learning and performance of any response which is
rewarded by a sudden reduction in strength of that fear. This is the
two-stage theory first elaborated by Mowrer (1947) and later refined
by Solomon and Wynne (1954).

The two stages of the theory can be illustrated by a rat which is
receiving shocks from the floor of its cage. After a few shocks it will
show fear whenever it is placed in the cage. This is the first stage in the
development of fear and this fear reaction is called the conditioned
emotional response (CER). After a while the rat may learn to turn
the shocks off by repeatedly pressing a lever. This behaviour is the

second stage in the development of fear, and is called the instrumental avoidance response.

The first stage is the *acquisition* of a new fear through pairing of neutral and noxious stimuli. This is contiguity learning of a conditioned emotional response (CER), also called classical or Type 1 conditioning. Experiments confirm that many new fears are in fact acquired according to the rules of classical conditioning (Kimble, 1961; Miller, 1951):

1. The strength of the new fear increases with the number of pairings of neutral and noxious stimuli, and decreases when the neutral stimulus is presented alone.

2. The new fear generalises to other similar stimuli in much the same way as do other conditioned responses.

3. New fears show spontaneous recovery following extinction.

4. Intensity of the new fear increases with the intensity of the unconditioned stimulus, so that a single pairing of a very intense unconditioned stimulus with a conditioned stimulus results in a new fear—this is called single-trial learning.

5. New fears are more likely to develop when noxious stimuli are presented under conditions of undue confinement, and greater fear ensues when no control is allowed over the noxious stimuli received (Mowrer and Viek, 1948).

6. The strength of a conditioned fear varies according to the time elapsing between the unconditioned and the conditioned stimulus— commonly the optimum arrangement is for the conditioned stimulus to occur half a second before the unconditioned stimulus.

7. Summation of conditioned fear responses can be demonstrated. If two stimuli such as a buzzer and a vibrator have been separately associated with electric shock, the responses elicited when both of them are given simultaneously will be greater than when either is given separately.

8. Conditioned fear responses seem to be weaker than unconditioned ones. Similarly, higher order conditioned fear responses (secondary, tertiary, etc.) seem to be weaker than those of lower order ones. Higher order conditioned responses are those which are based on reinforcement by another conditioned stimulus and response.

9. Fear responses like the conditioned avoidance response can be acquired in dogs even when their skeletal muscles have been paralysed by curare (Solomon and Turner, 1962). This suggests that acquisition of the fear involves classical conditioning. Whether peripheral autonomic, as opposed to skeletal, feedback plays a part is not clear.

Maintenance of fear after acquisition

How is fear maintained once it has been acquired? This involves the second stage of the theory. This part of the theory is unsatisfactory because it leaves important facts unexplained. Conditioned fear is thought of as a drive capable of motivating behaviour and this is reinforced by the drive reduction produced by avoidance and escape. As seen earlier, this process is variously termed trial and error or law of effect learning, or alternatively, instrumental, operant or Type II conditioning. It was Mowrer (1939) who first suggested that fear acts as a drive motivating behaviour, and that a sudden reduction in its strength acts as a reward to strengthen any immediately preceding response. In many experiments rats learned to switch off a shock by turning a wheel or pressing a bar, just as other rats learned the same actions for a different reward, such as food when hungry or water when thirsty. Since any reward can strengthen any response, the possibilities for reinforcement are considerably more flexible with instrumental learning than with classical conditioning, where the reinforcement is limited to those unconditioned stimuli which are able to elicit the response to be learned.

Fear is a strong drive which can be conditioned to new stimuli so that its occurrence depends upon the previous conditions of learning. If we did not know the special history of experimental animals we would find their wheel-turning or bar pressing abnormal. But this bizarre behaviour becomes clear once we know that such actions have reduced fear in the past.

Although it is well established that fear is a drive which leads to instrumental learning, two-stage theory fails to explain the great resistance to extinction of avoidance responses. In theory, as avoidance responses continue the classically conditioned CER is no longer reinforced and should extinguish. This should lead in turn to extinction of the avoidance response. But in practice neither the CER nor the avoidance responses are easily extinguished. Ingenious attempts to explain this problem have not yet met with success.

Animals can be trained to resist pain and fear by introducing electric shocks gradually into a situation in which they are rewarded for persisting in spite of receiving the shock. Mere exposure to electric shocks is not sufficient; the animals must be specifically rewarded for persisting despite the shocks (Miller, 1966).

Though avoidance conditioning usually emerges after escape training, the two are not synonymous (see e.g. Bancroft, 1966). Escape responses are less stable and easier to extinguish than avoidance learning. Chlorpromazine reduces avoidance learning but not escape learning. Hypothysectomy in rats interferes with avoidance but not with escape learning, and ACTH will partially restore the deficit. In goldfish removal of the forebrain, which contains precursors of the mammalian limbic system, enhanced extinction of a conditioned avoidance response but not of a conditioned escape response (Snowdon et al. 1966).

Effect of drugs and alcohol

Dollard and Miller (1950) showed that barbiturates reduce tension in an approach-avoidance conflict. They suggested that in such a conflict barbiturates reduce the fear motivating the avoidance more than the drive motivating the approach. Experiments with amylobarbitone confirmed this idea. It was found that barbiturates reduce fear and that fear reduction acts as a reward. Moreover, animals learn to press a switch which gives themselves an injection of barbiturates to reduce fear.

Alcohol also reduces fear in animals. Masserman and Yum (1946) subjected cats to severe emotional stress and then administered alcohol either intra-peritoneally or by stomach tube. When the cats were later again placed under stress they preferred a mixture of alcohol and milk to plain milk. As the animals became normal after the second week they lost this preference for alcohol. Alcohol could in addition cause frightened cats to resume manipulating an apparatus to secure food. Rats, too, who have learned to drink alcohol show an increased desire for alcohol when placed under increased stress (Ramsay and Van Dis, 1967).

In summary, once acquired, fear may be used as a drive to motivate instrumental learning and a sudden reduction in the strength of fear may be used as a reward to reinforce such learning. Animals learn to rotate a wheel or press a bar to secure the reward of escaping from a fear evoking situation; they will also learn to inject themselves with barbiturates or to drink alcohol to reduce fear. Animals may learn to react passively or actively to fear; they also may be motivated to learn to persist in spite of fear.

4. Extinction of fear

When the same response occurs repeatedly without reinforcement it gradually subsides and disappears. This phenomenon is usually called extinction with conditioned responses, and habituation with unconditioned responses. Extinction of fear depends upon repeated presentation of the frightening conditioned stimulus in the absence of noxious stimuli. Pairing of a frightening conditioned stimulus with pleasant stimuli enhances extinction. With this arrangement extinction can proceed fairly quickly where the fear is a conditioned emotional response acquired by classical conditioning. The same applies to conditioned escape responses.

In contrast conditioned avoidance responses are very persistent and hard to extinguish (Sidman, 1955). This resistance to extinction has been attributed to two mechanisms. First the avoidance response reduces the anxiety of the conditioned emotional response, i.e. the avoidance response is maintained by anxiety reduction. Second, avoidance occurs before fear can be fully aroused, thus protecting the new fear from extinction by preventing pairing of the new fear with further neutral stimuli. This explanation is supported by several experiments on "flooding" where rapid extinction of avoidance responses occurred in animals who were prevented from making an avoidance response in the presence of the fear stimuli (Masserman, 1943; Solomon et al. 1953; Baum, 1966).

In Baum's experiment 33 rats were trained to avoid shock from the grid floor of their cage by jumping onto a ledge. When a learning criterion had been achieved the rats were assigned to one of 3 groups: 1. normal control, where they went straight into the usual extinction procedure of putting them on the grid and allowing them to jump freely onto the ledge; 2. time control, where the rats spent a 5-minute interval on the safety ledge before undergoing the usual extinction procedure; 3. response prevention—the ledge was removed from the cage for 5 minutes while the rats were on the grid floor of the cage, after which the ledge was returned, thus starting the extinction procedure. Unlike the other 2 groups, all but one of the rats who were forced to remain on the grid floor without shocks showed rapid extinction of the avoidance response. That prevention of avoidance of fear stimuli produces extinction of the fear response supports the two-factor theory about the learning of fear.

Occasionally after one traumatic episode subsequent exposure to the same situation without any trauma does not produce extinction but instead increases fear or associated autonomic disturbances in that situation (Napalkov, 1963; Sanderson et al. 1962). The conditions governing this phenomenon are not yet understood.

Factors influencing resistance to extinction

1. *Strength of the fear.* On the whole, the stronger the fear the harder it is to extinguish, particularly if it began with a very intense and painful stimulus.

2. Another factor influencing resistance to extinction is the *type of fear response involved*, whether it is a conditioned emotional response, a conditioned escape or conditioned avoidance response. This has just been discussed.

3. The *interval between extinction trials* has an effect. Massed extinction trials reduce fear quicker than do daily trials, though this reduction may not be as lasting (Miller, 1951).

4. A feeling of helplessness intensifies fear, while *having something to do* reduces it, e.g. cats who were given control of their fear stimuli produced these stimuli repeatedly until they lost their fear (Masserman, 1953).

5. Specific *reinforcement of responses antagonistic to fear* helps to reduce fear (see below).

6. *Sedative drugs and alcohol* reduce fear, but do not extinguish it. Withdrawal is often accompanied by reemergence of the fear, unless the withdrawal is very gradual, as Sherman (1967) demonstrated in rats. The latter point has not yet been demonstrated in humans.

7. The *method of exposing the subject to fear-producing stimuli* may be important. One technique is to start with stimuli exceedingly weak, distant or remotely similar to the ones feared, and to approach the feared stimuli so gradually that only minimal fear is elicited, and antagonistic responses can then be applied. This is the method used in treatment by desensitisation. The opposite techique is that of flooding, in which subjects are exposed to the total frightening situation at once so that they experience maximum fear which is not reinforced and so gets extinguished. Desensitisation and flooding have both been used successfully in animals and humans, but have not yet been compared with one another systematically.

8. *Social situations* clearly influence fear. The presence of a trusted companion alleviates fear, while observing a model behaving fearlessly also reduces fear in humans (Bandura, 1968).

9. *Sympathectomy* in dogs causes avoidance responses to be learned more slowly and to be extinguished more quickly (Solomon and Wynne, 1950).

Responses antagonistic to fear

Fear can be reduced by repeated pairing of the fear stimuli with neutral stimuli. Pleasant situations are more effective than neutral ones in diminishing fear. We can all observe how anger, eating, companionship, familiar objects and sexual arousal help to allay fear. Angry men forget their fears in combat. Ardent lovers regularly engage in deeds of valour to impress their ladies. In dogs with experimental neurosis sexual stimulation can temporarily inhibit fear (Gantt, 1944).

In a classic case a boy called little Albert (Watson and Rayner, 1920) had a strong tendency to put his thumb in his mouth as soon as frightening stimuli were presented. Conditioned fear responses could not be elicited as long as he had his thumb in his mouth. Another child described by English (1929) showed no fear of strange objects as long as she was in her own familiar high chair, but became frightened when she was shown these objects while sitting on the floor.

Feeding is a useful method of reducing fear in animals. In chimpanzees Schiller (1952) systematically extinguished fear of snakes by repeatedly placing bananas on the lid of a glass box containing a snake. The most well known work on the reduction of fear by feeding is by Wolpe (1958). He experimented with 12 cats in a cage which contained a foodbox. Six of the cats were introduced into the cage and given shocks preceded by a hoot. The remaining 6 cats were first trained to approach the foodbox after hearing a buzzer. They were then shocked as they approached the foodbox. When tested on subsequent occasions, all the animals showed resistance to being put into the experimental cage, anxiety when inside the cage, and refusal to eat food anywhere in the cage, even after 3 days' starvation. Very gradually this fear was extinguished by placing food some distance away from the cage, sufficiently far for the approach tendency due to hunger to overcome the avoidance tendency due to fear. Gradually the food was placed nearer the cage and finally inside it, until eventually the cats again entered the cage normally.

In rats Gale et al. (1965) also showed that feeding responses help to extinguish fear. The conditioned fear response of freezing was induced in 18 rats by coupling a tone (CS) with a shock to the cage. After training freezing occurred to the tone alone. The rats were then divided into 3 groups. One group had no special treatment thereafter and showed no decrease of fear. A second group was simply presented repeatedly with the tone, without any shock. This second group showed some diminution of fear; however, this was less than that obtained in the third group, which had the same treatment, but with the addition of food at the same time as the tone was presented. A feeding response was incompatible with the freezing reaction. Gale et al. (1965) thus showed that pleasant stimuli were more effective in extinguishing fear than neutral ones.

Wolpe's experiments spurred him to devise an important technique for the treatment of human phobias (see page 182). Patients were relaxed and asked to imagine some aspect of their phobia which they could tolerate with slight anxiety. When this was done a few times in a state of relaxation this aspect of the phobia could generally be imagined quite comfortably. The patient was then asked to imagine a slightly more frightening phobic situation. The patient was relaxed repeatedly until this too could be tolerated, and so on until the phobia was extinguished in imagination. Over the same period the patient was taught to relax and then go out to practise these same situations in the real world until the extinction was completed in practice as well as in imagination.

Wolpe (1958) used the term "reciprocal inhibition" to describe the extinction of fear by coupling a pleasant with a frightening stimulus. The term was used originally by Sherrington (1952) in experiments on spinal cord reflexes of the cat to denote the reflex inhibition of one group of muscles occurring at the same time as the reflex excitation of another group, both inhibition and excitation occurring as part and parcel of one and the same reflex reaction. Sherrington's term described events of a different order to those noted by Wolpe, who was discussing a special form of extinction of fear. It is confusing to employ the same term for different phenomena, so it is best to speak of the psychological events as the extinction, counter-conditioning, or desensitisation of fear through its coupling with competing responses.

5. The notion of "conditionability"

It is often noted that people differ in the speed with which they form conditioned responses, including those of fear. One widespread assumption is that an individual's ability to develop and retain conditioned reflexes is independent of the reflex system being conditioned. On this view individual variability in fearfulness is the result of variability of conditionability.

In fact there is no evidence to support this notion of a general factor of conditionability (Franks and Franks, 1966). Franks and Franks subjected 50 normal men to a partial reinforcement conditioning procedure involving the following reflex systems: eyelid conditioning to sound, GSR conditioning to light; salivary conditioning to sound; and finger withdrawal to a complex light pattern. Although different measures of conditioning for any one reflex system tended to correlate significantly with each other, no significant correlations were obtained between the various systems. The results of this study indicate how we cannot assume a simple relationship between the speed of acquisition of a particular conditioned reflex and other variables.

Spence (1964) has reviewed studies of eyelid conditioning in subjects with high "anxiety" measured on the Taylor Manifest Anxiety Scale (Taylor, 1953). This form of anxiety is not quite the same phenomenon which patients complain of in anxiety states. In general, Spence noted that high anxiety tends to be associated with increased rate of eyelid conditioning, but only accounts for a small amount of its variability, and the intersubject variance is extremely large. A question of obvious clinical importance is whether patients with high anxiety in the clinical sense are predisposed to acquire new fears. The evidence from eyelid conditioning does not help us with this question.

6. Vicarious learning (modelling)

So far we have discussed aversive conditioning in which the subject acquires fear by direct exposure to the feared situation (to the UCS). This is direct conditioning, which deals with simple learning. Great caution is needed in using experimental results of this sort to explain the more complex forms of human phobia.

Informal observation often reveals that fears may be acquired by a person observing pain and fear reactions in other subjects exposed to aversive stimuli, without the person himself experiencing the direct trauma (the UCS). This is vicarious learning, alternative terms for which are vicarious conditioning, no-trial learning, social learning, modelling or imitation. This process enables complex fears in humans to be acquired quite readily in a short time.

Many variables influence the modelling of fears. Valentine's evidence cited earlier indicated that fears can be modelled more easily to certain situations than to others. Other variables include the overall timidity of the subject, the degree of emotion at the time fear is observed in others, and finally, the relationship between the subject and the model. If the model is a trusted parent a child will acquire the parent's fear more readily, whereas the child will less easily imitate the fear of a strange and younger child.

There is ample experimental evidence for the process of fear transmission through modelling, both in animals and in man. Much of the literature has been reviewed by Bandura (1965) and by Bandura and Rosenthal (1966). In rats, Church (1959) showed that animals which were shocked while observing other rats being shocked later displayed more emotional reaction to the pain cues of another rat than a group of animals which had been shocked in isolation. In monkeys, Murphy, Miller and Mirsky (1955) demonstrated that emotional responses could be vicariously elicited in monkeys not only by the sight of their experimental counterpart but also through stimulus generalisation by the sight of another monkey which had never been involved in the experiment.

In man, experiments of vicarious classical conditioning involve one person, the performer or model, undergoing an aversive conditioning procedure in which a formerly neutral stimulus is presented, after which the model displays pain cues supposedly as a response to an unconditioned aversive stimulus. An observer witnessing the model will also begin to show emotional responses to the conditioned stimulus alone, even though he himself has not experienced the unconditioned stimulus directly. In this way vicarious conditioning has been clearly demonstrated by Berger (1962), though there is wide individual variability in the rate of acquisition and maintenance of such responses.

Bandura and Rosenthal (1966) showed that vicarious aversive conditioning is directly related to degree of psychological stress in the observing subject. The relationship to additional physiological arousal by the injection of adrenaline is more complex. Vicarious aversive conditioning is not related at low and moderate doses, but is directly related at higher levels and, in contrast, is inversely related at still higher levels. Bandura and Rosenthal thought the disruptive effects of high levels of arousal may result from subjects trying to distract themselves when in an unpleasant modelling situation.

It is clear that fears can be acquired by modelling. We will later discuss how far this process applies to phobias seen in clinical practice.

7. Symbolic aspects of fear

We have just seen how new fears are acquired readily by social learning or modelling both in animals and men. However, man is unique in his capacity for intricate symbolic thought, and this forms a fertile source of new fears. The language used to describe the simpler type of conditioning experiment is inadequate when talking about complex thought processes. Pavlov coined the term "higher order conditioning" to describe long chains of conditioned events, and spoke of the "second signalling system" to denote speech and thought processes (Luria, 1961). Osgood (1953) coined the term "representational mediation process" to refer to similar events. In fact it is useful to think of ideas and thought as mediational or symbolic cues. These cues may become associated with anxiety to produce "higher-order-conditioning-like-progressions" (Paul, 1964)

Experimental work is badly needed in this area, though we can all relate anecdotes to illustrate the action of mediational processes in generating fear. A $3\frac{1}{2}$-year-old girl was happily going through a deserted Florentine courtyard until her parents mentioned that it was part of a palace. Immediately the girl wanted to leave and asked fearfully whether the king's soldiers would hurt her. For her the concept of "palace" at that moment included a king with frightening armed men, and this spontaneous and unexpected association made her apprehensive, though at other times the same child enjoyed passing other palaces where armed soldiers could in fact be seen. Clearly there were multiple determinants for the child's symbolism to arise at that particular time and place. Other children would probably have had very different associations.

Words act as symbols which can produce intense fear. A shout of the single word "fire" may cause extreme panic in a crowded theatre. Particular objects or situations are fraught with dread solely on account of their symbolic value. A gestapo uniform or a swastika would inspire alarm in entire communities during a certain epoch. Man's capacity for symbolism is infinite, and any cue may serve as a symbol for any idea. Any appropriate cue may therefore trigger fear through symbolic mediational processes.

This very plasticity of symbolism is a source of grave difficulty in studying the symbolism of human fears. We have no clear yardstick for saying when such processes are primary or secondary. Fears acquired by simple contiguity conditioning may be rationalised in terms of symbolic meanings attached secondarily to the frightening situation. For example, a woman became afraid to drive after a car accident and explained it as a fear of injuring people with the car; the explanation sounded plausible in terms of the symbolic value of the situation. The woman then regained confidence by gradually driving again and forgot about the symbolic meaning of the feared situation. On the one hand this was a fear acquired by one-trial learning in a setting of great anxiety, followed by gradual extinction through retraining. On the other hand, the symbolic aspect "makes sense" and is "understandable", even though it fell away during extinction. There may, of course, be interaction between levels of causation, conditioning mechanisms being more potent in a setting of guilt where symbolic conflicts are readily released.

Little systematic work is available on mediational cues in fear production. Agras (1966) studied the generalisation gradient of the GSR response to a hierachy of phobic stimuli imagined by several patients. He found discontinuities in the generalisation gradient at points of special significance to the patient. For example, when a patient with a fear of rabies imagined himself at different periods of possible exposure to infection, the discontinuity (a sudden increase in the GSR response) occurred at the imagined period of 10 days, which is the incubation period for the development of rabies after exposure.

Though mediational cues clearly affect fears and phobias systematic knowledge of this problem is sadly lacking. All we can say is that symbolism undoubtedly influences the production of certain fears in man, and that at other times symbolism appears as a secondary rather than as a primary phenomenon—here the fear produces symbolism, not the reverse, and in yet further cases a two way transaction occurs. This problem will be dealt with more fully when we come to discuss the phobias seen in clinical practice.

8. Experimental fear in children

For obvious reasons few experiments have tried to produce new fears in man by classical and instrumental conditioning. A classic case often cited is that of Watson and Rayner (1921), who produced fear of a white rat in an 11-month-old boy, Albert. Watson and Rayner presented him with a white rat to play with, and whenever he reached for the rat (CS) they made a loud noise by striking a steel bar behind his head (UCS). The sound caused him to cry (UCR). From the 5th trial onwards Albert showed fear in the presence of the rat (CR), and this fear generalised to other furry objects such as a fur neckpiece, a Santa Claus mask, cottonwool and a white rabbit.

Soon after Watson's work Mary Cover Jones showed how fears in children could be extinguished (1924 a and b). A 3-year-old boy whose fear of a white rat extended to a rabbit, a fur coat, a feather and cottonwool, was treated by direct reconditioning. The rabbit was associated with food which the child liked. In addition, other children attended who were not afraid, to foster social imitation.

Jones discussed 7 ways to eliminate fears in children. Three of these methods were ineffective—*disuse* (simple avoidance of the feared object), *repression* (by ridicule or teasing), and *verbal appeal*. Effective methods included *extinction* (negative adaptation), in which familiarity breeds contempt; *distraction* by playing with the feared object in the context of a desired goal—this is a variant of another method, *direct reconditioning*, in which the feared object is associated with a pleasant stimulus (a technique which Wolpe later called reciprocal inhibition). Finally, Jones noted the effectiveness of *social imitation*, in which the child watches other children enjoy playing with the feared object.

The cases of Watson and Jones have often been regarded as paradigms for human phobias (see e.g. Eysenck and Rachman, 1965). However, a neglected paper by English (1929) placed these cases in perspective.

English sat a 14-month-old girl in her own high chair in a laboratory and presented a wooden painted toy duck to her. As soon as the girl grasped it a large metal bar behind her head was struck a resounding blow. The duck was then withdrawn and was presented again at the next trial. Despite 50 trials no conditioned fear response was established to the duck because the noise itself failed to evoke fear. "The writer must confess his surprise—and admiration—at the child's iron nerves. In the later trials the metal bar was struck a tremendous blow with a two-pound hammer. Professors in remote parts of the building, students, and other children able to make a verbal report, all spoke of the distasteful and alarming nature of the sound". Yet a month later this same child showed fear of new patent leather boots when she saw them for the first time, and this fear generalised to objects next to it. English suggested that the child had become "unconditioned" to noise. "Since she has three older brothers, the means of this unconditioning may seem fairly obvious. Yet with the innately effective stimulus rendered ineffective, the fear response remains in excellent working order and can even be 'transferred' from one object to another". Yet usually conditioned responses require frequent association with unconditioned stimuli. English thought the differences between conditioned salivary reflexes, for example, and "unconditional emotional responses" made dubious the value of a single descriptive term. These observations antedate more recent workers like Franks and Franks (1966) who cast doubt on the notion of a general factor of conditionability.

One of the most systematic attempts to repeat Watson and Rayner's work was made by Bregman, a student of Thorndike's (see Thorndike, 1935). Fifteen babies of about the same age as little Albert were studied. A bell behind the baby's back caused startle. Instead of the white rat, 6 other objects were presented. Instead of the clang of the hammer on the steel bar, an electric bell rung behind the baby's back was used, which caused fear or startle. A rattle and the melody played by a little music-box was used to produce relief, contentment and interest. Bregman's technique largely failed to produce fear. Thorndike (1935) concluded that little Albert "was a special case and was definitely misleading concerning the probability of 'leaving on the infant's plastic nature a reaction pattern . . .' by any such quick and easy process of 'conditioning'. On the contrary, the influence of joint stimulation is so slight that we cannot demonstrate even its existence." Thorndike noted that these results "are like what parents usually get who try to shift attitudes (of children) toward fear of matches, knives, bottles, dangerous spots, and the like or toward tolerance and affection for uncles, aunts, physicians, cod-liver oil, green vegetables, keeping on mittens and the like. Progress is slow.

There are occasional sudden and dramatic shifts from a few associations (often only one), as when a child who is frightened and hurt shortly after being seated with a stranger in a railway car seat is extremely averse to being seated with any stranger in such a seat for months thereafter . . .", but these are rare.

Later writers like Kimble (1961) also pointed out that Watson's case was probably overstated. It took no account of the quality of the conditioned stimulus, and Valentine (1930) noted that fears might be much more easily conditioned to furry objects than to others such as a pair of opera-glasses. In fact English (1929) himself had noted ready conditioning of fear to a stuffed black cat despite his failure to condition fear to a wooden painted toy duck.

This point is relevant to recent findings in aversion treatment which further expose the inability of simple learning theory to account fully for the genesis of phobias in adults. Many adult patients with sexual deviations have now been shocked repeatedly while looking at or holding objects of their deviations. The objects included photographs of sexually deviant behaviour and an assortment of women's clothes. Although aversion reduces or abolishes sexual attraction to these objects, phobias rarely result (Bancroft and Marks, 1968), though they would be predicted by analogy with cases like little Albert. Phobias clearly involve more than simple associations between unpleasant and neutral or attractive stimuli. Fear can be conditioned much more readily to certain stimuli than to others.

Summary

Man is born with innate fear responses to a few unconditioned stimuli. Further innate fears take time to mature and manifest, but as he grows the child learns to fear many situations far removed from earlier frightening stimuli. These new fears develop by a complex learning process in which some of the principles are now understood from animal experiments.

The expression and learning of fear depend upon peripheral and neurophysiological mechanisms. Peripheral expression is effected through the sympathetic part of the autonomic nervous system. Autonomic responses reinforce emotional feelings produced by more central mechanisms. It is difficult to demonstrate a unique autonomic pattern of responses for fear, but some differentiation has been obtained from other emotional states such as anger. No single physiological variable is entirely satisfactory as an index of fear or anxiety, though measures of palmar skin conductance and to a lesser extent forearm blood flow have proved of some clinical value. Complex biochemical changes accompany states of fear, but these are not yet clearly understood.

Emotional states can begin as a non-specific increase in arousal to which cognitive cues are secondarily attached which help the subject to label the effect as fear, anger etc. depending upon the context of the emotional arousal.

Central physiological mechanisms underlying fear are largely situated in deep brain structures such as the hypothalamus, amygdala and other parts of the limbic system. Different aspects of fearful behaviour depend upon separate but interlinked central mechanisms. Epileptic attacks of fear suggest that both temporal lobes, especially the anterior portions, form part of the neurophysiological substrate of fear. They also can show separation of the experiential, cognitive and autonomic components of the fear response.

No single theory accounts for all the ways in which fear is learned. Fear can be learned easily as a response to previously neutral stimuli. Fear is a drive which motivates the learning and performance of new responses in the same way as hunger, thirst or other drives. Experimental paradigms of fear include classical conditioning situations, avoidance and escape conditioning, temporal pacing and punishment training. New fears may be acquired by a simple classical conditioning process in which a neutral stimulus is paired together with or shortly before a noxious stimulus—this is learning by temporal contiguity. The new fear increases with the frequency of the pairing, with the strength of the noxious stimulus, and when the pairing occurs in conditions of confinement or when nothing can be done to stop the noxious stimulation.

Once acquired, fear may be used as a drive to motivate instrumental learning, since a sudden reduction in the strength of fear serves as a reward to reinforce such learning—this is learning by drive reduction. Once fear becomes sufficiently strong it causes avoidance of the feared situation, often before fear has been fully experienced. This protects the fear from extinction by preventing its occurrence without reinforcement. When an avoidance response is prevented from occurring in the presence of fear stimuli, then rapid extinction of the avoidance response takes place.

Extinction depends upon repeated pairing of the frightening conditioned stimulus with neutral or pleasant stimuli or responses. Stronger fears extinguish more slowly than weaker ones. Some degree of control over the feared situation reduces fear. Sedative drugs and alcohol reduce fear but do not extinguish it. Subjects can be exposed to fear stimuli very slowly or very quickly—both methods can lead to extinction of the fear. Pleasant situations are more antagonistic to fear than neutral ones e.g. eating, companionship, familiar objects and sexual arousal.

The speed with which conditioned responses develop varies greatly between different reflex systems in the same individual, and between different individuals for the same reflex system. As yet there is no support for the notion of a general factor of conditionability for given individuals.

People can acquire fears rapidly by modelling or by simply being told that a given situation is frightening, without their ever experiencing any noxious stimulus themselves—this is vicarious learning. Objects or situations may also be frightening simply because of their symbolic value; mediational cues serve to attach fear to widely differing stimuli, but systematic data in this area is sadly lacking.

Section III. AETIOLOGY OF PHOBIAS

A. **Background features:**
   1. Phylogenetic influences: The prepotency of certain stimuli
   2. Epidemiological considerations
      a. Age incidence
      b. Sex incidence
      c. Overall incidence
          Fear Survey Schedules
   3. Individual genetic inheritance
   4. The varied disturbances associated with phobias
   5. Personality background
   6. Cultural influences inside and outside the family
   7. Physiological variables
   8. Biochemical factors

B. **Direct influences:**
   1. Trauma and stress. Forgetting and recall of the initiating trauma
   2. Modelling
   3. Sensory association (stimulus generalisation)
   4. Learning theory and the phobic disorders
   5. Symbolism: The psychoanalytic view

Summary:

A. BACKGROUND FEATURES

In assessing the aetiology of phobias in man we need to account for their general features. Phobias do not occur randomly with respect to all situations and people. Rather, phobias tend to occur in particular situations, at certain ages, with a sex bias, with other clusters of psychiatric symptoms, and in selected personality backgrounds.

1. Phylogenetic influences The prepotency of certain stimuli

Certain classes of stimuli are more likely than others to trigger off phobias, given that these different stimuli are all encountered quite frequently. Although in theory phobias may arise to any situation imaginable, most phobias in psychiatric practice are of a fairly limited range of situations with little reference to the frequency with which those situations are encountered in everyday life. For example, phobias of going into open spaces or of travelling by train are not often seen, yet all these situations are encountered frequently in daily life. Whether or not phobias develop depends in part upon the stimulus properties of a given situation.

It is not surprising that some stimuli have a prepotent ability to trigger phobias, since we have seen the same phenomenon in the normal fears of animals and man, and phobias are simply fears which are unusually intense. As Stanley Hall (1897) and Valentine (1930) pointed out, it is reasonable to expect that phylogenetic mechanisms in man make certain stimuli prepotent over others in the production of phobias, although naturally phylogenetic mechanisms in man play a subsidiary role to that of individual experience.

Phylogenetic influences concern, for example, the avoidance of perceived depth by many species including man as soon as they are mobile, the fear of strangers found in primates and man after the first stage of social approach, and the fear in older children of objects which move suddenly towards them in writhing or jerking fashion. Whether these fears become persistent phobias of heights, strangers or animals depends less on their innate basis than on the way such mechanisms are elaborated by subsequent experience.

This should be stressed. Innate mechanisms probably do not of themselves produce phobias, but make certain situations prepotent targets for phobias when other conditions are superimposed; the reflex mechanism can then be seen in certain aspects of the phobia. The point is illustrated by a woman who developed a phobia of heights for the first time at the age of 40. She suddenly felt dizzy and in danger of falling while on an escalator, shortly after a fenestration operation for deafness. The dizziness subsided but a phobia of escalators started and spread until she was unable to ascend a single flight of stairs. One traumatic episode had triggered the innate fear into a phobia which showed the same innate feature found in other adults with phobias of heights, viz. reflex increase of the phobias with any visual element which emphasises perceived depth. For example, the open well of a staircase triggers acute anxiety, and such patients feel quite comfortable looking through a glass window which only reaches down to their waist, but are frightened if the glass window extends from the ceiling to the floor. It seems likely that these phenomena depend upon opticokinetic reflexes which produce a healthy respect for heights in normal people. We have already seen that these reflexes appear in human infants as soon as they can crawl.

It is tempting to suppose a similar explanation for certain features in phobias of open spaces. Several writers (Westphal, 1871; Clevenger, 1890; Vincent, 1919; Weiss, 1964) have noted that such phobias are worse where there is no boundary to a large open visual field, and diminish as soon as a boundary is imposed, be this a hedge, fence, trees, undulations of the ground or simply an umbrella held above the head.

One seems to require an optimum amount of space around one's person for different purposes, and discomfort results if this is too large or too small. If a small dinner party is held in a vast hall, a sense of comfortable intimacy is preserved if a screen is placed between the dining section and the rest of the hall. Conversely, if this space is made too small a sense of oppression is felt, and we all have been in very small rooms which cause discomfort even though there is no actual physical limitation of movement. It is likely that the regulation of one s body space is based in part on innate mechanisms which are of course greatly modified by individual and cultural experience, and that such mechanisms help to shape the form of claustrophobia.

Traces of innate elements are seen in patients with phobias of animals. The same property which elicits reflex fear in primates, intensifies phobias of animals in patients. Such patients find that movement of the feared animal is especially frightening. Examples are the fluttering wings of birds and moths, the scurry of insects, the running of dogs and the stalk of cats.

Patients with social phobias complain that they are most afraid when subjected to the gaze of others, yet feel at ease in the same company when not under scrutiny. This is an intensification of the natural discomfort normal people feel when being stared at. It arises out of innate elements for which evidence has already been cited in man and in animals.

2. Epidemiological considerations

a. AGE INCIDENCE

Certain classes of stimuli are more likely to trigger off phobias at particular ages, regardless of the frequency of exposure to such stimuli. For example, sudden loud noises or movements trigger fear easily in very young infants, fears of strangers are the rule in older infants, fears of animals usually begin in preschool children, while fears of open spaces and social situations mostly start between adolescence and middle age (Marks and Gelder, 1966) and are rare in childhood (Rutter et al., 1968). The stage of development a person has reached thus influences the kind of phobia he is likely to develop.

The influence of age is a consequence of several factors. Maturation is important for the phasic emergence of fears of strangers in year-old infants. Maturation also helps to explain why, given constant exposure to animals at most ages, animal phobias start so commonly and spontaneously in early childhood, but only rarely after puberty. We have already seen that in preschool children animal phobias start with a trivial incident or none at all, though similar episodes at an earlier age had no remarkable result. Animal phobias which begin in adult life are usually initiated by a definite trauma involving the animal concerned.

In contrast, the age incidence of other phobias reflects not the influence of maturation but rather the effect of increased exposure to the situation in question. For example, school phobias not surprisingly occur only when children have had experience of school. Similarly, fears of death, heart disease or cancer appear increasingly in later life as the adult learns what these are and is exposed more to such experiences in his environment. A child with no concept of death will not express a fear of dying, though he may well fear ghosts, bogeymen and related horrors.

It is not at all clear, however, why the agoraphobic syndrome should be a particular feature of young adult life, when people of all ages are exposed to the rigours of going into open spaces and streets. It is possible that the cluster of phobias involved depends upon mechanisms which become prominent after puberty, but we have no firm clue to what these may be. It is relevant here that anxiety states have the same range of onset age as the agoraphobic syndrome, and that the two conditions overlap considerably in their clinical features, except that anxiety states occur with equal frequency in both sexes and by definition have few pronounced situational phobias—their anxiety is mainly generalised and not situational.

Finally, there are yet other phobias which arise with equal facility at any time of life. Such are the more isolated phobias of darkness, heights, enclosed spaces or thunder (Fig. 3.1)*

Fears in general have a higher incidence in childhood which falls off during adolescence and early adult life (MacFarlane et al., 1954; Agras et al., 1969). Only fears of death, injury and illness increase in the older age groups, with a peak in the 6th decade (Agras et al., 1969).

b. SEX INCIDENCE

Different phobias have a varying sex incidence. Before puberty both sexes seem equally liable to most fears (Macfarlane, Allen and Honzik, 1954), but after puberty most phobias are commoner in women (Marks and Gelder, 1966; Agras et al., 1969). The preponderance of women is less marked for social phobias (Marks and Gelder, 1966) and for isolated phobias such as those of darkness, heights, thunder or accidents. There are hardly any phobias which men manifest consistently more than women apart, of course, from those concerned specifically with their sexual role. A mixture of influences is again at work here, including greater masculine aggression due to androgens

---

* To introduce a wry note, phobic patients also find that their age influences the explanations their doctors offer as the cause of their phobias. Members of a phobic club noted the explanations to vary as follows: (The Open Door Newsletter, Nov., 1965).
"Teenagers—Adolescence—you'll grow out of it.
Early twenties—Sexual Frustration—find a husband.
25–35 (single)—Sexual Frustration—find a husband.
25–35 (married)—Effort of running a home and caring for your family.   'You'll feel better when the children go to school'.
36–65—THE CHANGE! This is the favourite explanation and dozens of women in their thirties have been told they've started early.
65 onwards—Old Age."

and social learning, differential exposure of the sexes to particular situations, and differences in their social obligations. All these will mould the opportunity for contact with the phobic situation, the quality of this contact and the vigour with which fear in that situation will be overcome.

c. OVERALL INCIDENCE

Little is yet known about the prevalence of phobic disorders in the general adult community. One of the few systematic studies was made by Agras et al (1969) in Vermont. They gave an interview schedule to 325 subjects who formed a 1 : 193 sample of Greater Burlington. Fifty phobic patients were also interviewed by two psychiatrists. The sample was carefully selected, but the total numbers were small, so the figures of this study should be regarded as provisional. The total prevalence of phobias was estimated at 77 per 1000 of the normal population, but severely disabling phobias were estimated at only 2·2 per 1000. Fewer than 1 : 1000 of the population was currently receiving psychiatric treatment for phobias, though 9 : 1000 had had treatment for phobias at one time or another. It was estimated that only a quarter of severely disabled phobics were being treated for their phobias.

Though agoraphobia formed 50% of clinical cases, its prevalence in the population was 6·3 : 1000. In contrast, phobias of injury, illness and death were five times more prevalent, but formed only 34% of the clinical cases. It is relevant here that in the Maudsley material shown later in Table 3.2 the commonest clinical phobia was also agoraphobia, with illness phobias as the next commonest group.

Recently fear survey schedules have been used to detect fear in normal populations, usually of students (e.g. Lang and Lazowick, 1963; Geer, 1965; Hannah et al., 1965; Grossberg and Wilson, 1965; Wilson, 1967) but these were not designed to study the incidence of phobias, and only measure self reports of fear, not the amount of avoidance. As was noted earlier, of 20% of Lang's students who reported intense fears, only 1–2% actually avoided snakes in a test, and Geer's male students who reported intense fears of dogs showed no avoidance of dogs. Of Geer's students, 38% reported one or more severe fears, and less than 2% reported no fears of any kind. A consistent finding with fear survey schedules is that women report significantly more fears than men (Manosevitz and Lanyon, 1965; Geer, 1965; Hannah et al, 1965; Wilson, 1967; Julier, 1967).

These figures, however, are no guide to the incidence of phobic disorders in the community, because most subjects who reported intense fears on the questionnaires were not so handicapped by these fears that they had to seek treatment for them. The fears of these subjects were interesting phenomena rather than disorders demanding treatment.

A rough estimate is possible of the frequency of phobic disorders in psychiatric practice. A survey of outpatient clinics in the United States by the National Institutes of Mental Health revealed that "phobic reaction" was diagnosed in 0·5% of males and 1·0% of females over 18 (Frazier and Carr, 1967). This was 2·6% and 3·2% of all male and female psychoneurotics. Terhune (1949) found phobic disorders in 2·5% of patients in his private practice, most of whom were psychoneurotics. Errera and Coleman (1963) noted 2·8% of patients in a Connecticut psychiatric clinic had phobic states. At the Maudsley Hospital in London 2 to 3% of all psychiatric outpatients had phobic disorders (Hare, 1965). The only study to report a higher incidence was that of Clapham et al (1956), who noted that 8% of psychiatric patients in a Glasgow hospital had "predominantly phobic illnesses".

Phobic symptoms are far commoner than phobic disorders and were present in 20% of Errera and Coleman's patients and in 20% of patients from several psychiatric institutions who completed Spitzer's standardized interview schedule (cited by Frazier and Carr, 1967). Paskind (1931) reported phobic symptoms in as many as 44% of all his cases in private practice, but he interpreted the term "phobic" very widely.

Spitzer found significantly fewer phobic symptoms in patients from a rural area of Kentucky than from New York City, and these differences were not accounted for on the basis of social class.

In summary, though phobic symptoms may be present in 20% of psychiatric patients, phobic disorders are found in fewer than 3% of all cases seen in psychiatric practice in America and England.

Fear Survey Schedules: Hall's was probably the first survey of fears in a normal population (1897). Few studies of fears in adults appeared subsequently until the last decade, since when many surveys have been made. In 1956 Akutagawa constructed a fear inventory which formed the basis for many later studies by Lang and Lazowick (1965), Wolpe and Lang (1964), Geer (1965), Manosevitz and Lanyon (1965), Hannah et al. (1965), Grossberg and Wilson (1965), Wilson (1967) and Rubin et al. (1968). The author constructed another fear inventory to assess the fears present in a phobic population, and this was also used by Julier (1967). A fear inventory for children was reported by Scherer and Nakamura (1968). Yet other inventories exist to screen for the presence of problems like stage fright, examination anxiety and the like.

Most fear survey schedules measure self reports of fear without testing the amount of avoidance of the frightening situations. The relationship between such self reports and avoidance behaviour was studied by Geer (1965) who found that women avoided dogs more as they reported more fear, but that men showed no avoidance

of dogs even when they reported intense fear. Lanyon and Manosevitz (1966) also noted that women's self reports of fear of spiders
correlated significantly with subsequent avoidance of spiders in a
test situation. They concluded that self reports of fear are valid,
if gross, indicators of fear in an actual situation.

Geer's finding that men showed no avoidance despite their report
of fear makes it unlikely that many men who avoid dogs conceal a
fear of dogs in their self reports. It suggests that the percentage
of men who report subjective fear is an overestimate of fear
behaviour amongst men. This is important because women
consistently report more fear than do men on fear schedules, and
this is true for most fears. Geer's result makes it less likely that the
sex discrepancy in self reports of fear is simply because men
conceal their fears in the belief that they are socially undesirable.
It makes it more likely that the adult males genuinely experience
less fear than women. Wilson (1967) noted that women report
more fears which a panel of judges rated as "silly" than do men,
but this may simply reflect their greater incidence of fears rather
than any concealment by men. Wilson also found (1966) that
16 males and 16 females showed similar changes in skin conductance when seeing a series of slides depicting snakes, spiders and
landscapes, and claimed that this supported the idea that men
express fewer fears than women because they regard fears as less
socially desirable. Unfortunately his sample was far too small to
allow any such conclusion, since the highest incidence of intense
fears reported for snakes and spiders in an undergraduate population is only about 3 % for males and 20 % for females (Hannah et al.,
1965). Before any conclusions are possible it is necessary to test at
least 100 members of each sex yielding parallel measures of subjective anxiety, skin conductance and overt avoidance.

Three mechanisms may be acting together to produce a lower
incidence of fears in normal men. First is the biological difference
between men and women in that men tend to be stronger, more
aggressive and less fearful—this difference is partly due to circu-
lating androgens. Next, from early childhood onwards environmental pressures are stronger on boys to be brave than on girls, and
this may later make men less susceptible to fear. Finally, men
may be less willing to admit fear than are women.

Several studies of fear survey schedules report significant
correlations between total scores on the schedules and other
measures of "anxiety" such as the Taylor Manifest Anxiety Scale,
the neuroticism score of the Eysenck Personality Inventory, the
emotionality scale of Bendig's inventory and Welsh's A scale
(Lang and Lazowick, 1965; Hannah et al., 1965; Geer, 1965;
Grossberg and Wilson, 1965). Manosevitz and Lanyon (1965)

failed to find a significant relationship in men between fear survey schedule scores and the Taylor Manifest Anxiety Scale.

Though several groupings of fears have been suggested, on the whole the range of fears covered in survey schedules so far is too small, and the relationship of the fears to other phenomena too ill-defined, to allow of meaningful conclusions from these groupings.

3.   Individual genetic inheritance

Though phylogenetic influences shape the form of phobias in man as a species, there is no firm evidence that genetic inheritance plays a significant part in the development of phobic states in particular patients. A minority of phobic patients have close relatives with the same phobia, but this might reflect the role of modelling rather than of genes. Genetic endowment could act through intermediary mechanisms such as constitution and temperament. For example, Shields (1962) has shown that on scores for "neuroticism" monozygotic twins reared apart resembled one another more than did dyzygotic twins. However, very few monozygotic twins are concordant for phobic disorders, and the author has not encountered any instance in the literature, unlike the occasional concordance for obsessive neurosis and obsessive fears (e.g. Marks et al., 1969) The Maudsley genetics unit has encountered five sets of monozygotic twins in whom one of the pair was phobic, but has no examples in whom both had a phobic disorder (Shields, personal communication).

It is interesting that few fat people appear to complain of phobias, the asthenic habitus seeming the commonest physical type amongst phobics. However, such impressions can be notoriously misleading, and a definitive study on the role of inheritance and constitution remains to be done.

4.   The varied disturbances associated with phobias

Certain phobias tend to occur alone as isolated problems, while other phobias are often found together in the same person and in association with other disturbances. For example, an adult with a marked phobia of cats is likely to have few other phobias and little else in the way of psychiatric symptoms. In contrast, a person who has marked phobias of going into open spaces is also liable to be afraid of going into crowds, trains, buses and into confined spaces; such a person is likely as well to have anxiety apart from these phobic situations, and to experience fluctuating mild depression, depersonalisation and perhaps obsessive thoughts and actions (Marks, 1967).

Different phobias thus have varying significance, some being a simple localised disturbance which is easily explained, whilst others are but one manifestation of a larger disorder whose aetiology is much more complex. This important problem is dealt with more fully elsewhere in this book, in the sections on classification and description of the different types of phobic disorder.

5. Personality background of phobic patients

Much has been written about the kind of *personality* which is predisposed to develop phobias. Most articles about this concern patients who are agoraphobics in the broad sense. In general the personalities of phobic patients have been described as timid, shy, dependent and immature, though this has been expressed in different ways by various authors; dependent personality disorder (Tucker, 1956); dependent, immature with a past history of childhood fears (Terhune, 1949); dutiful, reserved, high ideals, bottled up feelings (Diethelm, 1936); dependent, clinging and orally fixated (Weiss, 1957); dominant overprotection by mother with castration fear (Webster, 1953); emotionally immature and excessively dependent (Harper and Roth, 1962). Of these authors the only ones who had control groups were Webster, whose phobic women had significantly different personalities from women with anxiety neurosis or conversion hysteria, and Harper and Roth, whose patients with their phobic-anxiety-depersonalisation syndrome had significantly different personalities from a group of temporal lobe epileptics. A further control figure is available from Gelder, Marks and Wolff (1967): their phobic patients had high introversion scores on the Eysenck Personality Inventory which departed significantly from control norms.

It is thus clear that many phobic patients who see psychiatrists have unusual personalities. Nevertheless, it is important to note that phobic patients often have normally sociable outgoing and independent personalities before their phobias begin (Prince, 1912; Marks and Gelder, 1965). Statements like the following from a nurse who became agoraphobic are not uncommon: "I'd always been such an independent person before and I felt such an absolute idiot having to rely on somebody all the time. You feel so silly saying 'will you come with me, I don't like going on my own'." Though a dependent personality forms fertile soil for phobias, it is by no means a necessary condition for their formation. There is evidence (Klein, 1964; Marks unpublished data) that agoraphobics with a childhood history of separation anxiety or other fears develop their agoraphobia earlier in adult life than patients without a history of such childhood symptoms. It is possible that a dependent personality and agoraphobia both reflect the same constitutional make-up without being causally linked directly to one another.

6. Cultural influences inside and outside the family

The early family subculture of an individual plays some part in determining sickness phobias, as Ryle (1948) and Straker (1951) have noted. Sickness phobias can develop on the basis of childhood anxieties inspired when the threat of sickness is made as punishment for wrong-doing. The form of a particular phobia which develops depends upon the previous health history which may have fixated anxiety on a parti-cular body system, upon identification with illness in a close relative, and upon specific traumatic events during maturation and their signifi-cance on particular bodily symptoms. Like all symptoms, sickness phobias can be used to express a desire for dependence and sympathetic care.

Fears tend to run in families and are especially associated in mothers and daughters (Agras et al., 1969). Hagman (1932) found a correlation of ·67 between the number of fears reported by mother and child. Similarly John (1941) reported a correlation of ·59 between fears of air-raids shown by mother and child during the bombings of London in World War II. Finally, Marks and Herst (1969) found that 19% of agoraphobics in Britain reported that they had a close relative with the same kind of phobia.

Outside the family wider cultural factors also influence phobias of sickness. Zborowski (1952) showed that response to pain and to disease takes place within an elaborate cultural context in which the patient, his family and the community respond in socially patterned ways; for example Jewish and Italian Americans respond emotionally and tend to exaggerate their pain experience, while Irish and "old Americans" in contrast are more stoical. Clearly phobias based upon bodily symptoms will also depend upon cultural background.

Broad cultural influences affect the "popularity" of certain phobias (Laughlin, 1956), and these apply to situations both internal and external to the body. In the 16th century fears were prevalent about demons, witches and sorcery, whereas these are rarely met with in industrialised countries today. In this century we find fears of cancer, venereal and heart disease, fears of every kind of modern transport, and fears of atomic destruction or of outer space (e.g. Ashem, 1963; Kerry, 1960). As new objects and concepts evolve a few people are bound to develop phobias of these fresh situations and to express them in new ways. Other phobias persist unchanged across the cen-turies—Hippocrates and Burton described the same fears of heights, open spaces, animals, sharp instruments, death and insanity which we find so commonly today.

Laughlin (1956) suggested further that as civilization has progressed fear has changed from an originally simple response to external danger to become more complex, so that a manifest object of fear conceals a more latent hidden source of anxiety. "As the objects of fear have become more complex in modern life, responses of 'fight or flight' have done likewise". We will take up this problem of phobic symbolism later.

7. Physiological variables

Physiological variables are not the same in all kinds of phobias and anxiety states, which suggests that different mechanisms may operate in the genesis of different phobias. Four variables are relevant. Two are measures of the galvanic skin resistance (GSR) viz., the spontaneous rate of fluctuation of the skin conductance and the rate of habituation of the galvanic skin response to successive auditory stimuli. As noted earlier, spontaneous fluctuations increase and habituation decreases with high clinical anxiety (Lader and Wing, 1966). The third variable is forearm blood flow, which also increases as clinical anxiety rises (Kelly, 1966). The fourth variable concerns the rate at which eyeblink conditioned responses are acquired and extinguished. Data about this comes from Martin et al. (1969). Eyeblink conditioned responses (CR's) were measured with a puff of air as the UCS and a tone as the CS. The eyeblink CR acquisition rate correlates significantly positively with improvement in treatment by desensitisation, i.e. patients who improved most had the highest acquisition rates. Acquisition rates correlate significantly with extinction rates.

The physiological variables discriminate between different types of phobia and anxiety states as follows: Animal phobias have a normal GSR habituation rate, few spontaneous fluctuations of the GSR, normal forearm blood flow at rest and an increased rate of acquisition and slow rate of extinction of eyeblink conditioned responses (CR's). Agoraphobics have slow GSR habituation, many spontaneous fluctuations of the GSR, a slightly raised forearm blood flow at rest, and a normal rate of acquisition of eyeblink CR's. Patients with anxiety states are similar except that their forearm blood flow is much increased. Social phobics are like agoraphobics, except that social phobics have a raised rate of acquisition of eyeblink CR's. Improvement by a variety of treatments is greater when patients have few spontaneous fluctuations in the GSR. Improvement by desensitisation treatment is greater in patients with a GSR which habituates readily, and with a high rate of acquisition of eyeblink CR's.

Clinical features which will be amplified later help us to understand some of the significance of the physiological differences among phobias. We know clinically that patients with isolated animal phobias have little general anxiety, so it is not surprising that such patients as well as normal subjects had the physiological correlates of low general anxiety, viz. few spontaneous fluctuations and normal habituation of the GSR. What is rather surprising is that they should have shown rapid eyeblink conditioning, since this group had the fewest phobias and other symptoms. If one expected that phobias are acquired easily in patients who condition readily, then this group should have had the most not the fewest, phobias. But we have seen elsewhere that there is little evidence to support the notion of general conditionability across several functional systems, and we do not yet know the correlates of eyeblink conditioning. It is possible that eyeblink conditioning is related to learning at a particular sensitive age. This hypothesis fits our data that the majority of animal phobias began before the age of 7. One is tempted to speculate about facilitatory periods of learning, and the influence of conditionability during this period. This hypothesis is worth testing, although there is some preliminary evidence against it from our group of social phobias. These began mostly after puberty, yet their eyeblink conditioning rate was also raised.

We know that general anxiety is a feature of anxiety states and many agoraphobics, so it makes good sense that both these groups showed GSR and forearm blood flow correlates of general anxiety. It is gratifying that habituation rate should be related to improvement with desensitisation, since some of this therapeutic procedure involves a process analogous to habituation. Patients who did not habituate readily would not be expected to benefit greatly from this technique, and this is what was found. The association of many spontaneous fluctuations with poor response to treatment agrees with clinical observation that marked clinical anxiety makes treatment much more difficult.

The importance of general anxiety may lie in its association with sudden phasic panic attacks. A common event in agoraphobic patients is that months of arduous desensitisation are undone when the patient experiences a sudden panic attack in the street she has just become accustomed to again. This panic triggers off a fresh phobia of going into the street, and treatment has to start again. Desensitisation is then a Sisyphean task unless the anxiety and panic attacks disappear, as after modified leucotomy, after which desensitisation can proceed successfully (Marks, Birley and Gelder, 1966). It appears that during a panic attack a patient conditions rapidly to the prevailing environment, so although agoraphobics are not rapid eyeblink conditioners under most circumstances, they may well be rapid conditioners during the panic attack. This idea requires laboratory confirmation—panic attacks did not occur in our patients while they were being tested—but it would explain the discrepancy of normal conditioning rates in patients with high general anxiety and multiple phobias. Phobias may be conditioned only during moments of intense anxiety and panic. Patients with high general anxiety are susceptible to phasic panic attacks which are probably the crucial events in generating phobias. Lader and Wing (1966) have suggested that in normal persons a habituation mechanism damps down excessive arousal responses, while in anxious people minor arousal responses with many spontaneous fluctuations and poor habituation of the GSR are liable instead to go into a phase of positive feedback which we see clinically as a panic attack.

We are left with the question of origin of the general anxiety in agoraphobics. No one has yet answered this adequately.

8. Biochemical factors

No biochemical abnormality has yet been demonstrated in patients who have isolated phobias. However, in patients who have diffuse phobias together with anxiety at rest away from the public situation, certain abnormalities have been reported, though such patients have usually been included in a group of anxiety neurotics. Since many diffuse agoraphobics are clinically similar to anxiety neurotics apart from their additional phobias, this research in anxiety neurosis is relevant.

A number of abnormalities have been reported in patients with anxiety neurosis in response to standard exercises—decreased exercise tolerance, low oxygen intake, and increased blood lactate, though resting blood lactate is normal (Cohen and White, 1950; Pitts and McLure, 1967). However, it is not clear whether these findings apply specifically to patients with anxiety neurosis or whether they are the general signs of poor health, chronic illness, or poor state of physical training.

The effect of infusions of sodium lactate was recently investigated by Pitts and McLure (1967) in 14 anxiety neurotics and 10 controls. Three infusions were given of sodium lactate, lactate with added calcium ions and a control of glucose in saline. The lactate infusions produced anxiety attacks in 13 of the 14 patients with anxiety neurosis. The patients maintained that the symptoms were markedly similar or identical to those experienced in their worst attacks. The attacks began a minute or two after the infusions started and decreased rapidly once the 20 minute infusion was completed, but was often followed by 24–72 hours of exhaustion and symptom exacerbation. Only 2 of the control subjects experienced anxiety, and their symptoms were milder than those of the anxiety neurotics.

When calcium was added to the lactate infusion only a few anxiety symptoms were produced, and these were mild. Glucose in saline infusions caused no attacks.

Pitts and McLure noted that the symptoms of anxiety neurosis and of pretetanic hypocalcemia are identical, and that the infusion of sodium lactate produced some of these symptoms in all subjects and anxiety attacks in anxiety neurotics.   Since the addition of calcium ion to the sodium lactate infusion markedly decreased its effects, they suggested that there may be something highly specific about lactate ion in producing hypocalcaemic anxiety symptoms in humans.   They suggested that anxiety symptoms have a common determining biochemical end mechanism involving the complexing of ionized calcium at the surface of the excitable membranes in the interstitial fluid by lactate ion produced intracellularly.   Furthermore, they suggested that anxiety symptoms could be produced in normals under stress as a consequence of marked increase in lactate production in response to increased adrenaline release, and that the anxiety neurotic was especially subject to this by reason of chronic overproduction of adrenaline, over-activity of the central nervous system, a defect in aerobic or anaerobic metabolism resulting in excess lactate production, a defect in calcium metabolism or some combination of these.

This research adds to earlier observations that patients with anxiety neuroses react abnormally to many stresses of a psychological, physio-logical and biochemical kind. But we remain ignorant of the basic disturbance distinguishing anxiety neurotics from normals which lead to this abnormal reaction. This research may yield further clues to the pathogenesis of abnormal anxiety.

B. DIRECT INFLUENCES ON PHOBIAS

1. Trauma and stress

It is well recognised that sudden trauma can be followed by phobias of objects connected with that event. Phobias may be circumscribed when they follow a simple *physical* trauma—examples are fears of dogs after dogbites (Friedman, 1966b), a phobia of heights after a fall down stairs, and a fear of cars and driving after a car accident (Wolpe, 1962; Kushner, 1965; Kraft and Il-Issa, 1965). More subtle *psychological* trauma can have the same result when it evokes severe anxiety, guilt or impotent resentment. There is often a lag of a few days between the original trauma and the onset of the phobia. Once begun, the phobia may take a while to reach its full intensity. It is not clear what happens during the lag phase after the trauma: quite possibly during this period the patient rehearses the trauma in his mind and builds up associated emotions which increase and finally trigger the phobia. Tension is relieved once the patient begins to escape from or to avoid the painful situation, and this reduction in tension strengthens the tendency to further avoidance.

For example, a shy woman aged 42 had long felt sensitive to the stares of people. She was given the wrong change in a shop and was too uneasy to claim her proper change back. After a few weeks she gradually became first uncomfortable in the shop, then could not go into it, and later could not even pass the shop in the street lest she saw the man who had given her insufficient change. She was always able to remember the original trigger, and talking about it made no difference to the strength of her phobia.

In the war neuroses Kardiner and Spiegel (1941) suggested that the acute phase was the time when the neurosis became organised. To prevent this occurrence they recommended early therapy of the shell-shocked soldier as near as possible to the front lines and the sounds and smells of battle. Animal experiments bear this out. In rats Will-muth and Peters (1964) noted a critical period of about 3 days after the trauma of electric shocks during which re-exposure to the traumatic situation enhanced extinction of the newly conditioned fear.

Phobias may also begin after more general disturbance of the life situation, without a specific link between the disturbing event and the subsequent phobia. Agoraphobia (or in Roth's terminology, phobic-anxiety-depersonalisation) often starts shortly after major disruptions such as bereavement, marital separation, accident or severe physical illness, to the extent that it has been described as the "calamity syndrome". This event is an instance of a more general phenomenon, since other disorders such as depression, schizophrenia, asthma and coronorary thrombosis, to name but a few, may follow major upheavals of a similar kind. Massive physical and psychological disturbance renders an individual susceptible to a large variety of disorders. Hinkle and Wolff (1957) showed a close relationship between organic and psychiatric disorders within the same individual. Both classes of disturbance appeared to occur at the same period in an individuals' life history. Of equal interest are those many phobias which begin without any major change in the patient's environment.

In these instances the change appears to be within the patient rather than in his surroundings. One example of this kind is the spontaneous appearance of animal phobias in preschool children as they approach the age of sensitivity. A different mechanism is found in agoraphobia which starts out of the blue. A patient of this sort might give the story that "I was standing at the bus stop wondering what to cook for dinner when suddenly I felt panicky and sweaty, my knees felt like jelly, and I had to hold on to the lamppost and I was afraid I would die. I got on the bus and was terribly nervous, but just managed to totter home. Since then I haven't liked to go out in the street and have never been on a bus again". In such cases the primary event is anxiety which arose within the patient for no accountable reason. The phobia develops secondarily as the anxiety is attached to the immediate environment prevailing when the internal anxiety happens to surge. First comes the panic without relation to the surroundings, the surroundings are then attached or conditioned to the anxiety and agoraphobia has begun.

Severe depression is yet another change within the patient which can trigger an agoraphobic syndrome. In such cases the phobias start during a depressive illness and remain when the depression clears. Rarely the same occurs after a schizophrenic illness subsides. Finally, not a few phobias of all kinds begin without any obvious change either in the patient or in his surroundings. In these the origin of the phobia is obscure.

Forgetting and recall of the initiating trauma

Most phobic patients remember the onset of their phobia and discuss any precipitating trauma fairly openly. Occasional cases are found where the origins of the phobia are shrouded in mystery, but during treatment or chance events the patient will recall the original trauma which had triggered the phobia. In such cases recall of the forgotten events may herald disappearance of the phobia. In the early years of the 20th century such dramatic sequences were taken to support the prevalent view that neurotic disturbances resulted from repression of traumatic memories. This led to treatment designed to relieve phobias by obtaining recall of the original trauma.

Bagby (1922) was one of the authors who stressed the importance of trauma which caused intense fear, especially if it involved forbidden actions which prevented discussion and resulted in guilt with "protective forgetting" or repression. He cited two illustrative cases:

The first case was a 7 year old girl who went with her aunt on a picnic after she promised her mother to be obedient to the aunt. The two then went into the woods for a walk, and the girl, disobeying the aunt's instructions, ran off alone. The aunt followed, and after a search, found the child lying wedged among the rocks of a small stream with a waterfall pouring down over her head. She was screaming with terror. They proceeded to a farm house where the wet clothes were dried. The child expressed great fear that her mother would learn of her disobedience, but the aunt reassured her with the promise "I will never tell". They returned home and the aunt left the house next morning without seeing her niece. The child was thus left with no one in whom she could confide and had a period of anxiousness.

A severe phobia of running water developed shortly after this, and she became unable to hear a bathtub being filled without anxiety, might require three members of the family to give her a bath, was very frightened if she heard children using a drinking fountain near her classroom, and when she rode on trains had to have the window curtain down to avoid looking at streams over which the trains passed.

During her twentieth year the aunt came to visit her home, and the young woman saw her for the first time in 13 years. The aunt greeted the girl with the words "I have never told". This served to provoke recall of the original episode which had long been forgotten, after which the young woman found it possible to approach running water without discomfort. Gradually the special adjustments which her phobia had necessitated disappeared.

Bagby's second case followed the same pattern:

A young boy would often pass a grocery store on errands, and when passing would steal a handful of peanuts from the stand in front. One day the owner saw him coming and hid behind a barrel. Just as the boy put his hand in the pile of peanuts the owner jumped out and grabbed him from behind. The boy screamed and fell fainting on the sidewalk.

The boy developed a phobia of being grasped from behind. In social gatherings he arranged to have his chair against the wall. It was impossible for him to enter crowded places or to attend the theatre. When walking on the street he would have to look back over his shoulder at intervals to see if he was closely followed.

This phobia continued until the age of 55, when the man returned to the town of his childhood. He met the grocer, introduced himself and during reminiscences the grocer finally told him the story of the stolen peanuts. The man remembered the episode and the phobia disappeared after a period of readjustment.

These cases leave little doubt that phobias do sometimes clear after recall of a forgotten trauma which had initiated the phobia. The point is of sufficient import to warrant a final illustration (from Moss, 1960):

While a 4 year old girl was playing her pet dog knocked her little sister on the ground, causing a splinter wound in the cheek. The sister died a few days later, apparently of an infection. The mother openly accused the patient of knocking her sister down. The day of the sister's funeral the mother angrily accused the child again of causing yet other damage which in fact had been produced by the dog. Several days later the girl began to dislike dogs and soon developed a severe dog phobia which persisted until the age of 45, when the patient sought treatment as she wanted to give her daughter a puppy as a birthday present. Memories of the original events were recovered by the patient after four sessions of hypnosis. The dog phobia rapidly subsided and the patient remained well a year later.

Further cases like these have also been noted by Laughlin (1956), Galibert (1963) and Little and James (1964). Most of the cases which were cited experienced their traumas in childhood rather than in adult life, except in the dramatic cases of soldiers with war neuroses who obtained relief by abreaction. The histories are well documented and leave little doubt that in a minority of cases recall of forgotten traumas heralds relief from phobias connected with them. However, we must be cautious about the role forgotten traumas play in the genesis of phobias. Patients cited above recalled the original events decades after they had occurred, and it is not clear at what stage the incidents were forgotten, nor whether there were other equally important traumas which were never recalled although the phobia improved. Quite possibly the forgetting occurred long after the phobia had begun and included events unconnected with the trauma. The majority of phobics clearly remember the onset of their phobias and experience no relief from talking about it. Finally, hypnotic and abreactive sessions can alleviate anxiety non-specifically without the content of such sessions necessarily having much relevance to the original cause of the anxiety.

2. Modelling

Modelling or vicarious learning occasionally influences the production of phobias. We have seen elsewhere that this process can easily produce minor fears. Young children sometimes acquire persistent phobias from their parents, and in turn parents' existing phobias can be reinforced if the child develops the same phobia. Agoraphobic patients not infrequently have close relatives with the same disorder. Some agoraphobics also dread hearing fellow sufferers air their complaints, since this aggravates the listener's existing symptoms. On the other hand, yet other patients are simply relieved to hear that they are not the only people to have such problems.

On the whole the majority of phobics do not have relatives with the same phobias as themselves. Modelling experiences undoubtedly occur, but do not play a major role in the genesis of persistent phobias seen in psychiatric practice.

3. Sensory association

Sensory association plays an important part in the selection of a phobic object. Stimulus generalisations is an alternative term to describe the same process. Once strong fear has occurred in a particular sensory context it tends to reappear in other similar situations. The associations may be on the basis of simple sensory cues in any modality. The classical cases of Watson and Rayner (1920) and of Cover Jones (1924) involved auditory associations where little boys became afraid of animals which they had seen at the same time as they heard a loud noise. Tactile and thermal associations shaped a phobia of heat in a case of Ivey's (1959) who once fainted in hot weather. Multiple sensory associations influenced a case described by Lief (1955): this was a woman aged 38 who went to church unusually early one Sunday morning in order to visit her sick husband afterwards in hospital; in the hospital she surprised her husband holding the hand of a strange girl, and so learned of his long-standing extramarital affair. Thereafter the patient became anxious on Sunday morning, avoided church, the hospital, the dress she wore that Sunday, and made wide detours of the store where the girl worked and of the places where she knew her husband had been with the girl—motor courts, restaurants, and certain streets and highways. The fears abated quickly two years later when these relationships were made clear to the patient during treatment.

Ernest Jones (1953) described these mechanisms in Freud himself, although these were not elaborated into a phobia. Several times over a period of years Freud felt faint at meetings in the same room in the Park Hotel in Munich where he had had earlier arguments with Fliess, Jung and Riklin.

Many writers using different language agree about the role of sensory association. Writers with a psychoanalytic standpoint have clearly depicted the role of stimulus generalisation or sensory association. In 1895 Freud wrote (p. 136) that "in the case of agoraphobia, etc., we often find the recollection of a state of *panic*; and what the patient actually fears is a repetition of such an attack under those special conditions in which he believes he cannot escape it". Freud held this view even though he had already suggested with Breuer (1892, p. 26) the role of symbolism in some cases of hysteria where "the connection is not so simple, there being only, as it were, a symbolic relation between the cause and the pathological phenomenon, just as in the normal dream".

More recent writers with psychoanalytic views continue to note the importance of sensory association. Ivey (1959) wrote that "anxiety may be bound to a specific situation which aroused the first anxiety spell in the past", and Laughlin (1956) described sensory association as a primitive mechanism—"circumstantial, adventitious by association to the objects, locale or surroundings of the critical attack of anxiety". Lief (1955) commented that the selection of phobic object through sensory association "may merely be adventitious; if symbolism exists it is deeply hidden", but emphasised that symbolic associations could also be important, and that symbolic and sensory cues might be mingled in the same phobic object.

Writers who employ the language of learning theory have naturally termed sensory association "stimulus generalisation". In the words of Dollard and Miller (1950): "when a strong fear has been learned as a response to a given set of cues, it tends to generalise to other similar ones". Many experiments in animals have demonstrated stimulus generalisation in the learning of fear responses, and phobias in humans show the same phenomenon. One advantage of the term "sensory association" is its emphasis on the *sensory* cues which are generalised, thus implying a contrast with *symbolic cues*, which we will discuss later. "Stimulus generalisation" does not immediately convey this distinction.

4. Learning theory and the phobic disorders

It is convenient here to examine the important contribution of learning theory to our understanding of phobic disorders. This contribution has furthered knowledge not only by its explanation of some phobic phenomena but also by its exposure of our present points of ignorance about phobic disorders.

That phobias may be learned was recognised in the 17th century by Rene Descartes and John Locke. In 1650 Descartes analysed "from whence proceed the passions which are peculiar to certain men" ... "the smell of roses may have caused some great headache in the child when it was in the cradle; or a cat may have affrighted it and none took notice of it, nor the child so much as remembered it; though the idea of that aversion he then had to roses or a cat remain imprinted in his brain to his live's end".

A few years later in 1671, Locke wrote that "A grown Person surfeiting with Honey, no sooner hears the Name of it, but his Phancy immediately carries Sickness and Qualms to his stomach, and he cannot bear the very *Idea* of it; other Ideas of Dislike and Sickness, and Vomiting presently accompany it, and he is disturb'd, but he knows from whence to date this Weakness, and can tell how he got this Indisposition: Had this happen'd to him, by an overdose of Honey, when a child, all the same Effects would have followed, but the Cause would have been mistaken, and the Antipathy counted Natural".

In the present century experiments in animals have shown that new fears are learned readily according to well-known rules which were described earlier in this chapter. How far do these experiments aid our understanding of phobic disorders met with in clinical practice?

Many authors over the last 50 years have assumed that phobias can be described adequately as learned maladaptive habits which are acquired by the rules of conditioning and learning. This view has become increasingly prevalent in the last decade (see, for example, Eysenck, 1960; Wolpe, 1958; Marchais and Jason, 1962; Rigal et al., 1962; Rachman, 1968). Such authors regard experimental fears in animals and the well-known cases of Watson and Cover Jones as paradigms of phobic states in general.

According to the learning theory paradigm, phobias are acquired by classical conditioning in which the (future) phobic stimulus (the CS) is paired together with or shortly before a noxious stimulus (the UCS). Conditioning occurs through this temporal contiguity, and the phobia increases with the frequency of the pairing, with the strength of the noxious stimulus and when the pairing occurs in conditions of confinement or when nothing can be done to stop the noxious stimulation. Once there is sufficient fear to cause avoidance of the phobic situation, the phobia is maintained in part by drive reduction and is hard to extinguish—this is a form of instrumental conditioning.

This paradigm nicely fits those simpler phobias met with in clinical practice which were acquired in a traumatic setting. For example, in the case of Watson and Rayner (1921) the sight of a rat was the CS for the little boy, a loud noise was the UCS, and the fear reaction was the original unconditioned response (UCR) which became a phobia (conditioned response—CR) to sight of the rat. Experimentally pain and fear responses can build up conditioned reactions quite slowly (Solomon and Wynne, 1953) or in a single trial (Hudson, 1950; Sanderson et al., 1962; Napalkov, 1963). Phobias after a single trauma can be construed as instances of single-trial conditioning or learning. This is facilitated by the presence of extreme emotion such as anxiety and guilt. Marked affect might be regarded as a super-reinforcing situation, as Freud himself recognised in the genesis of hysterical symptoms when he wrote with Breuer about "ideas which owe their preservation to the fact that they originated during a severe paralysing affect like fright" (1892, p. 83). Where recurrent panics and chronic anxiety are present, as in severe agoraphobia, these help to maintain phobias through repeated regeneration of phobias. When panics and anxiety disappear either spontaneously or after modified leucotomy, fresh phobias are no longer generated and the original phobias can then be overcome (Marks, Birley and Gelder, 1966).

The simpler phobias often begin in a traumatic setting, remain localised to conditions which surround that setting, and tend to run a steady course unless they are aggravated by enforced contact with the phobic situation, or ameliorated by gradual retraining. These events fit the expectations from learning theory. Cases of this kind were cited earlier from Bagby, Moss and others, and similar phobias are found of heights, thunderstorms, animals or of driving after car accidents. However, there are many phobias of such situations where there was no apparent trauma to initiate the phobia. In these cases learning theory provides no adequate explanation of the onset.

Gantt (1962) evolved the concept of autokinesis to explain the spontaneous development of new symptoms in dogs, these new symptoms being assumed to be related to past stress. The concept of autokinesis assumes a change in internal relationships (visceral or somatic) triggered so firmly by excitatory stimuli in the past that repetition of the same stimuli is not necessarily required for the subsequent appearance of the symptom. After a trace is laid down in the nervous system it is not a lifeless "archive" item but has a degree of autonomy and may grow and recruit other traces and patterns to its service. Such a process could well be at work during the lag phase between the time of a trauma and the development of a phobia. When this lag phase lasts only a few days the connection between trauma and ensuing phobia is obvious. When the lag phase lasts months or years the connection is obscure and we speak of "spontaneous" symptoms. The concept of autokinesis has the drawback that it is difficult to test and could be invoked to connect any new symptom with any past stress. The concept of autokinesis will have limited utility until we have strict criteria to detect its presence.

Learning theory helps us to understand not only simple phobias but also certain features of more complex cases. In the case of Lief described on p. 89 we can clearly see stimulus generalisation in the patient's avoidance of the hospital where the trauma occurred and of the dress which she wore at that time. However, a learning model becomes strained in accounting for other features. For example, the long gap between the time the patient was in church (one of the CS) and the time she discovered her husband holding the hand of his mistress in hospital (the UCS) is much longer than that seen in simple conditioning experiments. The trauma itself is at a symbolic level, and generalisation of the phobia to places only remotely connected with the husband's mistress involves more symbolism than the simple sensory cues of conditioning paradigms. These could, of course, be called higher order conditioning processes which involve the second signalling system, but this seems a cumbersome way of stating that symbolic cues can be important. Yet another term—transmission by mediational cues—has been introduced by Osgood (1953) and used by Paul (1964) to describe the same process. In fact it is useful to describe as a conditioning mechanism the associations of a phobia with the conditions prevailing at its onset, and to call its spread "generalisation", as these features correspond fairly closely to those seen in experiments on conditioned fear responses in animals.

Learning theory also helps us understand how phobias recede after they have developed. Simpler phobias respond slowly but well to desensitisation procedures. Although several factors help to produce this effect, the main operative process in desensitisation is that of counterconditioning whereby the patient experiences the phobic stimulus in association with a pleasant opposing process such as relaxation (Davison, 1967). The gradual extinction of the phobia follows the same slow pattern as extinction of fear responses in animals by related methods.

However, the framework of learning theory does not account for those few cases where dramatic relief of the phobia has followed abreaction in which the initiating trauma was freshly brought back to awareness. The mechanism of relief by abreaction is still obscure.

In phobias seen in psychiatric practice other important phenomena are not encompassed by learning theory. Certain phobias, especially agoraphobia, are commonly found together with multiple other symptoms such as diffuse anxiety, panic attacks, depression, depersonalisation, obsessions and frigidity. Learning theory does not explain why these symptoms develop, why they occur together, nor why they are associated more often with agoraphobia than with any other type of phobia. One suggestion it might lead to is that panic attacks and depression act as super-reinforcers which facilitate phobic conditioning when a patient goes out while experiencing such affects. But the origin of the panics, depression and other symptoms is not indicated by learning theory, nor for that matter by any other theory at present.

Some of the symptoms may reflect physiological mechanisms. For example, depersonalisation may be triggered as a cut-off mechanism when anxiety reaches a critical level. In an agoraphobic patient of Lader's (1966) a panic attack developed while the GSR was being monitored. After a while the patient said she felt unreal rather than panicky. At that point the GSR tracing showed a sharp decrease in the number of spontaneous fluctuations.

5. Symbolism in phobias: The psychoanalytic view

Phobias may generalise not only by simple sensory associations but also through complex symbolic cues of special significance to the patient. From Freud onwards this was stressed by psychoanalytic writers, to the extent that phobias were regarded primarily as symbols for other hidden fears. This idea was elaborated into an extensive theoretical framework by Freud, Stekel, Abraham, Fenichel and many others. More recent accounts of this framework were given by Ivey (1959) and Friedman (1959). Since the psychoanalytic framework has been so influential, it is worth reviewing in some detail.

Freud originally suggested an organic basis for anxiety neurosis, that phobic anxiety "does not originate in a repressed idea, proves not reducible further by psychological analysis, and is also not amenable to psychotherapy" (1894, p. 84).

At this time* (1895, p. 135) he divided the phobias into two groups according to the nature of the object feared: 1. common phobias, an exaggerated fear of all those things everyone fears to some extent, e.g. night, solitude, death, illness, snakes, and 2. specific phobias, the fear of special circumstances that inspire no fear in the normal man, e.g. agoraphobia. Freud then regarded phobias as part of an anxiety neurosis. He thought anxiety neuroses were caused by "the accumulation of sexual tension, produced by abstinence or by frustrated sexual excitation".

Later he was persuaded by Stekel that some phobias had a psychological basis, for which he reserved the term "anxiety hysteria", and that other forms of anxiety rested on an organic basis for which he retained the phrase "anxiety neurosis". Under the influence of Stekel Freud put forward a psychodynamic basis for the classic case of a phobia of horses in a 5-year old boy called Hans viz. that the manifest phobia "was due to the repression of Han's aggressive propensities (the hostile ones against his father and the sadistic ones against his mother)" (1909, p. 281). The horse symbolised the feared retaliation from father. The phobia bound and concentrated the free-floating anxiety onto a convenient symbolic object which could easily be avoided, thus protecting the patient from excessive anxiety. This was regarded as a model of neurotic repression resulting from mental conflict.

---

* It is of interest that at the time Freud originally suggested that phobic anxiety did not originate in repressed ideas he himself had symptoms of this condition. Some years after these dissipated he formulated his concept of phobias as a symbolic facade displaced from other fears.

From the ages of 31 to 43 (1887–99) Freud suffered from anxiety about travelling by train. This was not sufficiently severe to deter him from travelling. Traces of it remained in later life in the form of slightly undue anxiety about catching trains. He was so anxious not to miss a train that he would arrive at a station a long while —even an hour—beforehand.

Later psychoanalytic writings assumed that all phobias disguised from the patient the real unconscious source of his anxiety. Lewin (1952) thought this resembled dream symbolism in which the manifest content of a dream is construed to be a facade behind which are concealed the latent thoughts which truly call forth the anxiety. Arieti (1961) spoke of phobias as "concrete representations of abstract anxiety-provoking situations and relationships". In psychoanalytic terms a forbidden unconscious wish produced a conflict between ego and id; this resulted in a conscious fear which became displaced to an apparently indifferent idea. Many writers proposed sources of anxiety for this conflict in forbidden wishes of different kinds, such as wishes about aggression (Deutsch, 1929; Sterba, 1935; Hitschmann, 1913—cited by Fenichel, 1944) prostitution and exhibitionism (Deutsch, 1929; Fenichel, 1944), promiscuity (Miller, 1953), masturbation (Bornstein, 1931), incestuous longings (Abraham, 1913; Katan, 1937) and desires to return into the womb (Lewin, 1935).

There is little doubt that symbolic cues play a part in the spread of phobias. This is not the same as saying, however, that all phobias are primarily symbols of fears displaced from other sources. Since anything can in theory be a symbol for anything else, we need strict criteria to judge whether a given phobia is symbolic of other fears or not. A useful critique of psychoanalytic symbolism and its criteria is given by Dalbiez (1941). Such criteria are generally rather loose or absent in articles about phobias as symbols for other fears, and the evidence is often open to different interpretations, even, for example, in the original case of little Hans in which Freud developed the idea of displacement (Wolpe and Rachman, 1960).

It is too easy to infer symbolism until one examines the evidence closely, as the following case shows:

Spider phobia in woman with sexual problems
    A married woman of 23 sought treatment for a phobia of spiders since early childhood—this had been recently aggravated when she

---

The travel phobia was accompanied by other signs of neurosis, to use the term Freud employed to describe his condition. This consisted of mood change fluctuating from elation, excitement and self-confidence on the one hand to periods of severe depression, doubt and inhibition on the other. In the depressed moods he could neither write nor concentrate his thoughts, except during his professional work.

During this same period Freud also had occasional attacks of dread of dying. In 1896 he wrote in a letter that "there came suddenly a severe affection of the heart . . . the maddest racing and irregularity, constant cardiac tension, oppression, burning, hot pain down the left arm, some dyspnoea of a suspiciously organic degree—all that in two or three attacks a day and continuing. And with it an oppression of mood in which images of dying and farewell scenes replaced the more usual phantasies about one's occupation".

Throughout all this time Freud never ceased to function and continued with his normal activities. (See Jones, 1953, Vol. 1, p. 14, 197–8, 335, 337, 340–2).

moved to a house infested with spiders. She had never achieved sexual orgasm. The phobia improved slightly during treatment with hypnosis, until she saw her husband kissing a friend, after which she left him for 3 days. During that time she saw a spider, screamed, and her spider phobia again increased. She became very tense during sexual intercourse because as soon as she became aroused she felt great tension, guilt and hate, hence sexual intercourse had to be carried out quickly before she could be aroused. Desensitisation of the phobia was then begun and the spider phobia improved considerably. The patient remained unable to reach sexual orgasm, though her hatred of her husband diminished after discussions with him.

One might have been tempted to infer sexual symbolism from the kind of phobic object and the conjunction of an increase of the spider phobia at the time of her problem about sex and aggression with her husband. However, the phobia long antedated the current problem with her husband, followed the typical natural history of animal phobias, and improved without change in her sexual capacities. Exacerbation of phobias during periods of special stress is a well known phenomenon which requires no symbolic explanation.

Even where symbolism can be shown satisfactorily, this does not prove its causative role—it might simply be a secondary effect of the phobia. If a child attributes his phobia of darkness to the presence of monsters the symbolism may be a genuine rationalisation of an irrational fear on the same lines that any posthypnotic suggestion is rationalised. This problem is met with in any psychopathological material—a patient with anorexia nervosa may have fixed ideas that her body is too fat; such ideas may produce anorexia or the same mechanism which produces the anorexia may cause such ideas. A patient with amphetamine psychosis can show fascinating symbolism in paranoid delusions, which in this case is due to a biochemical disturbance. Psychoanalytic writings assign a primary causal role to symbolism without taking adequate account of alternative possibilities; they generally require much tighter criteria for validating symbolism in given cases.

This important problem requires detailed illustration. Occasional agoraphobic patients express additional fears about their sexual and aggressive feelings, e.g. of exposing their genitals in public, or of soliciting or hurting men in the street. Psychoanalytic writings assumed that these additional fears were the primary disturbance from which the patient was protected by her agoraphobia. They regarded the agoraphobia as a displaced fear whose facade defended the patient against hidden sexual and aggressive impulses. In fact there are a number of possibilities. These additional fears may be 1. the original cause of the agoraphobia 2. a separate exacerbating factor after the agoraphobia began 3. simply some of a hundred fears agoraphobics often mention without reason to assign psychological primacy to any particular one 4. a secondary rationalisation of the agoraphobia or 5. totally irrelevant. The correct explanation probably lies with 2. and 3.

One of the commonest fears expressed by agoraphobics is that they will die, go mad or lose control. This could mean that they have strong unconscious feelings urging for release. Alternatively, we could say that in extreme tension of unknown origin the patient fears what is happening to him and what he may do under pressure.

Patients who are afraid of leaving home or their relatives are said to show separation anxiety. This may be symbolic of earlier childhood separation, but we can argue equally plausibly that the anxiety has an independent origin which the patients have learned is reduced in the presence of trusted people. The "separation" aspect of the anxiety is then a secondary conditioning effect. This point is well illustrated in the following patient:

Separation anxiety distinct from agoraphobia

A woman of 23 developed anxiety, sweating and shaking of the legs while travelling to work by train. She then changed to a slower train so that she could get out at any station she wanted. This slowly got worse until she was unable to travel to work and gave up her job. About this time she experienced frequent feelings of unreality during which she wanted to scream. She discovered that she felt better if her husband was present, took a job in the same firm as her husband and cycled to work with him, later travelling with him by car. Even with her husband, however, she remained unable to travel by train, plane or ship. After a few months she gradually became afraid of separation from her husband. At work she had to know exactly where to get in touch with him and would often phone him. If for any reason she could not contact him immediately she would panic, not know where to turn, feel completely lost, want to scream and fear that she would go mad. She became unable to remain alone at home unless she could phone her husband immediately. Her husband had to refuse to lecture abroad because she could not tolerate his leaving her even for a few hours where she could not get hold of him. Sexually she was always frigid. Ten years after her symptoms began she sought treatment after she developed depression with suicidal ideas.

As a small child the patient used to be frightened when her parents were out and once sent out her younger brother to find them. She had infrequent desires to scream which were hard to stifle. These disappeared in her late teens.

This extreme case clearly shows the sequence. First came the travel phobia and depersonalisation, then came the discovery of relief in the presence of the husband and after this he became indispensable. Finally the patient presented for treatment of separation anxiety, the first phobia only being mentioned in passing.   Earlier childhood psychopathology had already sensitised the patient to separation by the time her agoraphobia began in adult life.   The two pathologies then interacted.

Agoraphobia is not simply the outcome of separation anxiety. Rather, separation anxiety is a common complication of agoraphobia. Although a trusted companion is so often comforting in this condition there are important exceptions.   About 5% of agoraphobic patients are not helped by company and actually prefer to be alone when travelling (Marks and Herst, 1969).   They have agoraphobia with no separation anxiety.

Phobic patients, especially agoraphobics, often produce psychopathological material of great interest, richness and feeling.   The temptation is then strong to link this symbol-rich material to the origin of the phobia.   The temptation is even more powerful when disclosure of this material is accompanied by abreaction and temporary relief for a week or two.   Patient and therapist then strive in vain to produce the same effect once more.   The same sequence can be found during the treatment of other disorders such as obsessive states (Kennedy, 1960).   Patients with multiple phobias commonly find it difficult to express their feelings openly, and it was only natural to assume that the phobias were due to repression of such feelings, especially when expression of these feelings led to temporary relief of symptoms.   But this assumption may well be fallacious.   Relief from abreaction is a nonspecific effect.   It has been argued elsewhere (Marks, 1965, p. 95–97) that the relationship between the presence of symptoms and inhibited feelings can also be non-specific.   The two covary together but are dependent not upon one another but upon an anterior though unknown mechanism.   We can often see two reciprocating states in psychiatric patients.   In the inhibited or "repressed" state patients have severe symptoms such as phobias, depression and obsessions, and are also unable to show feelings, including aggression.   By contrast, in the released or "abreactive" state the symptoms diminish and patients talk about their feelings openly.   But our argument is that they can talk about their feelings *because of the same change which produced symptom relief.*   We are all familiar with patients emerging from retarded depression who "come alive" and talk freely as they improve. The same applies to patients in remission from severe agoraphobia. Such patients talk because they are better—they are not better because they have talked.

It is undeniable, of course, that there are many other psychiatric problems where "talking makes it better".   In certain forms of depression and abnormal personality improvement can only occur after patients have expressed their feelings freely, and treatment rightly aims to promote this process in psychotherapy. But this is not necessarily true for phobic disorders. We must distinguish in psychiatry between symbol rich material which is valuable in promoting change, and similar material which is an accompaniment of other more primary processes.

Since phobias may spread through the agency of mediating symbolic cues, we must always enquire of a phobic patient for hidden significances of his fear. But this is not to reduce the phobia to a mere "facade" for other fears. Whatever symbolic cues may have sparked off the phobia in the first place, once it has developed the phobia follows its own independent course. Dealing with the conflicts symbolised in a phobia is not enough to relieve that phobia. The patient has to face the phobic situation again before he can improve. This was in fact recognised by Freud (1919). Once begun the phobia is maintained by the anxiety-reducing mechanism of avoidance, and the phobia can then be properly overcome only when the patient faces the phobic situation again. In other words, regardless of the conflicts which may be symbolised in a phobia, the phobia itself becomes a learned habit which has to be unlearned, retrained, counterconditioned, deconditioned, or desensitised, to use the variety of terms employed to describe the same process. The idea of a phobia continuing independently of its original cause is that of the phobia as a "burnt out habit".

Though psychoanalytic writings have over-emphasized the role of symbolism in phobias, they have nevertheless been valuable in drawing attention to the way in which emotional conflicts influence the origin and maintenance of phobias. They emphasised that intense guilt and resentment catalyse traumatic events into producing phobias connected with those events, and that emotional factors obviously influence the course of phobias. For example, one woman developed her first symptoms when she rode on a bus to visit her rejected son dying in hospital. During psychotherapy a temporary remission of the phobias began after she had expressed her guilt about his death. However, she then relapsed and became housebound though she continued to ventilate her guilt without effect on the phobias, the guilt subsiding only when the anniversary of her son's death had passed. Clearly the expression of emotion influenced the patient's phobias, whether or not emotional conflict caused them in the first place.

Psychoanalytic writings also illustrated the secondary gains which result from phobias once they begin, as we find with any symptom in medicine. Secondary gains maintain symptoms and retard their resolution even though the symptoms originated in another way. This was shown by a man who contracted his second marriage when he was already agoraphobic, though he concealed this from his wife at the time. In the next few years he became totally housebound while his wife had to earn their keep, and sexual relations ceased. Intensive joint interviews showed the husband's passive dependency and the wife's contemptuous hostility.   After much enquiry two offers of employment were secured for the patient near his home, only to be frustrated each time when the wife phoned the doctor and employment officer to say that her husband was unfit for work.   The patient's impending rehabilitation proved too threatening for the precarious equilibrium established in the marriage once the phobia had reached its peak.   Emotional problems in the marriage clearly impeded recovery even though they were not present when the phobia first began.

In summary, psychoanalytic writings have been valuable in stressing the role of emotional influences and symbolic associations on phobias. However such writings assumed too readily that all phobias are merely symbols of other hidden fears, when in fact many phobias are acquired by conditioning mechanisms and have no symbolic meaning.

Summary I. Background features

Phylogenetic influences shape the form phobias take in man.   Certain stimuli have prepotency over others as triggers for phobias, given a similar frequency of exposure to all these stimuli.

The age of an individual influences the kind of phobia he is likely to develop.   This is due to the effect of maturation, frequency of exposure to the stimuli, and other factors.   Sudden noise or movement triggers fear in young infants, fears of strangers are the rule in older infants, fears of animals begin in pre-school children, while fears of open spaces or social situations usually start after puberty.

Different phobias have a varying *sex incidence*.   Both sexes are liable to most phobias in childhood.   After puberty animal phobias and agoraphobia are commoner in women, while social phobias and other specific phobias occur equally in both sexes.

Certain phobias are commonly associated with *other disorders;* Agoraphobia is often accompanied by diffuse anxiety, depression, depersonalisation, obsessions and frigidity.

Genetic endowment influences the *timidity* of a patient.   This in turn affects a patient's liability to develop phobias.   Agoraphobic patients who have a history of childhood fears develop their agoraphobic symptoms earlier in adult life than do other patients.   Patients with phobias often have a shy, dependent premorbid *personality*.   *Cultural influences* inside and outside the family also influence the kind of situations to which patients will show fear.

Phobic patients differ from normal subjects on several *psycho-physiological* measures.   The resting forearm blood flow is slightly raised in agoraphobics.   In agoraphobics and social phobics the galvanic skin resistance shows both an overall increase of spontaneous fluctuations and a slow rate of habituation to repeated auditory stimuli. Animal phobics and social phobics acquire eyeblink conditioning responses more rapidly than normal subjects.

II.   Direct influences

Sudden trauma is often followed by a phobia of objects connected with that event—this may occur only after a lag period of a few days. The trauma may be physical or psychological. Many phobias begin after more general stress in the life situation, while yet other phobias start spontaneously without an obvious trigger. A few phobias clear up rapidly on recall of a forgotten trauma which had initiated the phobia, but most phobic patients are aware of the circumstances in which the fear began without this influencing its course.

Once a phobia has begun to a given set of cues it tends to generalise to other similar ones in any sensory modality. This is stimulus generalis- ation, also called sensory association.

Learning theory is also useful in accounting for the onset, spread and course of the simpler phobias. It also helps the understanding of some features of more complex phobias. Learning theory does not account for the association of certain phobias with other psychiatric disorders, nor does it pay sufficient attention to their symbolic associa- tions. The response of phobias to desensitisiaton is partly a process of counter-conditioning, but no conditioning or learning paradigm explains those few cases which remit after abreaction.

Phobias may generalise not only by simple sensory associations but also by symbolic mediational cues of special significance to the patient This type of spread has been stressed by psychoanalytic writers. These writers have further suggested that phobias are the manifest symbolic facade which has been displaced from other hidden sources of anxiety. Criteria for the validity of symbolism are often too loose to be con- vincing. Symbolic material in a phobic patient may be a secondary effect of the phobia itself or relevant to problems other than the phobia. When relief occurs after abreaction of symbolic material, this does not necessarily prove the importance of that material in the genesis of the phobia. Psychoanalytic writings have usefully shown that emotional factors help to maintain phobias after they have developed.

Chapter 3

THE CLINICAL SYNDROMES

Section   I. Classification of phobic disorders
Section   II. The agoraphobic syndrome
Section III. Specific animal phobias
Section   IV. Social phobias
Section   V. Miscellaneous other phobias
Section   VI. Illness phobias
Section VII. Obsessive phobias
Section VIII. Autonomic equivalents to phobic disorders
Section   IX. Children's fears and phobias

Section I. CLASSIFICATION OF PHOBIC DISORDERS

As we saw earlier, from the time of Hippocrates to the 19th century occasional observations were made about phobias but phobic disorders were not clearly distinguished from other disturbances such as delusional fears. From 1870 onwards systematic descriptions of phobic disorders as such appeared with increasing frequency in the psychiatric literature, an example being the classic description of agoraphobia by Westphal in 1871. In 1895 Freud distinguished between common phobias of those things everyone fears to some extent, like death, illness and snakes, and specific phobias of circumstances which inspire no fear in the normal man e.g. agoraphobia. Also in 1895, Henry Maudsley castigated the current trend of allotting a special big sounding name to each variety of phobic situation since many phobias were often found together or successively in the same case. In 1913 Kraepelin included in his textbook a brief chapter on irrepressible ideas and irresistible fears, but he did not differentiate between phobic and obsessive phenomena.

Phobias achieved a separate diagnostic label in the International Classification of Diseases only in 1947, and in the American Psychiatric Association as late as 1952. Even by 1959 only 3 out of 9 classifications used in different countries listed phobic disorder as a diagnosis on its own (Stengel, 1959) and some recent textbooks still group phobias together with obsessive-compulsive disorders (e.g. Scott, 1966; Curran and Partridge, 1963; Henderson and Batchelor, 1962). Sub-division of the phobic disorders themselves has only just begun. The Camberwell Psychiatric Register now lists monosymptomatic phobias separately from other phobias (Wing, et al. 1967).

Two recent developments have led to increased knowledge about the phobic disorders. The first is the introduction of treatment by desensitisation, which led to greater interest in the natural history of phobias. The second development is the spread of psychophysiological measures in the study of neurotic disorders. Before we discuss a tentative scheme for classifying the phobias, it is necessary to examine briefly the purpose and pitfalls of any classification.

General problems of classification

Any condition may be classified in endless ways. Though classifications vary according to the purpose they serve, the most useful ones are those which "carve nature at the joints", and increase one's predictive powers.

To classify means to arrange phenomena systematically into classes possessing common attributes. In medical disorders these attributes may be a common set of symptoms and signs, or aetiology, or pathophysiology, or prognosis, or response to treatment. Ideally all these sets of common attributes should coincide. Few classifications approach this ideal, and perhaps the nearest we get to this in medicine is the classification of the more clearcut exanthematous infections.

At the other extreme are classifications which tell us only about one set of attributes and no other. These are of limited value. To take an absurd example, we could classify the phobias according to those in patients with and those in patients without an umbilical hernia. Such a division would not get us very far since it would not tell us anything more about other common attributes of the phobias.

Fortunately we can now tentatively pick out certain groups of phobias which are less arbitrary than this because they have clinical correlates to support their usefulness. Although they will have to be modified in future as knowledge advances, they form a useful frame of reference at the present time.

Special problems in the classification of phobias

In the delineation of these groups two problems had to be overcome. First, phobias can occur of almost any situation; second, phobias may be found together with practically any other psychiatric symptom. These difficulties are not unique to phobias and are found in other areas of psychiatry, for example in classifying delusions.

The problems are not insuperable. To take the first one, since a phobia can develop of virtually any object or situation it seems to follow that a classification dependent upon the feared situation will result in an endless terminology. Such a classification was in fact prominent until this century, and numerous Greek and Latin prefixes were attached to the word phobia to describe each of the situations which was feared. Table 3.1 shows a list of such terms, partly taken from Laughlin (1956). The table serves to slake curiosity rather than to inform and this type of classification can no longer be regarded as helpful. It is true, however, that certain phobias do tend to occur together and to have particular correlates. These clusters naturally overlap but are useful for purposes of description, aetiology and prognosis. The object of the phobia is therefore of some importance and should not be entirely ignored.

Table 3.1

Formal names which have been given to some phobias

Acrophobia	: height (Gr. *acro*, heights or summits)
Agora—	: open spaces (Gr. *agora*, market place, the place of assembly)
Ailuro—	: cats (Gr. *ailuros*, cat)
Arachno—	: spiders(Gr. *arachin*, spider)
Antho—	: flowers (Gr. *anthos*, flower)
Anthropo—	: people (Gr. *anthropos*, man generically)
Aqua—	: water (Lat. *aqua*, water)
Astra—	: lightning (Gr. *asterope*, lightning)
Bronto—	⎫ (Gr. *bronte*, thunder)
	⎬ : thunder
Keraunos—	⎭ (Gr. *keraunos*, thunderbolt)
Claustro—	: closed spaces (Lat. *claustrum*, bar, bolt, or lock)
Cyno—	: dogs (Gr. *cynas*, dog)
Demento—	: insanity (Lat. *demens*, mad)
Equino—	: horses (Lat. *equus*, horse)
Herpeto—	: lizards, reptiles (Gr. *herpetos*, creeping or crawling things)
Mikro—	: germs (Gr. *mikros*, small)
Muro—	: mice (Lat. *murmus* mouse)
Myso—	: dirt, germs, contamination (Gr. *mysos*, uncleanliness, abomination)
Numero—	: number (Lat. *numero*, number)
Nycto—	: darkness (Gr. *nyx*, night)
Ophidio—	: snakes (Gr. *ophis*, snake)
Pyro—	: fire (Gr. *pyr*, fire)
Thanato—	: death (Gr. *thanatos*, death)
Tricho—	: hair (Gr. *tricho*, hair)
Xeno—	: stranger (Gr. *xeros*, stranger)
Zoo—	: animal (Gr. *zoos*, animal)

The second problem is that phobias can occur either on their own or as part of a whole range of psychiatric disorders. Phobias include such contrasting states as the ephemeral fears of darkness which children go through, the multiple crippling fears of a housebound housewife, and the vague phobias found in some personality disorders. It is not surprising that some writers describe phobias as limited symptoms or "habits" which themselves constitute the disorder without any underlying cause, while for other writers phobias are but the visible aspect of deeper pathology. Each view may be correct in different cases and the varying significance of phobias is difficult to formulate only if we assume a unitary origin for all phobias instead of recognising that multiple factors play a role in their genesis.

Phobic symptoms and phobic states

Clinical observation reveals that phobic symptoms may be minor complaints in many disorders. Phobias occur as part of a depressive illness, waxing and waning at the same time as the more prominent depressive symptoms. Next, phobias may be a feature of obsessive neurosis, diffuse anxiety states, personality disorders and even schizophrenia. In all these conditions treatment of the phobic symptom depends upon management of the major condition in which the phobia occurs. This book will exclude such conditions. The distinction is not always easy to make in practice, but serves to define the field under discussion. Throughout this book on phobias our concern is with patients whose phobias are a main complaint and not a minor symptom which accompanies another major disorder such as obvious schizophrenia or severe depression.

When phobias occur as the patient's dominant symptom we call the condition a phobic state or disorder (or phobic reaction in the A.P.A. terminology). These phobic states are found in less than 3% of psychiatric outpatients (Hare, 1965; Errera and Coleman, 1963; Frazier and Carr, 1967), although there are many people with phobias who do not consult psychiatrists and may never seek any medical aid at all. Phobic states assume many forms from an isolated fear in an otherwise healthy person to diffuse extensive fears occurring together with other psychiatric problems. Their aetiology and treatment vary correspondingly. The phobias are thus a group of related disorders, and this has been recognised by their separate classification in Britain and America in recent years. Our present discussion centres on patterns emerging within this group of phobic disorders in adults. The emergent groups are necessarily incomplete and overlapping, and will have to be modified as we fill in the large gaps in our knowledge about them.

The Main kinds of Phobia in Adults

Table 3.2 shows the main groups of fears found in adult life. Commonest of all are normal minor fears which are present in most people. Fears sufficiently intense to be called phobias however, occur in only a small proportion of adults. In a student population, for example, most subjects might feel mildly squeamish in the presence of non-poisonous snakes, but only 20% reported intense fear, and only 1–2% actively avoided a snake to a degree which might get labelled a phobia (Lang, 1966).

Phobic states can conveniently be divided into Class I, phobias of stimuli *external* to the patient and Class II, phobias of stimuli *internal* to the patient. The most frequent phobias seen by psychiatrists are of stimuli external to the patient (Class I)—open spaces, heights,

birds, thunderstorms, social gatherings and so on. These situations
can be avoided when the fear becomes intense. Phobias of this kind
fall conveniently into 4 groups which will be described presently.
Phobias of stimuli *internal* to the patient (Class II) cannot be avoided

Table 3.2

The Main Fears in Adults

A. Normal fears
B. Abnormal fears: (phobias)

Class I: *Phobias of external stimuli:*	% of Maudsley phobics	Related Disorders
1. Agoraphobia	60	Anxiety states, "neurotic" depression
2. Social phobias	8	Sensitive personalities, conditioned autonomic disorders
3. Animal phobias	3	—
4. Miscellaneous specific phobias	14	—

Class II: *Phobias of internal stimuli:*		
5. Illness phobias	15	Hypochondriasis

6. Obsessive phobias — Classified separately under obsessive-compulsive neurosis.

Examples are palpitations thought to indicate heart disease, or obsessive impulses to kill one's child. Of course the distinction between
internal and external stimuli breaks down in certain cases as in agoraphobia which is accompanied by a fear of dying, or in an obsessive
phobia of harming one's child which leads a patient to hide any knives
at home far from temptation. Recent experimental work on phobias
has largely concentrated on Class I, phobias of stimuli outside the
patient, so far more is known about them, and this book will concentrate on these rather than on Class II phobias, about which little
systematic knowledge is available.

Each type of fear will be briefly described, and later sections in this
chapter will expand some of these descriptions.

A. Normal fears

Most children and adults have minor fears of one kind or another.
In children these include fears of parents leaving them, of noise,
strangers, animals and unusual situations. In adults such fears include

mild fears of heights, lifts, darkness, aeroplanes, spiders, mice, snakes, and taking examinations, as well as superstitions such as fears of houses said to be haunted by ghosts, of passing under ladders in the street, and other taboos which are quite elaborate in some pre-industrial societies. These minor fears do not lead to total avoidance of objects and can be overcome with explanation and persistence. They are within the cultural norm, and interest the psychiatrist only because they shed light on the nature of severe phobias.

B.   Abnormal fears (Phobias)

Class I. Phobias of external stimuli.   We will first describe the most clearcut varieties and then pass on to less well defined groups.

Animal phobias (Table 3.3)

The animal phobias are the most clearcut variety. They are also the rarest kind seen in hospital practice—only 24 presented at the Maudsley in the last decade, i.e. about 3% of all the phobics who came.   The vast

Table 3.3
Animal Phobias

Frequency:	Rare.
Sex incidence:	95% women.
Onset age:	Early childhood.
Phobic situation:	Monosymptomatic phobia of single animal species with little generalisation.
Associated symptoms:	Few. No general anxiety. Occasional depression or other phobias.
Course:	Continuous.
Psychological tests:	Normal low Cornell and Neuroticism score. Normal Extroversion score.
Pyschophysiology:	Eyeblink conditioning: acquired rapidly, extinguished slowly. G.S.R: few spontaneous fluctuations, habituates normally. Forearm blood flow not increased.
Response to treatment:	Good, though prolonged desensitisation may be necessary.

majority of animal phobias occur in women (Marks and Gelder, 1966). Though patients present for treatment in adult life, their phobias will generally have started in early childhood before the age of 8 (Figure 3.1) and have persisted fairly continuously thereafter.   Before puberty animal phobias are found quite commonly in boys and in girls (Mac-Farlane et al., 1954), so we presume that this group of adults is the residuum of the earlier and larger group. It is noteworthy that before puberty animal phobias are found in both sexes, while the few animal phobias which remain after puberty are usually found in women. These women usually have a monosymptomatic phobia of a single animal species with little generalisation despite persistence of the phobia

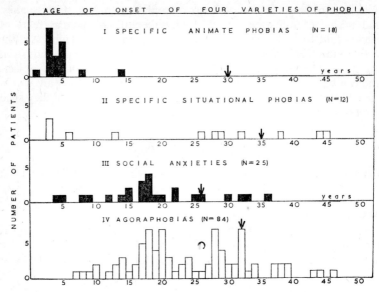

Fig. 3.1   Age of onset of four varieties of phobia

over decades. There is no tension or panic in the absence of the phobic object. Occasionally other symptoms may be present, but these are generally few. This is paralleled by a low score on the Cornell and Neuroticism questionnaire (Table 3.4).

The psychophysiological features are of particular interest (Table 3.4). Patients with animal phobias acquire eyeblink conditioned responses more rapidly and extinguish them more slowly than do normal subjects (Martin et al., 1969). Their skin resistance shows a normal number of spontaneous fluctuations and habituates normally to successive auditory stimuli (Lader et al., 1967). In the few subjects whose forearm blood flow has been tested this too has been normal. These skin resistance and blood flow measures are correlates of ratings of anxiety (Lader and Wing, 1966; Kelly, 1966), so that the physiological meaures confirm clinical observations about the absence of diffuse anxiety. Although animal phobias have usually been present for decades by the time they are treated in adult life, they show a good and persistent improvement with desensitisation, even though treatment may need to be protracted (Table 3.5).

The agoraphobic syndrome   (Phobic anxiety state)

We pass on to a very different group of phobias—the agoraphobic syndrome (Table 3.6). This is the commonest and also the most distressing variety seen by psychiatrists. They form roughly 60% of

Table 3.4

Summary of Clinical and Psychophysiological Data

	Anxiety States	Agora-phobias	Social phobias	Animal phobias	Normals
% Women	50	75	60	95	50
Onset age	25	24	19	*4	—
Treatment age	36	32	27	30	—
Overt anxiety (0–6 scale)	2·6	2·0	2·0	*0·4	0
Modified Cornell	—	34	21	*13	10
Neuroticism	**37	30	29	*21	20
Extroversion	**14	19	19	24	25
G.S.R.: spontan. flucs.	36	32	33	*12	6
G.S.R.: habituat. rate	29	39	39	*68	64
Resting forearm blood flow	**4·8	2·9	2·6	2·2	2·0
Eyeblink C.R. acquisition	11	15	19	***21	14

n Varies from 18 to 84 in different cells

* = differs significantly from other psychiatric groups

** =   ,,   ,,   ,,   all groups

*** =   ,,   ,,   ,,   all groups except social phobias

Data are composite of several studies, some unpublished. Main sources are:

Clinical variables: Marks and Gelder, 1966; Lader, 1966; Kelly, 1966

Questionnaire scores: Gelder et al., 1967; Kelly, 1966

Psychophysiological data: G.S.R.: Lader et al., 1967 and Lader, 1966

Forearm blood flow: Kelly (unpublished)

Eyeblink conditioning: Martin et al. (1969) and Martin (unpublished)

Table 3.5

Improvement of 4 kinds of Phobia after Desensitisation

(Maximum possible change = 3·5)

	Agoraphobias	Social Phobias	Animal Phobias	Mixed Specific Phobias
n =	31	11	13	9
Mean improvement:	0·9*	1·4	1·6	1·6

*Significantly less than the other three groups.

Data are from patients treated in trials of Marks and Gelder (1965), Gelder and Marks (1966), Gelder et al. (1967) and Marks et al. (1968).

Table 3.6

The Agoraphobic syndrome (Phobic anxiety state)

Frequency:	Common.
Sex incidence:	75% women.
Onset age:	After puberty: 15–35.
Phobic situation:	Multiple: going out alone, shopping, travelling, closed spaces, social situations—much generalisation.
Associated symptoms:	Multiple: general anxiety, panic attacks, dizziness, depression, depersonalisation, obsessions.
Course:	If persists longer than a year, fluctuating with partial remissions and relapses for years.
Psychological tests:	High Cornell and Neuroticism scores. Slightly introverted.
Psychophysiology:	Normal eyeblink conditioning: G.S.R. shows many spontaneous fluctuations, habituates slowly. Forearm blood flow slightly raised.
Response to treatment:	Variable. Poor in patients with multiple panic attacks and obsessions.
Comment:	Diffuse varieties overlap with anxiety states, affective disorders and obsessive neurosis.

all phobias seen at the Maudsley. The term agoraphobia is not an altogether happy one to describe this syndrome, since these patients have fears not only of going into open spaces but also of shopping, crowds, travelling, closed spaces, to name but a few of the fears which beset such patients. However, fear of going out is probably the most frequent symptom from which others develop, so the name has stuck since Westphal's lucid description. Many other different names have been given to this condition, e.g. phobic anxiety state, depersonalisation-phobic-anxiety-syndrome, locomotor anxiety, topophobia, kenophobia, platzangst. Each name highlights some aspect of the condition, but none is all embracing.

Most agoraphobics are women, and the majority develop their symptoms after puberty, usually between age 15 and 35 (Fig. 3.1). Multiple phobias occur which centre round going out alone but generalise rapidly to many other situations. Numerous other neurotic symptoms are commonly present including panic attacks and tension even at rest, dizziness, frequent depression, depersonalisation and obsessions. Once the syndrome has persisted more than a year it runs a fluctuating course with partial remissions and relapse over a long period. The diffuse symptomatology is reflected by high scores on Cornell and Neuroticism questionnaires (Table 3.4).

Unlike the animal phobics, agoraphobics acquire and extinguish eyeblink conditioned responses at a normal rate (Martin et al. 1969). Their skin resistance is abnormal in that it shows significantly increased spontaneous fluctuations and significantly slowed habituation to repeated auditory stimuli (Lader et al. 1967). The forearm blood flow is only slightly increased. These findings agree with the clinical features of diffuse anxiety so often seen in agoraphobics. Agoraphobics do not respond particularly well to desensitisation (Table 3.5) since they have a strong tendency to relapse repeatedly. Prognosis is poorer where patients have multiple panic attacks or obsessions. Alleviation of the diffuse anxiety is followed by gradual improvement in the phobias. Agoraphobics with diffuse anxiety may require large amounts of sedative drugs, and their management is much more difficult than that of more localised types of phobias.

Clinical evidence for the distinction of agoraphobia from other phobias was noted by Snaith (1968). He found that agoraphobics are more anxious, have a more remitting course and a different distribution of phobias from patients with other phobias.

Table 3.7

Agoraphobic Factor Based on Clinical Data From 275 Neurotic Patients
(Roth et al. 1965).

Loading
·80 Situational phobias (agoraphobic).
·76 Panic attacks.
·70 Depersonalisation and derealisation.
·56 Temporal lobe features.
·48 Marked precipitant.
·44 Sudden onset.
·40 Dizzy attacks.

Table 3.8

Agoraphobic Factor Based on Questionnaire Replies of 72 Phobic Patients
(Marks, 1967).
(Loadings are mean of analyses on test and retest).

Loading	Item
·73	(Diagnosis of agoraphobia).
·70	I sometimes have a fear of fainting in public.
·59	I feel nervous when I have to go on a train journey.
·51	I am nervous when I am left alone.
·51	I am uneasy when I am in a crowded place.
·48	I am uneasy when alone in a large open space.
·36	The thought of a surgical operation would terrify me.
·26	It generally makes me uneasy to cross a bridge or street.

The clinical features of agoraphobia are similar in widespread reports from Europe, America and Australia. Evidence for the unity of the syndrome also comes from statistical enquiries. Roth et al., (1965) managed to delineate a group of agoraphobic patients by factor analysis of the clinical features of 275 neurotic patients. Their resultant agoraphobic factor is seen in Table 3.7. Their own label for this factor was phobic-anxiety-depersonalisation. Further evidence was obtained from a factor analysis of answers to 239 questions of the Tavistock Phobic Inventory and the Cornell Medical Index given by a group of 72 phobics at the Maudsley Hospital (Marks, 1967). An agoraphobic factor emerged which concerned the usual complaints made by these patients, and correlated well with the clinical diagnosis made independently (Table 3.8). Finally, similar features were found to characterise 1,200 agoraphobics throughout Britain who completed a detailed questionnaire. Analysis of the replies yielded factors closely like that elicited by Marks, 1967 (unpublished data).

There is little doubt from clinical and statistical evidence that agoraphobia is a coherent clinical syndrome with a well-defined cluster of features which persist together over a long period of time. However, the more diffuse varieties of agoraphobia merge imperceptibly with anxiety states, affective disorders and even obsessive neuroses. In such cases more than one diagnostic label may be appropriate. During periods of depression or acute panic several of our agoraphobic patients have been labelled and treated as affective disorders.

Unlike agoraphobia, anxiety states do not occur much more in women (Table 3.4) (Hare, 1965) but their age of onset and clinical features are similar, except that anxiety states have more diffuse (free-floating) anxiety and fewer phobias. Anxiety states have higher Neuroticism scores and are more introverted. The skin resistance and blood flow measures indicate a higher level of diffuse anxiety. The eyeblink conditioning acquisition rate is marginally lower. In fact many agoraphobics appear to be anxiety states with superimposed phobias, and in cases where the anxiety and phobias are equally prominent allocation into one or other diagnostic group is purely arbitrary. We do not know why some cases with marked anxiety rapidly develop phobias which then dominate the clinical picture, while other cases with similar anxiety never show phobias. At our present stage of knowledge it is useful where possible to distinguish between the two conditions as the presence of agoraphobia produces a distinctive disability which requires a different emphasis in treatment.

Contrast of animal and agoraphobia

If we ever are tempted to think that all phobic states are a unity which reflect the same disorder and aetiology, we can quickly dispel this illusion simply by looking at the startling contrast between animal phobias and agoraphobia. These two conditions differ radically in onset, course, symptomatology, response to treatment and psychophysiological measures. No two syndromes can better illustrate the diverse conditions listed together under the same label of phobic state.

One might argue that the phobic situation is not of any importance, and that animal phobias and agoraphobias are but two ends of a continuum of phobias which are specific at one end and diffuse at the other. If this were true we should then find many animal phobias which are diffuse and many agoraphobias which are specific; we should not find that the phobic situation predicts the specificity of the disturbance.

In fact we do not find diffuse animal phobias in adults—the majority of animal phobias are discrete disturbances and more extensive symptoms are found only in those few cases where the animal phobia happens to be associated with another disturbance such as agoraphobia or a personality disorder. In this instance the phobic object predicts the specificity of the disturbance. The same usually applies in agoraphobia. Most agoraphobics have extensive symptoms, and it is exceptional to find a discrete fear of open spaces without other fears, except in the early stages of the disorder before there has been time for generalisation. The other exception is what we might call "burnt-out" agoraphobia, where after years of disability extensive symptoms gradually clear up to leave a few localised fears. The argument against a continuum is further strengthened by the fact that knowledge of the phobic situation is such a good predictor of physiological measures.

Social phobias   (Table 3.9)

Psychiatrists see a wide variety of social phobias in the form of fears of eating, drinking, blushing, speaking, writing or vomiting in the presence of other people. These differ from the fears of crowds found in agoraphobics in that the latter are more apprehensive about a mass of people together than of the individuals who make up the crowd. Not a few agoraphobics also have mild social phobias.

Table 3.9

Social Phobias

Frequency:	Not uncommon.
Sex incidence:	60% women.
Onset age:	After puberty: 15–30.
Phobic situation:	Restricted to social activities, e.g. eating, drinking or writing in company.
Associated symptoms:	Few. Little generalised anxiety. Occasional depression and other phobias.
Course:	Fairly continuous.
Psychological tests:	Slightly raised Cornell, raised Neuroticism, slightly introverted.
Psychophysiology:	Slightly raised eyeblink conditioning. G.S.R. shows many spontaneous fluctuations, habituates slowly. Normal forearm blood flow.
Response to desensitisation:	Quite good.
Comment:	Localised varieties merge with conditioned autonomic disorders. Diffuse varieties merge with personality disorders.

Social phobics form roughly 8% of the phobics seen in the Maudsley Hospital. It is interesting that their incidence is about the same in men and women. Social phobias usually start after puberty, with a peak in the late teens (Fig. 3.1). Their age of onset largely overlaps with that of agoraphobia, except that few social phobias begin after the age of 30.

This group of phobics is less coherent than the animal phobics or agoraphobics, and has characteristics intermediate to those two groups. Social phobics have rather more phobias and other symptoms than animal phobics, but fewer than agoraphobics. Psychophysiological measures are seen in Table 3.4. They acquire eyeblink conditioned responses quite rapidly (Martin et al. 1969). Their skin resistance is indistinguishable from that of the agoraphobics (Lader et al. 1967). In the few patients who have had their forearm blood flow measured, this has been at the same level as in agoraphobics.

Social phobics resemble agoraphobics except for their sex incidence, fewer symptoms and lower Cornell Scores. The more diffuse examples may have minor agoraphobic symptoms, but many are very specific phobias. We need to know more about social phobics before definitely classifying them on their own.

The groups seen together   (Table 3.4).

It is convenient at this point to summarise the evidence by looking at all the groups together in regard to each feature in turn. In preponderance of women the agoraphobics and animal phobics stand out. In onset age the animal phobias are distinctive. Treatment age does not distinguish the different groups of phobias. Overt anxiety is most prominent in anxiety states, least obvious in the animal phobics. Cornell and Neuroticism scores are normal only in the animal phobics. Anxiety states are significantly more neurotic and introverted than any other group. Skin resistance and forearm blood flow are again normal in the animal phobics and most abnormal in anxiety states. Eyeblink conditioned response acquisition is significantly more rapid and extinction more slow in animal phobics. Response to treatment is poorest in agoraphobia and best in specific phobias.

Miscellaneous specific phobias   (Table 3.10).

Our final group of phobias of external stimuli is a group of monosymptomatic phobias which start at any time in life and persist fairly continuously. Women do not have these phobias much more than

Table 3.10
Miscellaneous Specific Phobias

Frequency:	Not uncommon.
Sex incidence:	? 50% women.
Onset age:	Any time from early childhood to old age.
Phobic situation:	Restricted to specific locus: heights, thunder, darkness, travel, closed spaces, driving, etc.
Associated symptoms:	Few. No generalised anxiety.
Course:	Continuous.
Psychological and Psychophysiological:	Insufficient data, but resemble animal phobias.
Response to treatment:	Quite good. May need prolonged treatment.

men. The phobic situations vary from one case to another but are fairly specific for a given case. The phobic situations include heights, wind, darkness, thunderstorms, running water, and so on. Although agoraphobics frequently have fears of closed spaces such as lifts, tubes or aeroplanes, the reverse is not always found, as some patients with claustrophobia tend to have relatively isolated fears without the concomitants found in agoraphobia and these fall within this group of phobias. Such patients have limited phobias of travelling in lifts, trains, tubes or aeroplanes, and these may be an occupational hazard, for example in pilots.

Physiological data are not available for this group except that forearm blood flow has been normal in the few patients who have been tested. It is quite possible that this group will turn out to be indistinguishable from animal phobics apart from the age of onset and sex incidence. These cases respond quite well to treatment, and many of the successful cases in the literature about desensitisation come from this group.

Class II: Phobias of internal stimuli

In these phobias the feared situation is inside the patient, and there is thus no external situation which can be avoided to reduce fear.

Illness phobias

These are intense fears of illness which centre round specific disturbances like cancer, heart disease, venereal disease, death and so on. The phobia consists of endless ruminations about the possibility of suffering from any one of a host of diseases. The phobia resembles an obsessive thought except that there is no subjective feeling of resistance. Fears of this kind are often a prominent feature of depressive illnesses, in which cases they wax and wane with the depression. However, in a small group of patients these fears of illness occur and persist independent of any other symptom. They could be regarded as an extreme form of hypochondriasis, though in patients with hypochondriasis the fears are usually diffuse and not of any particular malady. Illness phobias occur in both sexes, the particular illness which is feared depending in part on what is fashionable in the culture. Little systematic work has been done on patients of this kind, as opposed to those with diffuse hypochondriasis. Their course is not clear, and series of patients with this problem have not been treated or investigated systematically. It is thus still too early to decide whether this group can be regarded as a separate syndrome.

Obsessive phobias

These are fears about one's own feelings "which come to consciousness in spite of and contrary to the will of the patient and which he is unable to suppress although he recognizes them as abnormal and not characteristic of himself" (Westphal, 1878).

Examples of such fears are fears of harming people or babies, fears of swearing or making obscene gestures, fears of contamination which lead to obsessive handwashing. These obsessions could strictly be called phobias because they are disproportionate to demands of the situation, cannot be explained away and are beyond voluntary control. However, they are generally found together with other compulsive phenomena, and so are best regarded as obsessive-compulsive disorders and omitted from the main rubric of phobias. Obsessive phobias are bound up with elaborate rituals and magical thinking, and are very resistant to treatment by desensitisation (Marks et al., 1969), to which phobias of external situations commonly respond.

Obsessive-compulsive disorders can start at any age and appear with equal frequency in both sexes.

Phobias in children

As in adults any object or situation can be the focus of a phobia in children, but overall patterns are rather different. Phobias of many kinds are more common and transitory events than in adults. Little is known by which we can classify childhood phobias usefully. As phobias in children present special problems, they will be dealt with in a separate section.

Discussion

The evidence suggests some general thoughts about the aetiology of phobias some of which were discussed earlier, but are worth emphasising again. Phobias do not occur randomly with respect to all situations, ages, or other psychiatric symptoms. Rather phobias tend to occur in particular kinds of situations, at certain ages rather than at others, and in association with well-defined clusters of other psychiatric symptoms.

One general point is that although in theory any situation may trigger a phobia, in practice certain classes of stimuli are more likely than others to trigger off phobias, given that these different stimuli are all encountered quite frequently. It is reasonable to expect that phylo-genetic mechanisms are at least partly responsible for this prepotency of certain stimuli to produce fear in man, just as they do in other species.

Another general point concerns the age incidence. At least in the animal phobias there may be a facilitatory period for the acquisition of such fears in childhood, since adults rarely acquire these fears for the first time in adult life.

The fact that agoraphobia starts after puberty may be linked to the fact that anxiety states also begin in the same age range. Similar mechanisms may be at work. Evidence from the effects of leucotomy indicate that agoraphobia is largely maintained by excessive diffuse anxiety. Remove this free-floating anxiety and phobias can then be unlearned without fresh fears being regenerated continually. The source of this anxiety is obscure.

Next, the kind of phobic object is of some importance. Not all phobic situations are equivalent, since by knowing the kind of situation which is feared we can often tell other likely characteristics of the patient.

It is not clear what the psychophysiological measures mean. Forearm blood flow, spontaneous fluctuations in skin conductance and habituation of the galvanic skin response, all correlate with anxiety. The habituation rate also correlates significantly with response to desensitisation that is, patients who habituate rapidly respond better to desensitisation.

Little is known about the correlates of eyeblink conditioning. It is surprising that the phobics with fewest symptoms were those who conditioned best and extinguished most slowly, and that phobic patients with the most symptoms only conditioned at a normal rate. If one assumed that the symptoms were due to rapid conditioning, then rapid conditioners should have many symptoms, and this is precisely the opposite of what we find. Similarly, if phobic symptoms were due to slow extinction of fear responses, then those patients who extinguished least should have most phobias, but again the opposite is in fact the case.

Conclusion

The phobic states are thus a series of related disorders with overlapping features. They range from very simple to very complex disturbances, and multiple factors contribute to their genesis. I have presented one way of classifying phobic states but there are other ways in which the clinical material could have been subdivided. The simplest classification would have been to describe two kinds of phobias —monosymptomatic and diffuse. It is true that such a classification is useful in predicting response to treatment. It does not predict symptomatology, onset age or sex incidence. Possibly the best classification would be the one which takes into account both the nature of the phobic situation and its specificity.

Summary

Phobic disorders were described increasingly from the middle of the nineteenth century onwards, and in recent years achieved a separate diagnostic category in Britain and America. The classification of phobic disorders must take into account the facts that phobias can occur of almost any situation and that phobias may occur together with practically any other psychiatric symptom. Phobic states are a series of related disorders which need to be differerentiated from phobic symptoms which are a minor accompaniment of another major psychiatric disturbance.

In adults mild fears are almost ubiquitous but intense phobias are uncommon. Phobic states are a series of related disorders which may conveniently be divided into Class I, those of external situations which can be avoided, and Class II phobias, those of internal situations which cannot be escaped. Amongst phobias of external situations, the agoraphobic syndrome is the commonest and most distressing phobic disorder in psychiatric practice. This is a cluster of fears which start in adult life and centre round going out alone, into open spaces, crowds and vehicles, occurring together in varying combinations, often with other symptoms as well. Animal phobias are rare monosymptomatic fears of a single animal species which start in childhood and persist into adult life. Social phobias are less rare, but evidence is lacking that this is a coherent group. Miscellaneous specific phobias are discrete phobias which start at any time of life. Amongst phobias of internal situations the status of illness phobias is unclear, while obsessive phobias are best classified separately with obsessive-compulsive phenomena.

Several groups of phobias of external situations can be differentiated from one another on the basis of clinical, questionnaire and psychophysiological variables.

Section II. THE AGORAPHOBIC SYNDROME

Autobiographical accounts

Natural history
    Prevalence
    Age of onset and treatment

Family, personality and background
    Sexual function

Precipitating factors

Clinical picture
    mode of onset
    clinical features
    fluctuations with internal and external events
    impact on the family
    non-phobic symptoms associated with agoraphobia
        depersonalisation
        depression
        obsessive compulsive phenomena
        organic disorder

Motivation: the role of willpower during different phases of agoraphobia

Note on survey of Open Door agoraphobics.

The Agoraphobic Syndrome (Phobic anxiety state)

The agoraphobic syndrome is the commonest and most distressing phobic disorder met with in adult patients. The term "agoraphobia" derives from the Greek root "*agora*" meaning an assembly, the place of assembly, and market place (OED). It was first used by Westphal (1871) to describe the ". . . impossibility of walking through certain streets or squares, or possibility of so doing only with resultant dread of anxiety". Today agoraphobia is still used to describe fears of going out into public areas such as streets, shops or vehicles in variable combination. Such phobias present a wide range of clinical pictures. At one extreme, for example, some travel phobias or claustrophobias occur as isolated symptoms; in such cases the term agoraphobia is overinclusive and actually misleading if taken in the strictly literal sense. At the other extreme, severe cases often have not only agoraphobia and other phobias, but also panic attacks, depression, depersonalisation, obsessions and other symptoms (Roth et al., 1965); in these patients the term agoraphobia is under-inclusive, and describes but part of their entire clinical picture.

It is not surprising that similar cases with multiple symptoms have been given several labels by psychiatrists; these include anxiety hysteria (Freud, 1919), locomotor anxiety (Abraham, 1913b), street fear (Miller, 1953), phobic-anxiety-depersonalisation syndrome (Roth, 1959), anxiety syndromes or phobic-anxious states (Klein, 1964), anxiety states, anxiety neurosis (Lancet, 1952, p. 79), severe mixed psychoneurosis, pseudo-neurotic schizophrenia and borderline states (Klein, 1964), non-specific insecurity fears (Snaith, 1968).

A frequent misconception is that agoraphobia is a fear of open spaces, and it is sometimes argued that agoraphobia is a misnomer for this condition, since streets and crowded shops are not open spaces. But the original Greek root chosen by Westphal denotes not open spaces as such but public places of assembly, and indeed it fits the clinical facts. However, since the cluster of phobias in this condition varies from one patient to the next, the reader will rightly wonder why agoraphobia is chosen as the label, especially since some patients give priority in their fears not to going out but to other features. The term is chosen because the commonest and most constricting elements of this condition are fears of going out into public places of various kinds. The syndrome is *not* characterised by fears of cats, dogs, thunderstorms, driving a car, running water or of having venereal disease. But simply knowing that a patient has fears of going out into the street and crowded places enables one to predict that many of the other features of the syndrome will be present in that patient, including the fact that he may indeed also be claustrophobic, be afraid of fainting, dying or going mad or losing control. The term does not denote only a fear of going into the open, just as the diagnosis of depressive illness does not imply that the patient is simply depressed in his mood. Indeed, a patient may have that disorder without ever admitting to feeling depressed at all, but if he expresses suicidal ideas, self blame, forebodings of disaster, has lost his appetite and cannot sleep most psychiatrists would regard such a cluster of features as a depressive disorder. Depressive disorder is a good label because depressive mood change is the commonest aspect of the syndrome, even though on occasion it is overshadowed by other features. Similarly, with the agoraphobic syndrome the most constant feature in the constellation of clinical events is a cluster of phobias centring round public places, which run a fluctuating course together through episodic exacerbations and partial remissions. Patients with borderline features could of course be classified differently, but the core symptoms appear so constantly together as to require unitary consideration.

There are alternative terms with the same literal sense as agoraphobia-kenophobia, platzangst in German, and peur des espaces or horreur du vide in French (Weiss, 1964). Agoraphobia, however, is now the accepted description for fear of open spaces. Certain writers point out correctly that the literal term agoraphobia describes such fears inadequately; Prince (1912) and Klein (1964) regarded the crux of this condition as the fear of lack of support, of suddenly being rendered helpless during panics, whereas Weiss (1964) singled out the sense of internal danger, "an unbearable feeling of illbeing to which they react with severe anxiety". Both descriptions fit many cases called "agoraphobic" in this book; the literal meaning of agoraphobia is extended here to include events closely linked to the central cluster of typical phobias. In this book "agoraphobia" is not meant in a purely literal sense. The term is unsatisfactory, but other terms suffer equal disadvantage. "Phobic anxiety state" does not draw attention to the most frequent phobias found in the syndrome, nor does "panphobic syndrome", while "phobic-anxiety-depersonalisation-syndrome" is rather long and clumsy.

Autobiographical accounts

Familiarity with agoraphobia comes readily by listening to patients' own words about their disorders. Several autobiographies illustrate the main features seen from the patient's point of view and help to show the hidden, enduring distress so often found in this condition. The following account describes the gradual onset of phobias which became increasingly restrictive as they spread to diverse but typical situations. Background anxiety is well described with the phobic anxiety as a special accentuation of this.

"My malady came upon me gradually and went through definite stages of development . . . I am now in middle life and I have not seen a well day since I was about 12 years of age. Before I experienced any of the symptoms of agoraphobia I recall that . . . I was taken suddenly with 'spells' which lasted about thirty minutes. During these attacks I was entirely conscious and rational —a sort of 'coldness' that produced a very unusual sensation, or perhaps a *lack* of sensation . . . I was more liable to these attacks during times of excitement; for example, one of the worst attacks I ever had came over me while I was attending the funeral of a relative . . . When my strange illness came upon me, I worried over it, fearing that I should die in one of the attacks . . .

(After a boy in the village was murdered) I almost feared to be alone, was afraid to go to the barn in the daytime, and suffered when put to bed in the dark . . . During the months which followed . . . I experienced the first symptoms of agoraphobia. There was a high hill not far from my home in the country where we boys used to coast in the winter time. One evening, while coasting, in company with other boys in the neighbourhood, I experienced an uncomfortable feeling each time we returned to the top of the hill. It was not a well defined symptom of this horrible . . . malady, but later experiences have taught me that it possessed the unmistakable earmarks. As the months went by I commenced having a dread of high hills, especially when the fields consisted of pasture land and were level with the grass cropped short like the grass on a well kept lawn. I likewise commenced to dread high things and especially to ascend anything high. I even had a fear of crowds of people, and later of wide streets and parks. I have outgrown the fear of

crowds largely, but an immense building or a high rocky bluff fills
me with dread . . . Ugly architecture greatly intensifies the fear.

The malady is always present . . . I am conscious of it during
every hour that I am awake. The fear, intensified, that comes over
while crossing a wide street is an outcropping of a permanent
condition" (Vincent, 1919, pp. 295–299).

Another autobiography describes spasmodic increase in agoraphobia
developing at the age of 30, after several years of intermittent anxiety
feelings unrelated to any particular situation.

"The brief trips to Bonn filled me with a surging sense of the
impossible and the far . . . a feel, especially as to distance, that could
convert a half mile, or even five blocks from home, in terms of subjective need and cowardice, into an infinity of remoteness, and at the
same time that it remains to be an estimate of exactly the same half
mile or two blocks it is . . .

(I developed) a strange new phobia of water. In rowboat, canoe
or launch I had for terror to hug the shore; I had always previously
crossed the lake from point to point over (miles) . . .of open water
. . . I tried to master these fears by the elementary device of 'try and
try again' to no purpose . . . Terror would drag me back, terror of
being so far from safety . . . The net result of this 'cure' was thereafter I found my normal rowing limit from shore reduced from 200
feet to 50 . . . (later after his wife's suicide) the panics subsided into
mere diffused dread . . . a relative relief . . . trying to fight back
another seizure . . . I have another seizure, I try to run it off . . . I
start a little walk down the street about a hundred feet from the
house, I am compelled to rush back, in horror of being so far away
. . . a hundred feet away . . from home and security. I have never
walked or ridden, alone or with others, as a normal man, since that
day. . .

At times this emotional effect remains merely a diffuse state of
terror, an intensity running the whole scale from vague anxiety to
intensest feel of impending death; . . . I am in terror of the seizure
of terror; and I fear seizure at a given distance; there are then
perfectly rational subterrors lest I may panic and make a public
spectacle of myself, or I am in front of an automobile, or actually
collapse from nervous exhaustion as soon as I get a certain distance
from home—a distance varying back and forth from yards to miles
—for the past 15 years I am overwhelmed with the feeling of insecurity, or terror that I can't hit back" (Leonard, 1928, pp. 238,
278, 302, 319).

In these two accounts there was no hint of precipitating factors at
the onset of the phobias, but once developed, the phobias were exacerbated by traumatic events—the first after a boy was murdered in his
village, the second after his wife's suicide. The initial anxiety symptoms

occurred out of the blue, and thereafter the original situations they occurred in became increasingly capable of provoking the same anxiety. The constant background anxiety was present even at rest, and secondary exacerbating situations were increasingly avoided to stave off sudden increases of this anxiety. The difficulties in these well-developed cases thus fell into two broad categories—background general anxiety not related to any special situation, and the particular phobic situations which exacerbated this.

Leonard's account contained a further important feature. After his phobias started he tried in vain to master them by self re-education, but the net result was the opposite to that intended. His "cure" simply restricted his activities further. At this stage of the disorder "willpower" alone could neither master the phobias nor affect the background anxiety.

Most agoraphobias fluctuate considerably, sometimes in response to minor occurrences in the environment, at other times with no obvious change internally or externally. In a later passage Vincent described this clearly, noting common stratagems which helped to alleviate his phobias—darkness, storms, changeable landscapes with a limited view, riding a bicycle, gripping a suitcase.

"At times my phobias are much more pronounced than at other times. Sometimes, after a strenuous day, on the following morning I find myself almost dreading to walk across a room; at other times I can cross the street without any pronounced discomfort. . . .

Usually I feel better in the evening than in the morning, partly because the darkness seems to have a quieting effect on me. I love a snow-storm, a regular blizzard, and feel much less discomfort going about the town or riding on the train on such days, probably because one's view is obstructed. In fact, I welcome stormy days . . . on such days I make it a point to be out and about the town.

I dread going on water in a boat, especially if the surface is smooth; I much prefer to have the waves rolling high. The most restful place in all the world for me is in a wood, where there is much variety in the trees and plenty of underbrush, with here and there little hills and valleys, and especially along a winding brook . . . I love quiet, restful landscapes . . . let the landscape be bold and rugged and bleak, and it strikes terror (into me) . . .

I ride a bicycle along the streets with comparative comfort where I should suffer agony where I had to walk. In walking I feel least uncomfortable in passing along the street if I carry a suitcase or travelling bag—something to grip . . .

I have such a dread of crossing a long bridge on foot . . ." (Vincent, 1919, pp. 295–299).

Much of the suffering in this condition is hidden, since agoraphobics can conceal their disorder for long periods if they manage to work. The first account by Leonard was published when he had been agoraphobic for 48 years—only closest relatives and friends knew of the disability, and he continued as professor of English at a university during this time, living very close to the campus. The second account by Vincent makes it clear that Vincent never sought medical aid for his fears and led an active public life while concealing his disability. These autobiographies showed what it feels like to be an agoraphobic. We will now pass on to the external features of the disorder as seen by psychiatrists. Other accounts by sufferers will be included later to emphasise important points.

Natural History

The literature shows impressive agreement about the natural history and clinical features of agoraphobia. Disagreement appears only when the boundaries of the disorder have to be defined, and when aetiology and treatment are considered.

PREVALENCE

The prevalence of agoraphobia in the general community was estimated at 6·3 per 1000 (Agras et al, 1969) in Vermont. It is larger than appears from psychiatric practice. After a B.B.C. talk about agoraphobia a journalist was asked to take on the correspondence arising from it; 300 letters were received, and a correspondence circle was formed; within a few months 1600 members joined from all over Britain (The Open Door, 1965). Some 5% of these had never sought medical aid for their complaints and 33% had seen general practitioners but never been to a psychiatrist (Marks and Herst, 1969). The author too, has encountered many stories about patients' neighbours, friends or relatives who were almost housebound but never sought treatment for their phobias. The total incidence is therefore appreciably greater than that seen by psychiatrists.

In psychiatric practice the incidence of phobias as a main complaint is ab ut 2–3% both in America and in England (Terhune, 1961; Errera and Coleman, 1963; Hare, 1965). Descriptions of those phobias indicate that the bulk of them are agoraphobias. Of course many more patients have phobias as part of another disorder such as a depressive illness, obsessive-compulsive neurosis or anxiety state. Paskind (1931), for example, found the incidence of phobias to be 48% in psychoneuroses, 65% in manic depressive psychoses and 10% in schizophrenia. He used the term phobia to include many minor fears which were a small part of the total clinical picture, and most of his cases would not be formally diagnosed as phobic disorders.

Nearly all descriptions show that about two-thirds of agoraphobics seen by psychiatrists are women (Table 3.11), and this is true both for America and Britain. The one exception is the 51% incidence of women in the series of Sim and Houghton (1966) with phobic anxiety. However

Table 3.11. Comparative features of published series of phobias

	Terhune (1949, 1961)	Friedman (1950)	Tucker (1956)	Roth (1959)	Bignold (1960)	Errera & Coleman (1963)	Warburton (1963)	Klein (1964)	Roberts (1964)	Marks & Gelder (1965, 1966)	Sim & Houghton (1966)	Snaith (1963)
Main symptoms	Phobias	Travel phobia	Agora-phobia	Phobic anxiety deperson-alisation	Agora-phobia	Phobias	Agora-phobia	Agora-phobia	Agora-phobia	Agora-phobia	Phobic anxiety	Agora-phobia
Number of patients	86	50	100	135	10	19	53	32	41	84	191	27
% incidence in psychiatric practice	2·5	—	—	—	—	2·8	—	—	—	†2–3	—	—
% female	67	64	89	70	100	74	89	81	*100	89	51	63
% married	85	—	74	—	100	94	—	—	*100	73	—	—
Mean age at treatment	20–40	17–53	28	36	37	31	37	34	20 40	32	36	38
Mean onset age	young adult life	9–42	—	20–40	33	—	—	—	—	24	30	—
Premorbid personality	"soft" passive anxious	—	dependent	dependent anxious shy	—	—	—	50% dependent	anxious	mixed	—	—
Home background	stable	stable	—	stable	—	—	—	—	—	stable	—	—

* artefact through deliberate selection
† Hare (1965)
— not given

only half of this sample were agoraphobic, and here the excess of women was indeed evident. Men predominated amongst their other patients who had work and social phobias. The preponderance of females amongst agoraphobics is surprising in view of the sex incidence in certain other neurotic disorders, e.g. in anxiety neurosis and social anxieties, men and women are usually about equally represented (Hare, 1965); Marks and Gelder, 1965) while four-fifths of patients with writer's cramp are men.

AGE OF ONSET AND TREATMENT

Agoraphobia usually begins in young adult life between 18 and 35 (Table 3.11, Figure 3.1) and is rare in childhood (Rutter et al., 1968). The mean age of onset was 24 in the Maudsley Hospital series and 28 in the Open Door sample of agoraphobics throughout Britain, which agrees with that of most other writers. Figure 3.1 shows the spread of the ages of onset of several neurotic conditions. Very few agoraphobics begin in childhood; the great majority start after puberty, with peaks at 20 and 30; this condition seldom starts de novo after 40. Agoraphobia starts at about the same age as anxiety states and social anxieties. However, it differs sharply in this respect from specific animal phobias, which nearly all start in early childhood, and from writer's cramp, which start about a decade later in the thirties.*

Most series report that patients come for treatment in their thirties. Mean age at treatment of the Maudsley sample was 34, a figure not dissimilar from that obtained for other "neurotic" disorders such as specific animal phobias, anxiety neurosis and writer's cramp, but slightly later than that for social anxieties. Of the Open Door sample the average time to elapse before the patient was handicapped was 15 months. The time it took to seek help from different agencies after the phobia began was 17 months from general practitioners, 34 months from psychiatrists (as outpatient or inpatient) and 57 months from religious and spiritual healers (Marks and Herst, 1969).

Compared to other agoraphobic patients, agoraphobia begins and leads to treatment 6 to 12 years earlier in patients with a history of childhood fears of leaving parents, or fears of the dark or excessive night terrors (Klein, 1964; Marks, unpublished data). It is not clear whether such childhood fears were causative or simply the expression of a predisposition already present in early childhood.

Family, personality and background of agoraphobics

In this section little systematic work can be quoted; figures of different workers depend on varying criteria and are not equivalent, nor are they easily compared with control populations.

---

* It is of historical interest that Freud's phobia of trains lasted from the age of 31 to 43 — Jones, 1953, p. 14.

Several workers agree that phobic patients come from stable families (Terhune, 1949; Roth, 1959; Marks and Gelder, 1965). Terhune found that the family was overprotective and Roth noted that the families of phobics were unusually stable and closeknit. Although Webster (1953) found that the mothers were overprotective he was exceptional in finding that fathers were absent from the home with unusual frequency. The stable family background of phobics differs remarkably from that of psychopaths, in whom broken homes are the rule rather than the exception (Marks, 1965).

The birth order of phobics is not remarkable (Terhune, 1949; Marks and Gelder, 1965). The incidence of psychiatric disorder reported in the family ranges from 21% to 40% (Roth, 1949; Roberts, 1964). The only available control is the phobic series of Harper and Roth (1962) who found the incidence of neurosis in the families of phobics (33%) was significantly higher than in a control group of temporal lobe epileptics.

Several reports quote an incidence of childhood enuresis, fears and night terrors of up to 55% (Marks and Gelder, 1965). Harper and Roth's phobics had a significantly commoner history of childhood phobias (60%) than their control. No reports find much aggressiveness of truanting in childhood.

The premorbid personality has been variously described as "soft", passive, anxious, shy, dependent (Terhune, 1949; Tucker, 1956; Roberts, 1964; Roth, 1956). Many agoraphobics do indeed have such personalities before their symptoms begin, but in a minority agoraphobia undoubtedly begins in active, sociable, outgoing persons. As Prince (1912) noted, such phobias "occur in people of all types and characteristics, amongst the normally self-reliant as well as amongst the timid".

Agoraphobic patients are not unusual in intelligence, education or occupation. Terhune's (1949) patients who were above average in these respects were not representative. The Open Door sample of agoraphobics throughout Britain was average with respect to education, occupational status, income and religious affiliation.

Since agoraphobics are generally young adults, most series naturally show them to be married, to spouses of average age (Webster, 1953; Marks and Gelder, 1965) and the marriages tend to be stable. Though it has been suggested that women who later become agoraphobic tend to marry passive husbands, this remains as yet to be demonstrated.

SEXUAL FUNCTION

Sexual disorder, especially frigidity, is not uncommon in agoraphobic women. This usually antedates the onset of the phobias, but occasionally starts secondarily with the phobia. The frigidity therefore does not run parallel with the agoraphobia, and a few patients who are severely agoraphobic have always had regular satisfying orgasm during intercourse. Terhune (1949) found no demonstrable connection between sexual maladjustment and phobias but gave no figures about this. Roberts (1964), Marks and Gelder (1965), and Webster (1953) respectively found 53%, 55% and 92% of agoraphobics to be sexually maladjusted. Roth (1959) found total frigidity in 60% of his phobic women, the difference from normal controls being significant. The incidence of sexual disorder in agoraphobic women is of the same order as that found in women in anxiety neurosis (Winokur and Holeman, 1963), obsessive-compulsive inpatients (Marks, 1965) and hysteria (Winokur and Leonard, 1963).

Several mechanisms contribute to the association of sexual dissatisfaction with agoraphobia. Anxiety from any cause reduces capacity for sexual enjoyment, and panic attacks and background tension are indeed a feature of agoraphobia. Agoraphobia often develops in anxious, shy people with personality problems which themselves are accompanied by frigidity and other sexual maladjustment. Since agoraphobia is often found with normal sexual enjoyment, sexual disorder is not a sine qua non for the development of agoraphobia.

Sexual disorder is less common in agoraphobic men than women. In the Open Door sample regular sexual enjoyment and orgasm was reported in 83% of the agoraphobic men but in only 60% of the agoraphobic women. When sexual disorder is present, the complaint is generally of impotence or premature ejaculation.

Precipitating factors

Figures given about the frequency of precipitating factors at the onset range from 10% (Friedman) to 83% (Roth), which reflects disparate interpretations about what should be regarded as a precipitant. Nevertheless, a substantial number of agoraphobics clearly start after a major change in the patient's life situation, e.g. serious illness in the patient or relative, acute danger or discomfort, leaving home, bereavement, engagement, marriage, pregnancy, miscarriage, childbirth, or after an unpleasant scene in a shop, street or bus. As with almost any other condition, agoraphobics often regard some trivial event as the trigger to their disorder, even though such events might previously have occurred without undue mishap. The presence and nature of a precipitant does not have much relevance to the subsequent course of the agoraphobia.

Since a multitude of events can precede agoraphobia it is likely either that such precipitants act as non-specific stressors in a patient already liable to the disorder for some reason, or that the disorder was already present but hidden until the stressor elicited or exacerbated it. In conclusion it should be emphasised that not a few phobias start suddenly without any obvious change in life situation of the patient.

Clinical picture

The characteristic features of agoraphobia appear unchanged in autobiographical and clinical accounts of the condition since Westphal's earliest description a century ago. The main features are fears of going out into the open, into streets, shops, crowds, closed spaces such as lifts, theatres, cinemas or church, or travel on tubes, trains, buses or coaches, ships and aeroplanes (but not usually cars), fears of going on bridges, into tunnels, having haircuts or hairdo's, and of remaining alone at home or of leaving home. These fears occur in many combinations over a variable period of time, and, at least in cases seen by psychiatrists, are associated with other symptoms such as general anxiety, panic attacks, depression, obsessions and depersonalisation. Certain social fears are also found in this condition—fears of trembling, blushing, eating or writing in front of other people or fears of being stared at. In yet other patients with agoraphobia, there are fears of vomiting or of seeing other people vomit. Many agoraphobias disappear

Table 3.12

The main phobias and other problems of 900 agoraphobic female patients from The Open Door

Phobias	% scoring 3 or 4	Mean for all patients	Other problems	% scoring 3 or 4	Mean for all patients
Speaking to audiences	60	2·36	Exhaustion	42	2·16
Tube trains	50	2·23	Tension	38	2·09
Trains	47	2·07	Obsessive thoughts	37	1·90
Crowds	28	2·04	Depression	29	1·73
Buses	38	1·91	Loneliness	32	1·68
Heights	36	1·91	Fears of fainting	31	1·52
Theatre	39	1·81	Giddiness	26	1·50
Hairdresser	31	1·76	Panic	24	1·50
Street, open spaces	23	1·76	Irritability	19	1·45
Tunnels	36	1·73	Headaches	22	1·40
Lifts	30	1·69	Depersonalisation	22	1·32
Dentist	28	1·65	Palpitations	20	1·31
Parties	21	1·46	Fears of dying	22	1·26
			Overchecking—tidiness	22	1·22
			Suicidal ideas	15	0·83
			Fears of disease	9	0·71

Anchoring points on rating scale for:

Score	Fears	Other problems
0	Almost no fear at all	Very little
1	Makes me uneasy but I don't avoid it	Occasionally
2	Makes me particularly uneasy—I avoid it when possible	Often
3	Frightens me even to think of it—I always avoid it	Very often
4	Terrifies me so much that every moment of my life is miserable	Nearly all the time

For fears of open spaces and streets, % for each score was:
0—12%, 1—32%, 2—33%, 3—14%, 4—9%

without the patient ever receiving treatment but these are seldom seen
by psychiatrists, who tend to see the more persistent varieties. This
account naturally dwells on the latter, but it must be recognised that
many people have minor phobias out of the list detailed above without
any other major complaint.

The central cluster of phobias in agoraphobia is impressively similar
in most cases, although naturally there is individual variation from case
to case. This was recognised by Prince in 1912 when he wrote of ". . . the
fear of travelling in trains, going into lonely places, walking along the
street alone, or entering places like a church, theatre, etc. Some of these
fears have been called agoraphobia, claustrophobia etc. Almost all, if not
all, patients suffering from phobia have fears of this kind". Most of these
items correlated well with the diagnosis of agoraphobia in a study of 72
phobic patients described earlier (Marks, 1967). They were similar
to those obtained in an independent study by Dixon et al. (1957) in
300 psychiatric outpatients. Items from an "exhaustion" factor also
correlated highly with agoraphobia. The same items appeared promin-
ently in the features of the Open Door sample of agoraphobics. A
detailed breakdown of their phobias and other problems appears in
Table 3.12. Autobiographies, psychiatric accounts and questionnaire
studies thus tend to agree on the central cluster of clinical features in
agoraphobia, and this cluster has physiological and prognostic correlates which were described earlier. The physiological correlates are an
increased number of spontaneous fluctuations of the galvanic skin
resistance at rest and slowed habituation of the galvanic skin response to
successive auditory stimuli.

MODE OF ONSET

The onset can be sudden within a few hours, more gradual over a few
weeks, or develop slowly over several years after a prodromal stage of
vague intermittent anxiety. Cases of sudden onset may start with an
acute sustained panic attack which is followed by phobias causing disability relentlessly increasing to housebondage within a few weeks;
others begin with vague intermittent anxiety which merges into fluctuating agoraphobia over many years. The period elapsing between the
first symptoms and maximum disability varies correspondingly, as does
the duration of symptoms before treatment is sought. Many patients
are for decades uneasy about going out alone, but dexterously manage
to conceal their fears until the anxiety increases rapidly in new situations,
when they seek treatment because the family cannot cope any longer.
The type of course possible between the two extremes is legion, and as
yet no prognostic or other value follows from classification on such
lines.

The following two case histories illustrate the extremes possible in
mode of onset, and incidentally of personality before the disorder
manifests.

Sudden onset of agoraphobia in a sociable person:

A girl of 19 suddenly came home from her work as shop assistant and screamed that she was going to die. She spent the next two weeks in bed and thereafter refused to walk beyond the front gate of her home. She did not improve after four months as a psychiatric inpatient and after discharge left her home only twice in the next seven years. She spent her time gossiping with neighbours, listening to the radio, and with a boy friend by whom she had a child at 27, though she continued to live with her mother. She was readmitted to psychiatric hospitals at the ages of 20, 25 and 31 for depression and increase in her phobias and anxiety. From the age of 32 until last seen at 36 she made a gradual partial improvement and was able to go on short bus rides and shopping expeditions.

As a child she had had a good relationship with her parents, but her mother had been in hospital with depression. One sister was agoraphobic. The patient had encopresis and enuresis until age 12; before her phobias started she was a good mixer, had many friends, and often went dancing. She was sexually frigid until she was 32, after which she said she achieved normal sexual satisfaction with her boy friend.

Slow onset of agoraphobia in dependent personality:

A girl of 17 gradually developed fears of leaving home; these improved at 20 when she attended a psychiatric clinic but became more marked when her son was born at 26, and she became afraid of meeting people and getting lost in a crowd. For the next two years she was limited to travelling by bike or car to her mother's home one mile away, and thereafter she could not go beyond her own home and stopped all shopping. She improved again after psychiatric admission at 29, became pregnant after discharge, and made further small gains after the birth of her second child. For the next six years until last seen she was able to do only local shopping, to fetch her child from school and to go out with her husband.

She was dominated all her life by her mother; she had enuresis and fears of the dark until 9, and was always a shy and dependent person. The marriage was unremarkable except for her sexual frigidity.

CLINICAL FEATURES

Typically the disorder starts with discrete episodes of anxiety outside the home. The patient suddenly feels ill, anxious, weak, has palpitations, lightness and dizziness in the head (as opposed to true vertigo), feels a lump in the throat and weakness in her legs, and has an illusion of walking on shifting ground; she feels as though she can't breathe although there is no dyspnoea, or she may breathe rapidly to the point of hyperventilation; she fears she may faint, or die, or scream out loud, or "lose control", or "go mad". This nameless panic can become so intense that she will be rooted to the same spot for some minutes until the intensity diminishes, after which she may just want to run to a haven of safety—a friend or her home.

"At the height of a panic I just wanted to run—anywhere. I usually made towards reliable friends ... from wherever I happened to be. I felt, however, that I must resist this running away, so I did not allow myself to reach safety unless I was in extremity. One of my devices to keep a hold on myself at this time was to avoid using my last chance, for I did not dare to think what would happen if it failed me. So I would merely go nearer my bolt-hole and imagine the friendly welcome I should get. This would often quieten the panic enough for me to start out again, or at least not to be a nuisance or use up any good will. Sometimes I was beaten and had to feel the acute shame and despair of asking for company. I felt the shame even when I hadn't to confess to my need" (Lancet, 1952).

Once the panic attack is over the patient may be reluctant to return to the scene of the attack for several months.

The seizure lasts from a few minutes to several hours. It can pass off leaving the patient feeling as fit as before, and many months may go by before another such episode occurs. This too can be followed by normal activities and a succession of such episodes may occur for years before the patient begins to restrict her activities. Such episodes will lead to consultation with a doctor, to whom the symptoms might vaguely suggest a cardiovascular or vestibular disorder, but physical examination will show no abnormality except for the signs of anxiety. At this stage before there is obvious phobic avoidance of many situations the disorder is indistinguishable from an anxiety state.

Phobic avoidance develops especially following a stuttering series of anxiety attacks. First avoidance is of situations in which the panic attack was experienced, and this gradually spreads to include novel situations for fear that they too might precipitate further panic. When a patient finds she cannot get off an express train immediately a panic starts and she restricts herself to slow trains; when these, too, become the setting for a panic attack she restricts herself to buses, then to walking, then just to walking across the street from home, until finally she becomes unable to go beyond the front gate without a companion. In rare instances the patient becomes bedridden for a while as bed is the only place where she finds the anxiety bearable. Patients who are severely restricted in their activities usually experience a chronic background of tension regardless of where they are, and acute panic attacks punctuate this backdrop.

Not uncommonly agoraphobia develops without obvious major panic attacks. In such cases the story is one of increasing avoidance of the same situations as above, but with less associated anxiety in the situations or at rest.

The course is typically punctuated by remissions and relapse of varying duration. In the earlier stages a brief episode may clear up completely after a few days or weeks, but in cases seen by psychiatrists once severe phobias have been present for a year or more, partial rather than total remissions seem to be the usual outcome without treatment until later life is reached. In the Open Door sample only 20% reported periods of complete remission after the initial onset of the phobias. Complete recovery is rarely described in autobiographical accounts of phobic states (Landis, 1964). The course after treatment is described more fully in Chapter 4.

FLUCTUATIONS WITH INTERNAL AND EXTERNAL EVENTS

It has long been recognised that agoraphobia fluctuates readily with certain changes in patients and their environment. Already Westphal had noted that the

"... agony was much increased at those hours when the particular streets dreaded were deserted and the shops closed. The subjects experienced great comfort from the companionship of men or even an inanimate object, such as a vehicle or a cane. The use of beer or wine also allowed the patient to pass through the feared locality with comparative comfort. One man even sought, without immoral motives, the companionship of a prostitute as far as his own door ... some localities are more difficult of access than others; the patient walking far in order not to traverse them ... in one instance, the open country was less feared than sparsely housed streets in town. One case also had a dislike for crossing a certain bridge. He feared he would fall into the water. In this case, there also was apprehension of impending insanity".

Westphal's observations in 3 male patients apply equally to cases seen in the last two decades. Agoraphobics generally feel easier in the presence of a trusted companion, be this human, animal or inanimate, and in such cases become dependent upon the relative, pet or object for their peace of mind. Many agoraphobics become afraid of being left alone or in any situation where they cannot reach "safety" with speed and dignity. In severer cases a patient's need for constant company places strain on relatives and friends. Exceptionally, patients find it easier to travel alone. Of the Open Door agoraphobics, 65% felt better when accompanied, while only 5% felt it was easier to go out alone. Stratagems which are useful include the grip of walking sticks, umbrellas, suitcases, shopping baskets on wheels, perambulators, folded newspapers under the arm, or a bicycle to push rather than to ride to work. Strong sucking sweets in the mouth divert a few from their fears. Deserted streets and vehicles are much preferred. Trains are easier to go on if they stop frequently at stations, and if they have a corridor and a toilet. Some journeys are easier if they pass the home of a friend or a doctor, or a police station, when the patient feels that help is at hand if they get panic stricken. In such instances if patients know the friend or doctor is not at home their journey becomes more difficult. It is the *possibility* of aid which helps them in their acute anticipatory anxiety before the journey. One patient was able to go on a particular bus route because it passed a police station outside which she would sit if the tension got too much for her. Agoraphobics usually find it easier to travel by car than any other way and may comfortably drive themselves many miles even though they cannot stay on a bus for one stop.

Agoraphobics often feel easier in the dark, and move more freely at night than in the daytime; even wearing dark glasses affords relief. 34% of Open Door agoraphobics reported their fears were better in the dark, and 23% felt their phobias were aggravated by daylight. Some agoraphobics also find their fears abate during rain or storms (26% of Open Door sample). Conversely hot weather often aggravates agoraphobia (35% of the Open Door sample).

If agoraphobics go to a cinema, theatre or church they feel less frightened in an aisle seat nearby the exit so they can make a quick dash away if seized by sudden panic. A telephone at hand to call a trusted person may afford similar relief. A ground floor flat near the main entrance to the block is preferable to one many storeys up to which access can only be had by lifts or several flights of stairs.

One popular writer conjured together many of these features in an archetypal figure called Aggie Phobie: a woman walking at night up a dark alley in the rain while wearing dark glasses, sucking sweets vigorously in her mouth, with one hand holding a dog on a leash, the other trundling a shopping basket on wheels.

Other stratagems have been noted in particular patients: Weiss (1964) described a male patient who had to remove his belt whenever he had an anxiety attack; a woman patient of his had the urge to rid herself of all clothing when she panicked, and could wear only garments which could be closed in front by zippers, and who had to carry a pair of scissors and a bottle of beer in her purse when she left home; Legrand du Saulle (1895) spoke of an army officer who felt anxious in crossing a square when he was in civilian clothes, but not at all when he wore his uniform with his sabre at his side. A man with a fear of crowds for example was able at times to face crowds when he clutched a bottle of ammonia in his hands to be used in case he felt he was about to faint (Errera and Coleman, 1963).

Minor visual features of the environment affect the intensity of agoraphobia. These features vary from one patient to another, but usually the wider and higher the space walked in, the greater the fear; if a vista can be interrupted by trees, or rain, or irregularities in a landscape, the phobia diminishes. One account claimed that ugly architecture intensified the phobias (Vincent, 1919). A patient described by Weiss (1964) felt anxious during a party on a private lawn and would have been relieved if he could have broken down the surrounding fence. A clergyman described by Westphal (1871, pp. 219–222) felt dizzy as soon as he went into the open, but obtained relief by creeping round hedges and trees or as a last resort, by putting up his umbrella.

Certain patients cannot tolerate confinement in a barber's or dentist's chair, or at the hairdresser, since the possibility of immediate escape is blocked. This can be so pronounced that cases have been labelled " the barbers' chair syndrome" (Erwin, 1963). The anxiety produced by confinement in these cases is relevant to Cook's (1939) observations that experimental neurosis in animals is produced successfully while the animal is restrained from making gross bodily movements either by mechanical devices or by previous training to be quiet.

Again because of the difficulties in making an immediate exit, some patients may be unable to take a bath in the nude. This fear is quite apart from the obsessive sexual thoughts of some people in such situations. When standing in the street or on a railway platform, the patient may feel drawn to jump beneath an approaching bus or train and therefore have to look away from the oncoming vehicle. This fear is related to the impulse normal people often have to jump when looking down from a great height, a fear which is also found in some agoraphobics, and is countered by withdrawal from the edge of such heights, or by avoiding them completely. Fears of bridges come into a similar category—long narrow bridges with open sides high above a river are especially difficult. Let there be a parapet waist high between the patient and the edge of the cliff or bridge, and the fear is diminished.

Just as anticipation of pleasure can be better than its fulfilment, so the converse applies in agoraphobia. For weeks before a planned journey a patient dies a thousand deaths from anticipatory anxiety— let the same journey be sudden and unexpected and the patient can do what she cannot if forewarned. Patients can board a bus if they don't have to wait for it at the stop, but should there be any delay, panic rapidly builds up and can prevent them from boarding the vehicle when it finally arrives. This is, of course, an exaggeration of a normal phenomenon.

When agoraphobia has been stable for some time it can be exacerbated suddenly by as many factors as those which might have precipitated the original episode. Again, remissions may coincide with similar sudden changes in the life situation. In the second case cited on p. 131 the birth of her first child coincided with an exacerbation, the birth of her second child with a minor remission.

Any stressful situation might intensify agoraphobia. *Depression*, particularly, often increases agoraphobia, and produces "decompensation" to major disability until the depression clears, after which the patient reverts to the previous level of phobic disability. A few agoraphobias start for the first time during a severe depressive illness and remain as residual symptoms when the depression lifts. Fatigue and physical illness exacerbate agoraphobia. So does confinement of the patient to bed, since this results in loss of practice at going out which makes it harder for the patient to resume her former activities when she is ambulant again.

As with any anxiety, alcohol and sedative drugs alleviate the phobias for a few hours, depending on duration of action of the drug. With the help of drugs patients can temporarily break new ground, but usually no lasting benefit accrues once the drug effect has worn off. Patients often find it helpful to carry a stock of sedatives which they take shortly before a journey or some other anticipated stress. A small minority of agoraphobics eventually get addicted to barbiturates or alcohol but most cases dispense easily with drugs or alcohol once the anxiety dissipates.

Any event which heightens motivation allows the patient to extend her activities for a while. Intense rage under certain circumstances can help a patient to go out again—this occurred in one patient who was openly enraged against a therapist she identified with her dominating husband. At other times, however, this same patient quivered with resentment she could not express against another patient in the ward—at such times she was less able to go out (Shapiro et al., 1963).

IMPACT ON THE FAMILY

Most agoraphobics live with their families. As the patient's restrictions increase her family inevitably becomes involved; she may require an escort to and from work, or give up her work; her husband and children have to do her shopping; social activities are restricted or abandoned. Sometimes a constant companion is required when the patient cannot remain alone at home without anxiety. The husband may lose time from work to remain with his wife—in such an event a doctor may be rapidly consulted. When a patient drives a car the disability may remain hidden for a long time, as even severe agoraphobics can feel safe in a car despite distress with any other mode of travel. If the patient's work can be done at home and there is help at home, again the agoraphobia can be concealed for years.

The response of patient and family to the symptoms depends largely on their personality and circumstances. In a well-adjusted and well-off patient and family, restrictions will be coped with by providing increasing help with a minimum of friction, and the patient will only accept restrictions after battling unsuccessfully to extend the range of her activities. Where a patient has few personality or economic resources and comes from a family with existing friction, the agoraphobia becomes a new source of argument and is used by each party in their own interests, as any symptom would be, and the patient may restrict herself more than the anxiety warrants.

NON-PHOBIC SYMPTOMS ASSOCIATED WITH AGORAPHOBIA

An important aspect of agoraphobia in psychiatric practice is its frequent complication by other symptoms such as general anxiety, panic attacks, depression, obsessions, depersonalisation and sexual disorders. Evidence for this comes from numerous clinical reports and from a factor analytic study by Roth et al. (1965). They studied the main clinical features of 275 cases of neurosis and isolated a distinct cluster of items which included situational phobias of agoraphobic type, panic attacks, depersonalisation and derealisation, and dizzy attacks.

The features of *general anxiety* are closely linked to those of the phobias and are partly described together with them; the term denotes free floating anxiety experienced regardless of the situation the patient is in, forming a pervasive background of tension which might be constant or fluctuate considerably for no obvious reason. Lasting general anxiety merges into the more acute, abrupt phasic disturbance of *panic attacks* which form the most distressing symptoms found with agoraphobia. Panic attacks may occur with or without the background of general anxiety; they may be few and far between, or repeated in intense staccato over a variable time. Acute panics last from a few seconds up to an hour. When these are pronounced, patients suffer considerably and urge their doctors for relief by drugs or any other means available—admission often results. Vivid portraits of panic attacks have already been given. Such panics increase the patient's phobias and can in a few minutes undo the gains patients have slowly and painfully made by repeated efforts in preceding months of rehabilitation. Panic attacks are akin to the diffuse autonomic reaction experienced by any normal person during an acute unexpected fright, but differ in that they go on longer and come repeatedly without the external stimulus apparent in normal fright; nor are internal stimuli obvious, though some writers trace the panic to unconscious feelings of diverse kinds. In a minority of panic attacks an understandable link is indeed present between a patient's personality problem and the panics; whether such problems constitute sufficient explanation is an open question, and they do not apply to most panic attacks, which come at any time of day or night, but can be precipitated by stressful tasks.

Response to medication suggests a distinction between panic attacks on the one hand, and background and phobic anxiety on the other. In agoraphobics Klein (1964) found that imipramine radically decreased panic attacks, but did not affect expectant or anticipatory anxiety. He emphasised the role of panic attacks in the origin and maintenance of agoraphobia.

General anxiety and panics in agoraphobia are no different from those in anxiety states. In agoraphobia these occur together with the typical fears of going out, travelling or remaining alone. Given the same degree of general anxiety, agoraphobics are more restricted in their activities by virtue of their phobias, and while a patient who suffers only from anxiety attacks readily resumes his normal life once the anxiety and panics cease, in an agoraphobic at this stage the phobias have acquired an impetus of their own which require further treatment. There are also agoraphobics who do not complain of much general anxiety or panics. Anxiety states and agoraphobic therefore merge in some cases so that both labels can be applied, while at the extremes of divergence only one or other label would be appropriate. The terms deserve separate recognition because we do not yet know whether the two conditions have the same aetiology, there are certain clinical differences, e.g. their sex incidence and type of restrictions, and they require rather different management outside the acute phase.

Depersonalisation: Depersonalisation and derealisation occur at times in many agoraphobics, e.g. in 37% of the series of Harper and Roth (1962). The patient feels temporarily strange, unreal, disembodied, cut off or far away from her immediate surroundings, or feels the same change has occurred in her environment. Change referred to herself is called depersonalisation, while the same change referred to the surroundings is termed derealisation. Depersonalisation and derealisation are equivalent, and the word depersonalisation will be used here to cover both phenomena. Depersonalisation is a temporary phasic phenomenon which lasts a few seconds or minutes, though rarely it lasts several hours. Its onset and termination is generally abrupt. In mild cases the symptoms may not be easy to distinguish from certain anxiety symptoms such as floating, dizziness or feeling cottonwool in the head. The onset can follow some situation of extreme anxiety, e.g. one agoraphobic woman provoked repeated arguments with her boy friend during which he threatened to leave her; each time these precipitated acute anxiety followed by severe depersonalisation. Lader (1966) described an agoraphobic patient who was severely anxious for some minutes during a continuous G.S.R. tracing and then complained of feeling strange and unreal; the G.S.R. tracing then displayed a more relaxed pattern. One might speculate that sometimes depersonalisation is a switch or cut-off mechanism which is triggered when anxiety reaches a given level. In phobic patients depersonalisation can fluctuate independently of the phobias, but together with anxiety and depression.

Roth (1959) described a phobic-anxiety-depersonalisation syndrome usually following a sudden change in the patient's life situation. 80% of his cases had phobias, and the majority closely resembled agoraphobics with fairly prominent depersonalisation. Roth also found other symptoms thought to indicate disturbance of temporal lobe function.

There is no doubt that depersonalisation does occur in temporal lobe disturbances, but it would be premature to conclude that agoraphobics with depersonalisation have temporal lobe dysfunction. It is also important to note that many agoraphobics do not experience any depersonalisation at all. As with depression, the two groups of symptoms are often found together and often are totally separate.

Depression: Psychiatrists often see repeated episodes of depression in agoraphobics. Patients complain of depressive mood, crying spells, feeling hopeless, irritability, increased anxiety and panic attacks, lack of interest in their work, difficulty in falling asleep; mild retardation and suicidal ideas may occur but severe retardation, nihilism and bizarre delusions are not a feature. At the same time as the depression the agoraphobia tends to increase—this might result in several ways: increased panic attacks sensitise the patients to formerly comfortable situations, and lack of interest lowers motivation to cope with tasks hitherto managed with difficulty. As the depression clears so the patient reverts to her previous level of phobic disability. This concurrent improvement of phobias with depression sometimes gives the impression that the chronic agoraphobia is merely a "marked" or "latent" depression. It is better formulated simply as agoraphobia which is aggravated during a depressive episode.

The frequent association of depression with agoraphobia may be spurious through self-selection, since agoraphobics without depression might simply seek less aid from psychiatrists. Suffice to say that agoraphobia and depression interact but are separate disorders which run largely distinct courses: an opinion recorded in 1621 still holds: "Some indeed are sad, and not fearful; some fearful and not sad; some neither fearful nor sad; but both . . ." (Burton, 1621).

Obsessions: The term "obsession" will be used here to refer to both obsessions and compulsions. Many obsessions are fears disproportionate to their apparent stimulus and can then strictly be called phobias, but when subjective resistance is felt to such ideas they are more accurately described as obsessions, and their clinical features usually differ from those of phobias in general.

Any obsession may be found in agoraphobics. These mostly play a small role, but at times they are as crippling as the phobias. Commonest are minor checking compulsions and rituals, or obsessive thoughts of harming others with knives, by strangling, or by other means. When they become pregnant, agoraphobic women may fear that they will eventually strangle their infants, and after delivery fear being alone with their babies. Other obsessive thoughts occur as sexual fears of exposing their bodies in public, or of soliciting men; Deutsch (1929) regarded these as important in producing agoraphobic anxiety—in fact such obsessions are often entirely absent in agoraphobics.

Related phenomena are fears of jumping from heights or in front of an oncoming train or bus—at such times patients feel drawn down against their will. These fears are more closely stimulus bound than the obsessions mentioned earlier.

In summary, as with depersonalisation and depression, obsessions of varying severity may be found in agoraphobics, but they fluctuate largely independently of the phobias. Marked obsessions, however, affect the prognosis adversely (Gelder, Marks and Wolff, 1967).

Organic Disorders: No clear organic disease has been demonstrated more in agoraphobics than in controls. Some agoraphobias start after a major organic episode, e.g. subarachnoid haemorrgage, encephalitis, brain tumour, multiple sclerosis, hypothyroidism, miscarriages or major operations. The evidence suggests, however, that these organic disorders play a role similar to that of other stressors such as bereavement, separation from home, family illness or other emotional crises—a host of traumata can trigger the onset of agoraphobia, and it remains to be demonstrated whether any organic disorder plays a special role in this condition.

Motivation: The role of 'willpower' during different phases of agoraphobia

In the active stage of their disorder, agoraphobic patients try to master their phobias by forcing themselves into the very situations they dread. These manoeuvres not only fail but may aggravate the phobia as they produce further anxiety and make the next foray in that direction more difficult. This is described by patients who are pressured to proceed beyond their limits of tolerance. Anything which heightens motivation increases patients' level of tolerance while the motivation continues. The limits of tolerance fluctuate readily in many circumstances—in an acute emergency such as a house on fire or an accident, patients can temporarily overcome their phobias and venture forth. Once the emergency subsides the phobia reappears in pristine form. A Viennese Jewess could only walk a few blocks from her home in Vienna; when the Nazis came to power she had the choice to flee or be placed in a concentration camp; she fled, and for the following two years travelled half-way around the world until arrival in the United States; after she settled in New York City she developed the same phobia of travel as she had in Vienna (Laughlin, 1956).

Similarly, enthusiastic "total push" treatment in hospital produces temporary improvement in the range of patients' activities. This improvement is short-lived as long as the patient continues to experience marked anxiety during such activities. As one patient said "I'm doing more now, but it isn't any easier to do—I feel just the same as before". She became housebound again a few weeks after discharge. Once the pressure is off, motivation drops and the patient returns to her original state.

The fluctuating nature of agoraphobia makes it difficult for family and friends to accept that it is an illness and not the result of laziness, lack of willpower, or a way of getting out of awkward situations. The logic runs: if they can master their phobias in an emergency then they simply need to exert themselves more when there is no emergency, and so the patient just needs to be forced to go out. In fact a patient cannot be expected to muster her energies so that she treats every minor shopping expedition as she would a fire in the house. Not only agoraphobics but everybody can perform unexpected feats in an acute crisis; it would be unrealistic to demand such feats constantly of everybody as a matter of routine, and in an agoraphobic who has much anxiety, any minor sally outside the house requires great effort, trivial though it would be for a normal person.

At present we have few indices to the activity of agoraphobia. As long as there is repeated acute panic, or marked depression, or a plethora of other symptoms, the patient is not likely to show sustained improvement and undue pressure on her to go out will make her worse. This phase was clearly depicted by a woman of 31:

"I could barely get myself to the office or stay in it until it was time to go. I was always exhausted, always cold; my hands were clammy with sweat; I cried weakly and easily. I was afraid to go to sleep; but I did sleep, to wake with a constricting headache, dizziness and tachycardia. To these now familiar symptoms were added waves of panic fear followed by depression. The panics almost overwhelmed me. I felt very much more frightened when I was alone and but little less frightened with other people. There were only three with whom I felt at all safe and able to relax, though even with them I was behind the screen of my fears" (Lancet, 1952, p. 74).

Unfortunately we also have few ways of telling when this phase is past and the patient is ready for successful rehabilitation. One way, of course, is to watch for enduring freedom from the symptoms of the acute stage, when the patient feels perfectly well away from the phobic situations. However this state is no guarantee that further acute panics will not develop again. Once the patient finds that the effort and anxiety diminishes steadily each time she goes out, then remission can be expected with further graduated efforts. A chance occurrence may show this. One woman had a leucotomy for severe agoraphobia; she felt more relaxed thereafter but remained housebound for a year, until one afternoon a friend who had just visited left a handkerchief behind inadvertently; the patient rushed into the street to return the handkerchief and to her surprise felt quite relaxed in the street she had previously dreaded; she proceeded systematically to do more and more, and remained relatively well when last seen four years later.

The same phenomenon is described in an autobiography by a professional writer; in her case, as in many others, no explanation is obvious for the sudden new ability to master her phobias after she had had so much unsuccessful treatment.

Her first panics started at the age of 25, and increased until she was housebound by day through "fears which continually kept me in a state of anxiety so severe as often to practically paralyse me for hours as I lay wracked and tortured on my couch . . . the core of (my phobias) was an abject fear of light . . . so overpowering that I darted out into the daylight only to be driven back as if by an unseen force into the darkened room where I could find the comparative peace and feeling of safety, although even there I had to fight off periods of intense fear" (Mrs. F. H., 1952, p. 162). Over the next 22 years her treatment included Christian Science, a stay in two sanatoria and two psychiatric clinics, 6 months psychoanalysis with Sandor Ferenczi, and further visits to another five psychiatrists. At the age of 47 she slowly began to increase her activities. "I had reached farther and farther in my wanderings . . . I decided to get on a bus . . . I boarded the dread thing . . . I realised I had to go over and over the same trail again in order to do a good job . . ." (p. 163). She managed to take up her life again without crippling fears; though she attributed her improvement to the self-analysis she attempted at this time, she commented honestly: "Shrouded in mystery (is) why and how I reached the point where my unconscious self was willing to begin to let me see underneath the surface. I had always had the world to see, but what it was that had to be added to give me the final fiat for the task of laying bare the things beneath the surface, I cannot say . . . Why I was able to look at all my fears unaided and at the particular time I did I cannot say" (Mrs. F. H. 1952, p. 176).

Once anxiety has diminished, motivation is thus of some importance in rehabilitation. One might invoke the concept of "burnt out habits" to explain the failure of efforts of willpower and retraining procedures while many acute symptoms are present, even though such methods are of some use at a later stage when symptoms other than phobias have subsided. This expresses in different words the same idea as before, that agoraphobias can pass through an acute phase of variable length when motivation and retraining have little effect on the distressing symptoms, to enter a more quiescent phase when the factors maintaining the phobias are no longer active, and they can be very gradually reduced by careful rehabilitation. What these factors are that have been "burnt out" is unknown, as are the processes which allowed these factors to subside. The concept does draw attention however to the possibility of helping some agoraphobics whose symptoms have been present for many years.

Indirect evidence for the role of motivation comes from a study of the effect of modified leucotomy in patients with severe agoraphobia (Marks et al., 1966). Leucotomy was followed by an immediate sustained drop in anxiety while phobias improved more gradually. There was greater improvement in those patients with sociable outgoing personalities than in those with shy solitary personalities, which suggested that the greater efforts of the former contributed to their more rapid rehabilitation. Further indirect evidence comes from the effects of desensitisation and psychotherapy in mixed phobic patients (Gelder Marks and Wolff, 1967). Patients with traits of depression, hopelessness and selfconsciousness had a poorer prognosis and it seemed this was because they did not fully utilise opportunities for rehabilitation. This is not surprising when we learn the great effort needed to diminish agoraphobia even in a more quiescent phase. It is best described by the same woman who portrayed her state during the acute phase years before.

"For three years I had been unable to make a train journey alone. I now felt it was essential to my self-esteem to do so successfully. I arranged the journey carefully from one place of safety to another, had all my terrors beforehand, and travelled as if under light anaesthesia. I cannot say I lost my fears as a result, but I realised I could do what I had been unable to do.

Soon after this I had to learn to drive. I passed the driving test without difficulty. . . . The vagaries of an old car ensured that the therapy was occupational. Waiting in traffic blocks brought at first a return of panics—and there was no running away . . .

Now, like others who are disabled, I have my methods. The essentials are my few safety depots—people or places. The safety radius from them grows longer and longer. I am still claustrophobic; that rules out underground trains for me, and I use the District Railway. I find it difficult to meet relations and childhood friends, and to visit places where I lived or worked when I was very ill. But I have learnt to make short visits to give me a sense of achievement and to follow them when I am ready for it by a longer visit. Both people and places are shrinking to their normal size. Depression usually returns about a week before menstruation, and I have learned to remind myself that life will look different when my period begins . . . I am also learning that it is permissible to admit to anxiety about things I have always sternly told myself are trifles to be ignored. Many of them, I find, are common fears.

If I am fearful of going anywhere strange to meet my friends I invite them home instead, or meet them at a familiar restaurant

... Strangers, too, can be more helpful than they know, and I have used them deliberately: a cheerful bus conductor, a kindly shop assistant, can help me to calm a mounting panic and bring the world into focus again. If I have something difficult to do—to make a journey alone, to sit trapped under the drier in a hairdresser's, or to make a public speech—I know I shall be depressed and acutely afraid beforehand. I avoid trying myself too high meanwhile. When the time comes I fortify myself by recalling my past victories, remind myself that I can only die once and that it probably won't be so bad as this. The actual experience now is not much worse than severe stage fright, and if someone sees me to the wings I totter on. Surprisingly, no-one seems to notice ...

I dare not accept my sickness—fear—because it never stays arrested. My very safety devices become distorted and grow into symptoms themselves. I must therefore, as I go along, break down the aids I build up; otherwise the habits of response to fear, or avoidance of occasions of fear, can be as inhibiting as the fear itself" (Lancet, 1952, pp. 81–83).

No further comment is needed on the value of motivation in agoraphobia, and the difficulty of its maintenance.

To sum up: High motivation alone ("willpower") is not enough to cure this disorder, but it is an asset to an agoraphobic, as in any disability; it is but one of many factors leading to improvement, and is of the greatest value once anxiety and other symptoms have subsided.

Note on Survey of Open Door Agoraphobics

A correspondence club for agoraphobics in Great Britain— The Open Door—afforded a unique opportunity to sample the characteristics of a nation-wide sample of sufferers from this disorder. This sample must be biased in terms of features leading people to join such clubs, but where comparisons are available with clinical populations the clinical features are very similar. It is therefore of some interest to summarise the findings in this large sample.

1,500 questionnaires were sent by post to all members of the Open Door, and 1,200 replies were received—an 80% response rate. Non-responders were similar to responders in terms of age, onset age of phobias, marital status, and percentages who were female. They differed only in that more non-responders had never sought medical aid (14% v. 5%). A psychiatric social worker interviewed 15 responders and their relatives to check the validity of questionnaire replies, and found the questionnaire reflected the responders' situation accurately. 95% of the responders were women, a bias which reflected the publicity given to the club's activities in magazines and broadcasts for women.

Mean age of the responders was 42, mean age of onset of the symptoms was 28, and mean duration of symptoms was 13 years. The patient became handicapped on average 15 months after the phobias began, and once the phobias began 80% of the patients were never again completely free of them. Most subjects rated their condition as "a nuisance, but I can cope". The time it took to seek help from each agency from the time the phobias began was 17 months to the G.P. (general practitioner), 34 months to see a psychiatrist (or be admitted) and 57 months to a "spiritual healer". On average the G.P. had last been visited 18 months earlier, and the psychiatrist 32 months earlier.

Features leading to psychiatric treatment

These were increasing severity of phobias and associated neurotic symptoms. Compared to club members who had only seen G.P.'s, those who had had psychiatric treatment had phobias which were more severe and incapacitating, and accompanied by more other neurotic symptoms. Those who had had in-patient treatment were the most severely disturbed group of all as regards severity of phobias, number of phobias and other neurotic symptoms, such as tension, depression, obsessions and exhaustion. Their fears hampered them more in their daily activities, they needed more help and most couldn't get it when necessary. Despite the greater social timidity and anxiety of the in-patients, they could nevertheless confide in other people.

The most important feature of phobics who had never had any treatment at all was their social timidity combined with difficulty in confiding both in intimates and in other people. Surprisingly, the severity of their phobias and other problems was similar to those in members who had seen G.P.'s.

Employment

Only 22% of the women were employed, a total much lower than would be expected in a normal group of women of similar age. Only 20% of the women were contented to remain as house-wives, the remainder (the majority) expressing a desire to do outside work when their phobias subsided. Those housewives who wanted to do outside work (58% of total sample) had more severe phobias and other problems than the employed or "contented housewife" group. They were also more lonely, and more afraid when left alone. Their desire to work was thus partly an expression of desire to escape their psychiatric problems. Socio-economic pressures also seemed to play a part, since those expressing a desire to go out to work were of lower income and socio-economic status than the contented housewives.

Of the women who were employed outside the home, most (68%) were hampered in their job by their fears. Although 78% of the men were employed, fully 80% felt their fears hindered them in their work.

The phobias also impaired the performance of the housewives. It hampered the housework in 40%, and 68% could not manage their shopping alone because of their fears. 31% needed daily help because of their fears, and only 20% could manage without outside help. Nevertheless, help was usually available, 50% being able to get help whenever necessary.

Section III. SPECIFIC ANIMAL PHOBIAS

These are isolated phobias of animals or insects such as birds (or feathers), cats, dogs, frogs, spiders, moths, bees and wasps—the commonest of these encountered by psychiatrists are of birds and spiders. Such phobias are only included in this category where there is clear fear and avoidance of animals in their own right rather than a fear of contamination by them—the latter fears have different clinical correlates, have more the character of obsessions, and will be dealt with separately. Specific animal phobias in adults are a distinct group from agoraphobias. They cause a more localised disturbance, are associated with but few other psychiatric symptoms, start generally in early childhood even though they may present for treatment in adult life, run a steady rather than a fluctuating course, have different psychophysiological correlates and respond quite well to desensitisation techniques. In all these respects they differ from agoraphobias, although a few cases are seen with both types of phobias and show a corresponding mixture of clinical features.

In contrast to the wealth of literature on agoraphobia, only single case reports of this phobia have appeared in the literature—Freud (1909), Sterba (1935) and Kolansky (1960) described such phobias in children while Paskind (1931), Laughlin (1956, p. 37), Wolpe (1958), Moss (1960), Freeman and Kendrick (1960), Clark (1963), Malan (1963), Wolpin and Pearsall (1965) and Friedman (1966b) described animal phobias in adults. No collection of these cases has been made, nor have their characteristics as a group been described in adults, except in a brief report by Marks and Gelder (1966). Detailed characteristics of 23 cases from the Maudsley Hospital will form the substance of this chapter.

Mild fears of spiders, mice, dogs and other animals are extremely common in our culture, but such fears are rarely strong enough to be called a phobia and bring the patient for treatment. Psychiatrists see far fewer adults with these phobias than with agoraphobia and social anxieties, which probably reflects a smaller incidence in the community. Far more animal phobias are found in young children than in adults, but most of these subside before puberty; those seen in adult life are usually the persisting remnant of these childhood phobias.

Age of onset and at treatment

The great majority started before the age of seven and very few began after puberty, though such cases do occur, for example after dog bites (Friedman, 1966b). Agoraphobias provide a striking contrast—most of these started from age 15 to 40, and social anxieties started mainly from age 15 to 30. Nevertheless, the age at which the animal phobics came for treatment was similar to the age at which other phobic patients sought psychiatric help. The salient point is that of phobias seen in adults very few animal phobias began for the first time after puberty whereas most other phobias did, even though the age at which patients requested treatment for animal phobias resembled that found for other phobias. The selective age at which animal phobias began suggests a facilitatory phase for their acquisition, and once this is safely passed the mechanism which allowed these phobias to develop is no longer active.

Of four patients in the series with bird phobias, two also had agoraphobia and two had social anxieties. Significantly, in each of these patients the bird phobias started in early childhood while their other fears began after puberty. This supports further the view that maturational factors partly determine which phobias are acquired.

Two patients who were not included in this series expressed a fear of contamination from animals and developed handwashing rituals on this basis. Their fear was better described as part of an obsessive-compulsive syndrome, and it is noteworthy that these symptoms began in adult life rather than in early childhood.

Sex incidence

The few reports in the literature all concern women, and only one man was noted in a series of twenty-three patients from the Maudsley Hospital. This preponderance of women is even greater than in agoraphobia. Before puberty, however, animal phobias are commonly found both in boys and girls, though by age 10–11 they are already much rarer in boys (Rutter et al., 1968).

Reasons for seeking treatment

When such fears are found in adults they have generally been continuously present for decades since childhood. Why then do some patients only seek treatment as adults? Though such phobias tend to persist unchanged after puberty, there are various factors which affect the amount of disability which results.

A city dweller can cope easily by avoiding most animals and insects. Increased disability will occur if the patient moves to a new environment in which such animals are present. One woman managed well in a town flat, became anxious and sought treatment after she moved to a country cottage infested with spiders, but felt better again on moving to a house which was free of spiders. Another woman began treatment when she could not take up a residential art scholarship in an old spider-infested hostel and her career became jeopardised. A young woman moved from a town with a few pigeons to another city where they were ubiquitous—she had to ask for treatment when she became unable to walk to work through streets which contained pigeons.

Other patients came on hearing for the first time that treatment could be offered. Yet others came for fear of passing on their own phobia to their young children. Some patients saw a doctor originally for different psychiatric symptoms such as depression, and their doctor then spotted the phobia and suggested that it be treated. During depression pre-existing symptoms are often magnified and cause the patient to seek help with a minor disability they could tolerate easily before. Finally, certain patients ask for treatment of a simple phobia with the silent hope that other problems they find hard to talk about will also be dealt with. Patients who are leading lonely lives are probably more likely to come with a minor complaint, and social contact with a hospital can provide as much satisfaction in an empty life as relief of a mild isolated symptom. Mechanic (1962) has shown that given the same disability patients who are lonely seek medical aid significantly more than do other patients.

Mode of onset

In adults the origins of such phobias are usually lost in the mist of early childhood memories, but a few can be dated to specific incidents. A cat phobia began when one little girl watched her father drown some kittens, dog phobias began after dog bites, a bird phobia began after a child posing for a photograph in Trafalgar Square took fright as a bird alighted on her shoulder and she couldn't move—the resultant photograph preserved the record of the origin of her phobias; another feather phobia began when an infant strapped in a pram took fright when a strange woman with a large feather in her hat bent down to look at the baby.

For the rest we know little more about the onset than Freud wrote in 1913: " The child suddenly begins to fear a certain animal species and to protect itself against seeing or touching any individual of this species. There results the clinical picture of an animal phobia, which is one of the most frequent among the psychoneurotic diseases of this age and perhaps the earliest form of such an ailment. The phobia is as a rule expressed towards animals for which the child has until then shown the liveliest interest, and has nothing to do with the individual animal. In cities, the choice of animals which can become the object of phobia is not great. They are horses, dogs, cats, more seldom birds, and strikingly often very small animals like bugs and butterflies. Sometimes animals which are known to the child only from picture books and fairy stories become objects of the senseless and inordinate anxiety which is manifest in these phobias. It is seldom possible to learn the manner in which such an unusual choice of anxiety has been brought about".

In children such fears remit rapidly without any apparent reason or because the patient has been exposed to gradual relearning situations. Equally they can be stamped in when other children tease the child repeatedly with the feared object. We do not know why a small fraction continues after puberty.

Family, personalities and background

The following details are reported from the Maudsley series of patients, since no other collection of animal phobias has appeared in the literature.

Patients with animal phobias tend to come from stable families. 85% had formally intact homes before the age of twelve, and they had no special birth order in their sibships. Most of the homes were reasonably happy; 15% reported a dominant or overprotective mother, and 20 % described frequent parental quarrels. It is noteworthy that only 15% had first degree relatives with the same phobia as the patient; 10% had parents with psychoses, and 20% thought their mothers were "nervous".

Half the cases were fearful as children, manifested as excessive crying, shyness and fears of various kinds. Enuresis had occurred in 10%. Half the cases had a history of a normal childhood personality. Their schooling was unremarkable, and afterwards their occupations ranged over most social grades.

Only 20% of the patients were never married, 15% were divorced or separated, and 40% had fairly happy marriages. Sexually 30% were satisfactorily adjusted, 20% had always been frigid and 20% became frigid after initial responsiveness. Over half the patients had children, and 90% of patients were living with their family. The personalities of patients were described as anxious, dependent or shy in 35%, and as sociable in 35%. Only a small minority had had previous psychiatric treatment for their phobias before coming; 22% had had outpatient and 6% inpatient treatment for depression, frigidity, aggressive outbursts or phobias, and psychogenic blepharospasm. One patient had had hysterical paraplegia in her youth without psychiatric treatment.

Without adequate controls any small differences of this population from normals will have been missed. Failing such a study, it is fair to say *in summary* that the families of these patients were stable and fairly happy without many phobias. The childhood work and marital records were unremarkable, and there was wide variation in personality and sexual adjustment. The backgrounds of animal phobias thus resemble those of agoraphobics, and do not depart grossly from accepted norms in most aspects.

Clinical picture

The patient complains of long-standing phobia of an animal or insect and appears to be free of other symptoms. Practically any animal or insect may be involved. Of the Maudsley series ten phobias were of birds and feathers—in every instance pigeons were amongst the most feared birds, whilst the smaller budgies and canaries could be tolerated more readily. Six phobias were of spiders, two of dogs, and one each of cats, worms and frogs. Patients with fears of one kind of animal did not usually have fears of other species. Seven patients had additional minor fears—two of these patients had social fears sufficiently intense to prevent them from eating in restaurants and two had agoraphobia.

Other symptoms were present in a minority; three patients had had recent depressive episodes severe enough to require psychiatric help, and two had abnormal personalities.

The degree of distress caused by the phobia will depend upon the intensity of the fear and the prevalence of the animal involved. In milder cases the phobia is a nuisance rather than a psychiatric disability, e.g. a woman living in the country could not go near ponds where frogs abounded nor look at pictures of frogs in books. In intense phobias of ubiquitous animals the distress can be great and sustained, as in a woman with a fear of birds who could not go to work through the streets of London since they abounded in pigeons, and she had to give up her job and remain indoors all day, only venturing out at night when pigeons no longer flew about.

It is surprising how seldom these fears are found in other members of the patient's family, because one might expect these fears to be modelled after the behaviour of close relatives. In fact in the Maudsley series this was only true of three patients—one each had a father, mother or sister with the same fear. One of these three patients transmitted the fear to her daughter, which then reinforced her own fear and they both came for treatment. Patients do sometimes ask for help lest they pass on the phobia to their young children.

Though a localised phobia might seem a trivial problem, striking distress does result from contact with the phobic object. A woman with a fear of spiders screamed when she found a spider at home, ran away to find a neighbour to remove it, trembled in fear and had to keep the neighbour at her side for two hours before she could remain alone at home again; another patient with a spider phobia found herself on top of the 'fridge in the kitchen with no recollection of getting there—the fear engendered by sight of a spider had induced a brief period of dissociation. If in treatment sessions patients are brought too close to the animal, an acute panic ensues immediately in which they sweat and tremble and show all the features of terror which will wake them even from a deep hypnotic trance. This fear subsides when the object is removed.

Recurrent nightmares of animals plague a few patients—they dream they are surrounded by large spiders or swooping birds from which they cannot escape. As treatment is followed by improvement these nightmares disappear.

Patients search for the feared object wherever they go. The slightest evidence of its presence will disturb them where any normal person may never have noticed it. One sign of improvement during treatment is diminished awareness of these animals in the environment.

Patients with simple phobias of animals can of course have other problems which complicate the phobia for which they first sought treatment. This is true of any condition.

Dog phobia with depression of independent cause

A married woman of 24 complained of a dog phobia. This began at the age of 18 months when she was bitten and dragged from the room by an Alsatian dog, since when she always ran away from dogs. If there was a loose dog in the street she had to cross the road to go the other way, and this would make her late for appointments. She could not go alone for walks for fear of meeting dogs. She came for treatment of the phobia as she was afraid of passing it on to her young infant. She felt herself neglected by her husband and at time of referral was in the middle of an affair with a younger man. Shortly after she began treatment by desensitisation her lover broke off the affair. The patient became severely depressed, made a suicidal gesture, and eventually was referred for group psychotherapy. The dog phobia continued through these events.

Section IV. SOCIAL PHOBIAS

Minor degrees of social anxiety are, of course, perfectly normal and compatible with excellent function. This has been recognised since ancient times, for Burton (1621, p. 143) described fear which

"amazeth many men that are to speak, or show themselves in publick assemblies, or before some great personages, as Tully confessed of himself, that he trembled still at the beginning of his speech; and Demosthenes that great orator of Greece, before Phillipus .. .."

Prominent public figures commonly experience qualms before major public appearances, even if these occur daily. Indeed, some anxiety is often regarded as better than none at all since mild anxiety is alerting and facilitates function.

Only when social anxiety becomes excessive does it begin to disrupt activity, as in a case of Hippocrates' described by Burton (1621, p. 272) who:—

"through bashfulness, suspicion, and timorousness, will not be seen abroad; loves darkness as life, and cannot endure the light, or to sit in lightsome places; his hat still in his eyes, he will neither see, nor be seen by his good will. He dare not come in company, for fear he should be misused, disgraced, overshoot himself in gesture or speeches, or be sick; he thinks every man observes him . . ."

Many patients complain of phobias in a variety of social situations, the fears being of the people themselves or what they might think, rather than of a crowd "en masse" in which the constituent individuals seem anonymous. Agoraphobics commonly have some fear of crowds, but usually express this as a fear of being crushed or enclosed or suffocated by the crowd, rather than a fear of being seen or watched by people in the crowd. In contrast, social phobics are very conscious of being observed, and are able to engage in certain activities only as long as nobody's eyes are on them. A glance from another person will precipitate the phobia concerned.

Clinical features

Though social phobias are not uncommon and make up about 8% of all phobics at the Maudlsey Hospital, only Kraupl Taylor (1966) has described their clinical features in any detail. Most of the following description is based upon analysis of 23 cases seen at the Maudsley Hospital.

Patients with social phobias may be afraid of eating and drinking in front of other people; the fear may be that their hands will tremble as they hold their fork or cup, or they may feel nauseous or have a lump in their throat and may be unable to swallow so long as they are watched. One patient noted "when I go out to eat in strange places I cannot eat, my throat feels a quarter of an inch wide, and I sweat". The fear is usually worst in smart crowded restaurants, and least in the safety of the home, but a few patients even find it impossible to eat in the presence of their spouse alone. Such patients become unable to go out to dinner, or to invite friends home because they are afraid that their hands will tremble when drinking tea or handing a cup to a friend. Social life then becomes very restricted.

For fear of shaking, blushing, sweating or looking ridiculous patients will not sit facing another passenger in a bus or train, nor walk past a queue of people. They are terrified of attracting attention by behaving awkwardly or fainting. Some may only leave their house when it is so dark or foggy that they cannot easily be seen. They will avoid talking to superiors, and stage fright will prevent them from appearing in front of an audience. They may cease swimming as it involves exposing their bodies to the gaze of strangers. They will avoid parties and be too embarrassed to talk to people. "I can't have normal conversation with people. I break out in a sweat, that is my whole problem even with the missus" said a man who was nevertheless performing normally sexually with his wife. In some patients the fear appears only in the presence of members of the opposite sex.

Patients of this kind are often afraid to write in public, will not visit a bank or shop because they are terrified their hand will tremble when writing a cheque or handling money in front of someone else. For fear of shaking a secretary may become unable to take shorthand dictation or to type, a teacher may stop writing on a blackboard in front of a class and cease reading dictation, a seamstress will stop sewing in the factory, an assembly line worker will find it impossible to perform the manouvres necessary for assembling a package. Harmless activities like knitting or buttoning a coat can induce agonizing panic when done in front of other people.

Nearly always the fear is that their hands or heads *might* shake, yet it is rare for such patients to actually tremble or shake so that their writing becomes a scrawl, their teacup rattles against the saucer, soup is spilled when they raise the soup spoon to their lips or their head nods visibly when talking. This is in striking contrast to patients with organic tremors such as those due to Parkinsonism, who shake vigorously but unself-consciously, and have no fear of doing anything in public despite their disability.

Some patients have a fear that they might vomit in public, or that they may see other people vomiting. Normally this should not cause much incapacity but such patients also avoid any situation remotely likely to provoke vomiting in themselves or in others, e.g. travelling on a bumpy bus or coach, going on a boat, or the eating of onions.

In general social phobias occur without many other symptoms, and the following case history is fairly typical:

Social phobia as an isolated complaint

The patient was a 34 year old unmarried secretary with a fear of vomiting of 13 years duration. As a child her mother had not been able to help the children when they vomited and instead would ask the father to help. Although the patient remembered being concerned at other children vomiting when she was 5 years old, she did not develop the phobia until the age of 21, at which time she became afraid that other people or she herself would vomit on the train and she began avoiding various travelling situations. This fear became fluctuatingly worse in the last five years. The patient had woken at 5.15 a.m. daily in order to travel to her office in the City before the rush hour. She could, under duress, return during rush hours. In the previous two years she had drunk a bottle of brandy a week to calm her fear of travelling, in addition to the chlordiazepoxide which she took intermittently. She feared she was becoming increasingly dependent on the brandy. In the last 5 years she had avoided eating in public places, in restaurants, or in strangers' homes. She also avoided going to theatres with friends if she could help it because it was easier to leave the theatre if she was alone in the event of a fear of vomiting developing. In fact the patient had never vomited in public and had not seen anybody else vomit for many years.

Away from the phobic situation the patient had no anxiety and was not depressed. Her work was satisfactory. She had had practically no sexual experience.

The patient had four years group psychotherapy with the result that she felt more comfortable in the company of men and got on better with people generally, but her phobia remained unchanged during this period. Later, after 12 sessions of densitisation the patient became able to eat out in restaurants both by herself and in company without undue anxiety. She became able to travel in crowded tube trains and to enjoy social situations in general with less difficulty than formerly.

A smaller number of patients may have not only social phobias but also generalised anxiety and depression. Cases of this kind are similar to those with more severe forms of the agoraphobic syndrome, and could justifiably be included under the common rubric of "phobic anxiety state", as the following case illustrates:

Social phobia with diffuse anxiety

The patient was a 20 year old unmarried typist with social phobias of 3 years' duration which caused her to restrict her social activities. In the previous year she had not been out alone except to travel to work and since she stopped working 2 months previously she had not been out anywhere alone. She had to come to the hospital with her mother. Her fears were of people looking at her, of herself shaking while drinking in public, of walking out in public or of any social situation. In addition to the social fears, even when the patient was resting at home she was continually on edge, shaky and restless and occasionally had panic attacks superimposed on this background anxiety unrelated to any external stimuli. She was only free of tension when she had alcohol or sedative drugs. In addition the patient had been intermittently depressed and wanting to cry over the previous two years. This had been rather worse in the previous week.

Patients with the more diffuse varieties of social phobia and agoraphobia bear some resemblance to patients included in the Japanese syndrome of "*shinkeishitsu*". This term includes "much of what is covered under the several Western headings of neurasthenia, anxiety reactions and obsessive-compulsive reactions" (Caudill and Doi, 1963). The chief features of this syndrome are tense interpersonal relations, anthropophobia, fears of blushing and fears of light and sound (Caudill and Schooler, 1969). The word anthropophobia includes fears of blushing, a morbid fear of one's eyes meeting those of others and of one's facial expression giving displeasure to other people, inability to find topics of conversation and awkwardness when appearing before others, uneasiness when people are nearby, and reluctance to meet others because of the belief that one's own looks are ugly (Kora, 1964). An example of this condition was cited by Kora (1964). The patient was a 33-year-old man with the history since 26 of anthropophobia, insomnia, headache and the feeling that faeces remained even after evacuation. He felt it very painful to interview people and would often droop his head in the middle of the conversation, being unable to look the other party straight in his eyes any longer. As his condition worsened, he felt it painful even to talk to his children and the home became a dismal place to live in. Although he kept up going to work, the life at the office was extremely unpleasant. Since it became almost impossible to go out of the house except for going to work, he came to Tokyo for treatment.

Psychiatric symptoms additional to social phobias

Nearly half the Maudsley series of social phobics had some history of depression, and in 3 patients this was moderate or severe, requiring admission in 2 patients. Some general anxiety at rest was present in 22%, being moderately severe in 13%. Alcohol dependence or addiction was noted in 18% of the patients. Phobias additional to social anxieties were present in 2 patients (9%). This group of patients thus had not infrequent psychiatric problems accompanying the social phobias, so resembling less severe forms of the agoraphobic syndrome.

Age of onset and age at treatment

This was described by Marks and Gelder (1966), and was illustrated in fig. 3.1. Social anxieties started mostly after puberty between the ages of 15 and 30, with a mean onset age of 19 years. This onset age is not dissimilar from that for agoraphobia except that very few social anxieties start after the age of 30. Social phobias are rare before puberty, and no cases were found in a large survey of children aged 10 and 11 (Rutter et al., 1968). Mean age at treatment was 27 years in the series of Marks and Gelder (1966).

Sex incidence

Of the 25 patients of Marks and Gelder (1966), 60% were women. The female preponderance was smaller than in agoraphobia or animal phobias, and social phobias are among the commonest phobias to be found amongst men. No explanation for this is obvious.

Reasons for seeking treatment

Usually this was because of the social discomfort itself, but a minority of patients presented with complicating symptoms such as depression or increasing alcohol consumption to control their anxiety.

Mode of onset

Most social phobias developed slowly over a number of months or years, with no clear history of any precipitating cause. A small number began suddenly after trigger incidents, e.g. a young man at a dance felt sick at the bar and vomited before reaching the toilet, making an embarrassing mess. Thereafter he became afraid of going to dances, bars or parties.

Usually when the initial episode was described there was no clear cause for the embarrassment, though emotional situations might sensitise the patient. For example, fears of shaking in public began for the first time in a young woman at her wedding service while she was walking up the church aisle with her father, wondering if her future husband was really good enough for her. The fears became aggravated shortly afterwards when her husband was in hospital with tetanus, and she went to a restaurant to eat after visiting him.

In a few patients there was no sharply defined onset but instead there was a history of social sensitivity since early childhood which gradually increased after puberty.

Families, personality and background

Only 9% of cases had a first degree relative with the same phobia as themselves, and none had relatives with a different phobia. None had close relatives who had psychiatric treatment.

34% came from broken homes, a disproportionately large figure, though probably not significantly so. There was no particular pattern of parental upbringing. 18% of parents were reported to be strict and 9% to be indulgent, and the rest were not distinguished by any special feature.

Half the patients were fearful, timid or over-shy during their childhood. After puberty 45% of patients were relative social isolates, while 26% were sociable personalities. Education and subsequent working careers were unremarkable.

Half the patients were not married, but mean age was only 26. Only 1 was divorced, and most of the marriages seemed reasonably happy. Sexuality was normal in most of the men but in only 23% of the women, and 38% of the women were frigid. Only a quarter of the patients had children. Most patients were living with their immediate families.

Only one of the patients had had previous psychiatric treatment before coming for their phobias.

In summary, the background and personalities of social phobias are rather like those of agoraphobics and animal phobics, except that a larger proportion are men, and rather more came from formally broken homes. Very few of the close relatives had phobias.

Section V. MISCELLANEOUS OTHER PHOBIAS

The commonest phobias in clinical practice are those of the agoraphobic cluster (going out alone, shopping, crowds, travel) and social fears (eating, drinking, writing, shaking, blushing, sweating and vomiting in public). Next in frequency are probably the phobias of animals and insects, but these are quite rare. Phobias of other situations are also rare, and generally are monosymptomatic. They can begin at any age, occur in both sexes, and once they have persisted for a year tend to continue unchanged. The physiological characteristics of such cases are unknown.

There is little point in detailing the endless list which has been reported in the literature. Practically any situation can be involved. A few situations are worth particular note.

Phobias of natural phenomena are seen from time to time. A mild fear of *heights* is not uncommon in many people, but severe incapacitating phobias of heights are rare. Patients with phobias of heights emphasise that their visual space is important. They will not be able to go down a flight of stairs if they can perceive the open stairwell. They will be frightened looking out of a high window which stretches from floor to ceiling but not if the window is obscured to waist level or higher. They have difficulty crossing bridges on foot because of proximity of the edge, but may be able to do so in a car. Sometimes this fear is linked to an acute *fear of falling*, if there is no support within a few feet of the patient, and he may be afraid of being drawn over the edge of a height. This is slightly different from a similar fear expressed by many anxious agoraphobics. In the latter the fear of falling is but one of many phobias and appears to be secondary to acute anxiety. In a more primary fear of falling there is no anxiety if the patient is at rest, and only loss of visual support will induce the fear as in the following example:

Fear of falling in absence of support

The patient was a 49-year-old housewife who as a child had been afraid of the dark. At the age of 48 while running for a bus she suddenly felt dizzy and had to hold on to a lamppost for support. This recurred and gradually the patient became unable to walk anywhere without holding on to a wall or furniture to support her —she was "furniture bound". Removal of visual support more than a foot away from her induced terror and crying. Actual physical contact with the supporting object was not essential. The patient was perfectly calm when sitting or lying down. There was no sign of vestibular disturbance.

Patients with fears of heights and falling can be very resistant to treatment. This may be because their phobia is an intensification of a normal physiological mechanism present in most people which makes them uncomfortable on perceiving a sharply receding visual edge.

Phobias of *darkness* are perfectly normal in childhood but are rarely incapacitating in adults. The same applies to phobias of *thunderstorms and lightning*. Patients with this phobia may show generalisation of the fear to include listening to weather forecasts, and may become unable to venture out of doors when thunder is forecast in a few hours time. They may dread the approach of summer and long for the winter when thunderstorms rarely occur. Yet other patients have a phobia of any *wind or storms.*

Apart from fearing natural phenomena, patients may have a phobia of loud noises, of driving a car, e.g. after a car accident, or of other forms of travel. Much the commonest phobia of *travel* is part of the agoraphobic syndrome, but occasionally a monosymptomatic fear of travelling does occur especially in men. Many people avoid travelling by aeroplanes or by tube, but otherwise lead normal unrestricted lives. Other phobias complained of sometimes are of *dental treatment,* or of *injections.* In such patients severe dental caries may develop over the years due to their inability to go to a dentist, and appropriate medical treatment for other conditions may be delayed for fear of going to doctors.

Rarely patients may have a phobia of swallowing solid food which will force them to resort to a liquid diet. This can be understood as an intensification of the common symptom of anxiety known as "globus hystericus" where patients have a lump in their throat and find it difficult to swallow during intense anxiety. Fears of fainting, of collapse, of having a fit, of dying or going insane are generally not seen in isolation but are part of the clusters of symptoms found in anxiety states or the agoraphobic syndrome.

Other phobias seen by the author or reported in the literature are of being in the vicinity of anybody who smoked, of going through a door if voices could be heard on the other side, of running water or of being grasped from behind (Bagby, 1922), of reading books or even letters (Timpano, 1904), of dolls (Rangell, 1952) and of outer space or cosmic disaster (Kerry, 1960, Ashem, 1963).

Another rare phobia is that of *texture.* A prominent man had an intense dislike of fuzzy textures such as those of the skin of peaches, on new tennis balls, or on certain carpets, and could not enter a room containing a carpet with that particular texture. When playing tennis he would have to wear a glove to handle the ball until the fuzz wore off.

Sexual phobias

Many men who are sexually impotent are found on examination to be anxious in the presence of women, especially in a potentially sexual situation. Fear is not generally present in other situations, and the patient is usually normal apart from his sexual anxiety. Treatment of sexual anxiety by methods usually applied to other phobias, e.g. by desensitisation, has been reported to be successful (e.g., Wolpe, 1958), though controlled trials of treatment of series of patients with impotence have not yet been published.

Section VI. ILLNESS PHOBIAS

Fears of illness flit through the minds of most people at one time or another. Who has not looked at a spot on his hand and wondered whether it was not a form of cancer or other dread disease? Medical students habitually think they harbour the disorders they happen to be studying at the time, and experience a succession of illness fears as they progress through their medical curriculum. These, however, are transient phenomena which cause no handicap and require no treatment.

In some people fears of illness are so insistent that they may lead the person to seek medical advice, commonly not from the psychiatrist but from the general physician. A substantial proportion of out-patients in a general hospital require reassurance that they have not got a serious complaint they've been worrying about. Where the fears are about multiple bodily symptoms and a variety of illnesses the patient is said to have hypochondriasis. When the fear is persistently localised round a single symptom or illness in the absence of another psychiatric disorder one can talk of an illness phobia, or nosophobia, to use Ryle's term (1948).

Hypochondriasis itself is a feature of many different conditions. It can be a lasting personality trait, a response to anxiety and stress or part of a depressive or schizophrenic illness. Hypochondriasis was well recognised by the 17th century. Burton (1621, p. 272) wrote of

"... some are afraid that they shall have every fearful disease they see others have, hear of, or read, and dare not therefore hear or read of any such subject, not of melancholy itself, lest, by applying it to themselves that which they hear or read, they should aggravate and increase it".

A vast literature exists now on this subject, much of which has been reviewed by Ladee (1966). The current consensus is that hypochondriasis is not a clinical entity on its own but usually reflects some other disturbance in the patient.

It is not at all clear how nosophobias relate to more general forms of hypochondriasis, and whether they aren't simply a special form of it. Systematic study of nosophobias has rarely been attempted, and the definitive status of illness phobias awaits further clinical and psychophysiological study. It is undoubtedly true that numerous patients present with a single fear of disease which is part of a depressive illness, and that these fears wax and wane with the depression and should be regarded simply as a depressive concomitant. Yet others may be part of an abnormal personality, obsessive neurosis or other psychiatric disorder. It is not known how small the residue is of patients who have illness phobias as the main complaint without other complicating factors. Ryle (1948) also noted that fears of dying should be clearly distinguished from the alarming sense of dying which accompanies certain organic conditions like the constricting chest pain of angina pectoris, labyrinthine vertigo, anaphylactic shock, too large a dose of adrenaline, and vasovagal attacks. This sensation of dying is very distressing while it lasts, but once it has passed off the patient is not usually left with a persistent fear of death.

The incidence of prominent phobias of illness was 15% in the author's Maudsley material, but these patients were not studied in detail. Phobias of death, illness and injury formed 34% of a series of 50 phobic patients of Agras et al. (1969). In one survey of 155 healthy university students accorded the chance of a free health examination 10 had fears of disease (Ryle, 1948) but these were not severe enough to lead to psychiatric treatment.

To a certain extent illness phobias will reflect worries about disease which are fashionable either in the culture at large or in the family sub-culture. For example, Pope (1911) noted how a campaign to educate the public about tuberculosis caused many patients to present with fears of that disease. Nowadays tuberculosis is an unfashionable disease to fear, while cancer and heart disease are much commoner worries.

The causes of illness phobias are probably multiple and have been described by Straker (1951) and Ryle (1948). The previous health history may have sensitised the patient to a particular body system, e.g. a history of rheumatic heart disease makes the heart vulnerable psychologically as well as organically. The patient may identify with a parent or sibling who has a particular disease. Specific traumatic events during maturation may have significance for certain bodily symptoms. Fear of given illnesses may reflect relevant psychological problems e.g. fears of syphilis may occur in a person who is guilty about sexual adventures. All these factors may be potentiated by an upbringing in surroundings where undue attention was paid to physical disease, and when public propaganda is being disseminated about a given disorder. A patient may mistakenly misinterpret the silence of a taciturn doctor as an ominous sign that frightening information is being concealed from him.

The clinical picture in illness phobias is of a patient who is perfectly healthy but worries excessively that he might have one or other disease. The fear is constant and distracts the patient from his everyday activities, more than might be the case if he actually had the disease he feared. In Sir Philip Sidney's words ". . . fear is more pain than is the pain it fears". The patient will constantly search his body for evidence of disease. No skin lesion or bodily sensation can be too trivial for the keen senses of a phobic patient. He will misinterpret genuine physio-logical sensations. His anxiety itself may produce fresh symptoms such as abdominal pain and discomfort due to pylorospasm, and this will reinforce his gloomy prognostications.

Although in some cases a physical disorder does trigger the illness phobia, usually there is no history of physical disturbance to explain it. Indeed, cases are recorded where development of the feared disease in fact led to resolution of the fear. Rogerson (1951) cited the case of a man who was almost beside himself with venereophobia and soon required admission to a mental hospital. After discharge he contracted a primary syphilis with a typical chancre quite large enough to see himself. From that moment his mental symptoms disappeared and the patient happily attended for regular antisyphilitic treatment.

Illness phobias are fears of a situation from which the patient cannot escape as the problem feared is internal to him. For this reason the pattern of avoidance of situations which is so characteristic of phobias of external stimuli is not a feature of illness phobias.

Very few series of patients with fear of a given disease are described in the literature. Ryle (1948) described 31 cases of cancer phobia, 21 of whom were women. Mean age was 50, with a range of 33 to 75. There was a high incidence of other psychiatric problems; 13 patients were "nervous or had a breakdown previously". The physical symptoms were those usually associated with anxiety—e.g., colonic spasm, flatulence, globus hystericus. Twelve of the patients had lost a near relative or acquaintance from cancer or had intimate knowledge of such a case.

MacAlpine (1957) outlined a series of 24 patients with syphilophobia seen in a dermatology department of a general hospital and in a mental hospital. All except one patient were male, and MacAlpine noted a similar male preponderance was found in another series of syphilo-phobics described by Schuermann. Mean age at treatment was 38 with an age range from 17 to 55. There was thus no direct relation between syphilis and syphilophobia, as the highest incidence of syphilis is in the third decade. There was a high proportion of batchelors—only 11 of the 23 men were married.

A large proportion also had a history of previous psychiatric break-down—10 had been psychiatric in-patients before, while 4 were "so severely disturbed . . . as potentially to require admission to mental hospitals".

Thirteen of the patients were only seen once. All the 10 patients who were seen repeatedly showed some improvement after 3 to 6 interviews.

All the patients had had repeated investigations for syphilis, and on average had had 6 negative Wasserman reactions without being re-assured. One patient had had no less than 22 negative Wasserman reactions over the previous year. Most patients had a lengthy history of their fear. All patients gave a history of "exposure", but on close questioning more than half of them revealed this to be misconceived or even delusional, e.g. patients recounted exposure in terms of "strange looks, drinking or eating from utensils that may previously have been used by a syphilitic, the inevitable lavatory seat, and sleeping in strange beds". Four patients who gave lurid accounts of sexual experience were later found to have been impotent at the relevant times. In these patients ideas of exposure derived from their conviction that they had syphilis.

MacAlpine regarded syphiliphobia as analogous to two complaints in which women predominate—the delusion of parasitosis and the delusion of growing or losing hair. The excess of men with syphili-phobia might be due to cultural and anatomical factors. Men are more promiscuous, know more about venereal disease, and can freely observe their genitals for minute changes.

Section VII. OBSESSIVE PHOBIAS

In the course of obsessive-compulsive neurosis the appearance of certain fears is not uncommon. Obsessive phobias usually have a compelling quality which is absent in other phobias. The ideas intrude into the patients' consciousness despite all attempts to banish them from his mind. When present, obsessive phobias are usually of contamination or of harming other persons or oneself. Some writers also include illness phobias under the rubric of obsessive-compulsive disorders, though in the author's view these are best kept separate for the present as they are not so constantly accompanied by other features of obsessive-compulsive disorder.

Obsessive fears of contamination are generally found together with compulsive washing and rituals of avoidance. For example, patients may feel contaminated each time they micturate or defaecate, or after being near dogs, and may have to bath and wash for hours after every such occasion. One woman felt that her son was contaminated and developed complicated rituals of washing his clothes, his room and everything connected with him. Another patient felt that dogs are dirty and spent much of his life avoiding any possibility of contact with dogs, dog's hair, or even buildings where dogs may have been, giving up his job if he heard that a dog may have been on another floor of his office building. Intense washing of his hands and clothes would follow the remotest possibility that he might have been "contaminated". Strikingly, he was as afraid of the hair plucked from a dog as of the dog itself. This illustrates the hallmark of an obsessive phobia, that it is *not a direct fear of a given object or situation, but rather of imagined consequences arising therefrom.* This patient would rather touch a dog with his hands than let it touch his clothes, because hands were easier to wash than clothes. Similarly, a woman obsessed with the idea of possible injury from glass splinters was more afraid about fragments she suspected but could not find at home than of the glass splinters she actually found and removed with her bare hands.

Obsessive phobias of harming persons include fears of killing, stabbing, strangling, beating or maiming, and may lead to avoidance of potential weapons and to complicated protective rituals. A housewife may have to hide sharp knives in her kitchen far out of reach to remove temptation, mothers may need to have constant company for fear they will strangle their babies if left alone, and so on.

Sometimes patients are afraid of swallowing pins, broken glass or other sharp objects, and go to ridiculous extremes to guard against the remotest possibility of this occurrence.

The risk of translating obsessive ideas into terrible actions is in fact very small. It is rare for obsessive-compulsive patients to actually perform the murders, stabbings and stranglings which they dread.

Obsessive phobias tend to have distinctive features. First they are usually part of a wide variety of fears of *potential* situations rather than the objects or situations themselves, and because of the vagueness of these possibilities the ripples of avoidance and protective rituals spread far and wide to involve the patient's life style and people around him. Next, clinical examination usually discloses obsessive rituals not directly connected with the professed fear, and it is clear that the obsessive fear is part of a wider obesssive-compulsive disorder. Furthermore, the emotion is commonly less one of fear than one of disgust. Finally, obsessive phobias are much more resistant to treatments which make an impact on fears of external situations. Desensitisation is very slow in reducing anxiety, the effect is highly specific and the generalisation gradient is steep, so that hardly any improvement generalises to untreated situations. The patient often resists progress at every step. Moreover, removal of anxiety to a situation does not necessarily lead to avoidance of that situation, as is exemplified by the following patient and fig. 3.2.

The patient had obsessive fears of contamination by dogs and was already referred to earlier in this section. At the time the recording shown in fig. 3.2 was obtained he had had 39 sessions of systematic desensitisation to dogs hairs on his arms, and claimed that now he felt completely calm in that situation. Measures of skin conductance confirmed his subjective report that anxiety was absent during the fantasy of the desensitised obsession but present with the others. Fluctuations in skin conductance were normal during the treated fantasy (fig. 3.2B) but increased during fantasies of the untreated obsessions (fig. 3.2 A and C). This demonstrated the specificity of the change. In addition, the patient continued his compulsive handwashing to this situation despite the absence of anxiety i.e., the compulsions were not maintained simply by the anxiety alone. In contrast, with phobias of external situations, treatment of the anxiety is the essence of successful treatment, despite the fact that phobic avoidance does not correlate perfectly with subjective anxiety. In obsessive fears treatment of the associated anxiety achieves less than in phobias of external situations. Correspondingly, administration of sedative drugs reduces obsessive rituals far less than it does avoidance in conventional phobias.

Further description of obsessive-compulsive states is outside the scope of this book and has often been detailed elsewhere (see Lewis, 1938; Pollitt, 1960; Ingram, 1961; Marks, 1965).

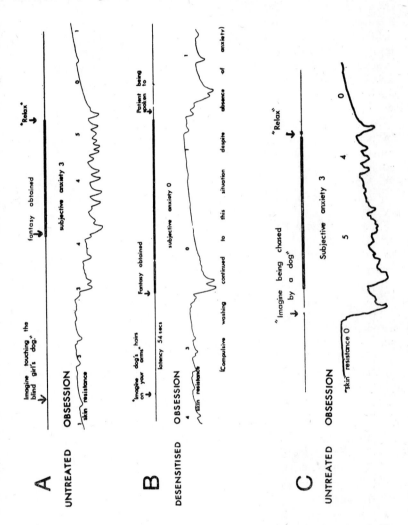

Fig. 3.2 Contrast of anxiety accompanying treated and untreated obsessive phobias

Section VIII. AUTONOMIC EQUIVALENTS TO PHOBIC DISORDERS

Occasional patients present with specific autonomic disturbances which are triggered by special situations. The disturbances resemble specific phobias in that an autonomic equivalent of fear occurs each time the patient enters certain situations although he may not experience much subjective fear, the patient learns to avoid the situations concerned, and treatment of the condition can be effected along lines similar to those for specific phobias.

Patients of this kind may present with urinary urgency or desires to defaecate whenever they are in social situations. They may run to the lavatory dozens of times a day in consequence, or avoid social gatherings instead, or choose only those gatherings where they can easily reach a lavatory. In contrast some men may be unable to urinate in front of any other person, and may waste much time at work and other places waiting for the urinal room to be empty before they can perform.

A minority of asthmatics notice that their bronchospasm is triggered by particular psychological situations, and if these are avoided they remain free of attacks. Hyperhydrosis—excessive sweating—may be a source of embarrassment when it is stimulated repeatedly by social situations, and blushing can cause similar difficulties. Nausea and vomiting are occasionally contingent specifically on certain environmental events.

Some of these patients closely resemble social phobics who were described earlier, and indeed in many cases the distinction from them becomes rather arbitrary and perhaps fruitless. Systematic clinical and physiological comparisons have not yet been made between series of patients with conditioned autonomic disorders and specific phobias.

Several authors have reported successful treatment of conditioned autonomic disorders by desensitisation. In a controlled investigation of asthmatics Moore (1966) found desensitisation to be significantly superior to hypnosis or relaxation alone. In an uncontrolled study Cohen and Reed (1968) found desensitisation to be effective in a variety of conditioned autonomic disorders, including functional diarrhoea.

Section IX. CHILDREN'S FEARS AND PHOBIAS
(written by I. M. Marks and M. G. Gelder)

Incidence
    Sex incidence
The objects feared
Changing incidence and objects of fear with age
Influence of social setting
Disturbances associated with fear
Aetiology
School phobia
    Clinical features
    Mode of onset and precipitants
    Age and sex incidence
    Family setting
    Separation anxiety or fear of school?

Fears in children are partly described elsewhere in this book in the sections on aetiology and treatment. However, childhood phobias display features of their own which merit separate consideration. Fears are much commoner in childhood than in adult life, start often with no apparent cause, and subside again with as little reason. They are more volatile and more intense than in adults. This is true of course for most childhood emotions, which are generally more labile and more keenly expressed. Maturation plays a clearer role in young children, and the home evironment is more influential. Because of the intensity of childhood fears, it is even more difficult to differentiate between the normal fears and abnormal phobias of children. Less systematic research has been done on childhood phobias, and the gaps in our knowledge are even greater than for phobias in adults.

Incidence

No data are available for the frequency with which children present for psychiatric treatment of a phobic disorder. Studies so far have not usually distinguished between mild fears and severe phobias in the children's lives. Fears occur frequently in young children, but the incidence of total fears and the nature of the feared object both change as children grow older, so the picture is complicated. Furthermore, the incidence varies according to the source of information, parents tending to underestimate the number of fears their children have (Lapouse and Monk, 1959).

Several studies show specific fears to be a perfectly normal occurrence in children, and to decrease as the child gets older. The behaviour of 1096 normal children over 14 years was surveyed by MacFarlane, Allen and Honzik (1954), based upon mother's reports. The children were a sub-sample of every third child born in Berkeley, California over an 18 month period from 1928–9, and were over-represented by families with a higher educational level. At least one specific fear was reported for 90% of the children at some stage between the ages of 2 and 14. The frequency of fears diminished with age. The peak was at age 3 when 56% of boys and 67% of girls showed specific fears. The incidence slowly declined with age. Further peaks appeared at age 9 and 11 for boys and at 11 for girls and for boys.

In Leicester, England, 142 school children aged 2 to 7 were studied by Cummings (1944 and1946) , on the basis of teacher's reports. 38% of the girls and 23% of the boys showed specific fears. The incidence declined with age, being 33% before age 4, 22% in the next 2 years, and only 13% from age 6 to 8. The fears were fairly transitory. After 6 months follow-up 72% of the fears had decreased, while by 18 months follow-up 75% of the fears had decreased and 17% had disappeared completely. Although the younger children showed more fears, these were also transitory. Unlike specific fears, generalised anxiety did not decrease with age.

In Buffalo, New York, 482 normal children aged 6 to 12 were studied by Lapouse and Monk (1959). The sample was selected from the city telephone directory, and mothers were the main source of information. 43% of the children were reported to have 7 or more fears out of the 30 about which mothers were questioned. Mothers reported 41% fewer fears in the children than did the children themselves when interviewed. There was no significant relationship between the amount the mother worried and the number of fears she reported in her child. Girls showed significantly more fears than boys (50% vs. 36%) and Negro children had significantly more fears than white children. There was no significant correlation between fears and tension phenomena such as nightmares and bedwetting.

All these studies were of reported fears. The incidence of fear may not be same when the child is confronted with the situation. Holme's (1935) work illustrates this point (in Jersild and Holmes, 1935). She studied fear reactions experimentally in about 50 children who were confronted with various situations and stimuli. A strange person elicited fear in 31% of 2-year olds, 22% of 3-year olds, 7% of 4-year olds and none of the 5-year olds. Fear reaction to being left alone, darkness and loud noises also diminished from ages 2 to 4 and disappeared completely by the age of 5. On the other hand, snakes were feared by 34% of 2-year olds, 55% of 3-year olds, 43% of 4-year olds and 30% of 5-year olds, while the corresponding percentages for fears of dogs was 69%, 43%, 43%, 12%.

Handicapping phobias are much less common than the fears reported in the studies so far. Rutter et al. (1968) screened the total child population of the Isle of Wight aged 10 and 11 for psychiatric disability. Of the total 2,193 children aged 10 and 11, 118 had psychiatric disorder. 16 of these had clinically significant and handicapping phobias. This figure was a minimum estimate, as it did not include subjects with monosymptomatic disorders, which their screening procedure would tend to omit. In no case was the phobia the only symptom and only in very few cases was it the most marked symptom. 6 of the phobias were of animals (all in girls), 6 were of darkness, 3 of school and 1 of heights (7 in girls and 5 in boys). No cases of social phobia or of agoraphobia were found. Disease or dirt phobias were found in 3 boys and 2 girls.

Phobic disorders are also uncommon amongst referrals to child psychiatrists. Graham (1964) found only 5 cases of school refusal and no other specific phobias in a group of 162 cases referred to a local authority clinic, and only 10 specific phobias in 239 consecutive new cases to the Maudsley Hospital Children's Department.

Sex incidence

Most workers report that girls have more fears than boys, (Hall, 1897; Cummings, 1944; Pratt, 1954; Lapouse and Monk, 1959; Grant, 1958;

Dunsworth, 1961; Scherer and Nakamura, 1968) but there are exceptional findings such as those of MacFarlane et al. (1954) whose sample showed no sex difference in the incidence of fears until age 11, after which boys showed a more rapid loss of most fears, leaving girls on average with more fears than boys after puberty.

The objects feared

The situations which children fear are very varied, and as in adults, nothing is gained by elaborate systems of classification. There are, however, certain fears which occur more frequently than others, in particular fears of animals and of natural phenomena such as darkness, storms and thunder. These fears occur in most children, and indeed in Pratt's study of 570 rural school children aged 4 to 16, based on their self-reports, all but 9% of fears were shared by others in the group. Many of these fears were cultural stereotypes, such as fears of lions and tigers which were not present in the area.

In Hagman's (1932) study of 70 children between 2 to 6 years of age, information was obtained from the mothers. The most common fears were of doctors, dogs, storms and darkness. In Jersild et al's (1933) interviews of 398 children aged 6 to 12, the greatest incidence of fears was of mysterious supernatural events and occult phenomena. The second largest cause of fears was animals, often beasts with which the child had never had any direct experience. At all ages children reported many fears of dangers that had never actually threatened them. Bodily injuries, which all these children had experienced to some extent, did not frighten them.

Changing incidence and objects of fear with age

The common fears change as the child grows. As Thompson (1962, p. 289) noted "almost every parent has observed the sudden onset of a fearful response as the child moves forward in perceptual growth. Yesterday the 2 year old child was not afraid of the roar of the vacuum cleaner, today he is terrified—and he has had no intervening experience with either the vacuum cleaner or other loud noises. This type of fear often disappears just as suddenly. We can only infer that the child's perceptual response to the vacuum cleaner is undergoing change as a result of the joint interaction of maturation and learning".

Fears of animals are commonest at age 2 to 4, but by age 4 to 6 they have been supplanted by fears of the dark and imaginary creatures (MacFarlane et al. 1954; Jersild, 1950). The great majority of animal phobics found in adult life give a history of its onset before the age of 9 (Marks and Gelder, 1966), suggesting that children over that age are resistant to such fears. Agras et al. (1969) found that fears of snakes usually start in childhood. Angelino et al. (1956) showed that fears of animals diminish very rapidly in both sexes between age 9 and 11, as judged from the self reports of 1100 children aged 9 to 18 in varied socio-economic groups.

Jersild (1950) and Angelino et al. (1956) give interesting curves for the relative frequency of different specific fears at different ages. The incidence in fears of animals increases from about 6% to about 18% at about 3 years, while fears of darkness reach a peak by about 4 years. On the other hand, parents' reports indicate that fears of noises, and strange people decline from about 25% at $\frac{1}{2}$ to 2 years to 10% at 4 years.

Influence of social setting

The commonest objects of fear vary somewhat in different social settings; for example 75% of the fears of rural children aged 4–11 years are of animals (Pratt, 1945), while those of urban children of about the same age range amount to only about 15% of their fears (Jersild and Holmes 1935 a & b). On the other hand, a survey of Dakota Indian children of about the same age range living in rural conditions gave an incidence of about 50% (Wallis, 1954). Thus the environment in which the child lives is important, as well as the culture in which he is brought up. Of the fears of animals, 95% were of vertebrates and only 4% of arthropods—usually spiders—and 3% of birds.

The objects of fears other than those of animals were spread more widely. Pratt found that 12% were of natural phenomena such as wind, storms, thunder and lightning; 11% of guns and explosives, 10% of cars and trains; 9% of darkness; 8% of diseases and illness; 7% of water and drowning; and 5% of supernatural phenomena such as ghosts. Girls reported significantly more fears of illness, diseases and darkness than boys, while fears of illness increased with age. These surveys are based on the children's reports of what they fear, so they may include some fears which are adaptive and proportionate to the real danger involved, e.g. some of the fear of snakes and large animals. But Pratt (1945) concluded that only a small proportion are of this kind and that in most children the amount of fear appeared disproportionate to the danger. It is also important to note that many of the fears were of animals which were not even met with in the region; thus the fears must have been learnt in some way other than direct conditioning or modelling. Presumably they were passed on verbally by parents. In this context, it is of interest that there is a significant tendency for children to report the same kind and number of fears as their mothers (Hagman, 1932). The correlation between the total number of fears by children and mothers was 0·67 in Hagman's study, while May (1950) reported a correlation ranging from 0·65 to 0·74 between siblings. An apparent exception to this is the study of Lapouse and Monk (1959) which showed no relation between the worries of the mother and the number of fears she reported in the children. However, only the worries of the mother were reported, not her fears.

In relation to learning by modelling it may be noted that Jones (1924) found that children are less likely to develop fears if a trusted reassuring adult is with them, than if they meet the same stimulus alone. Equally, more fears developed in the presence of other children who were afraid than in the presence of children who had no fear. Conversely John (1941) found that pre-school children were more afraid of air-raids if their mothers showed fear than if they did not. Fear evinced by the child correlated 0·59 with that experienced by the mother. An observation of Hagman's (1932) is also relevant here: in an experimental fear situation, children tended to look at the adult who was with them at the moment the fear stimulus was presented.

Disturbances associated with fear

These are often remarkably few. MacFarlane et al. (1954) reported that at the age of 3 years fears were significantly but lowly correlated with physical timidity and, in girls, temper tantrums. Fears were also correlated significantly negatively with overactivity. By the age of 5 the correlates of fear in both sexes were irritability, tantrums and timidity, but girls also showed overdependence, mood swings, poor appetite and timidity. John (1941) also noted that fear, in this instance during air raids, correlated significantly with other signs of maladjustment. In contrast Lapouse and Monk (1959) found no significant relationship between either children's or mothers' reports of fears and any other problems in the child. Dunsworth (1961) considered that when specific fears have led to a child's referral to a child psychiatrist, it is common to find that the mother herself is anxious and the child is overdependent on her.

Aetiology

Wider questions about the aetiology of phobias were considered in detail in an earlier chapter. Here we shall simply summarise some of the main features relevant to fears in children.

Fear is an inborn response to certain stimuli which becomes differentiated from other emotions in the first year of life. The startle reaction which is present at birth is probably a precursor of the later fear response. Startle is elicited by intense, sudden, or unexpected stimuli of many kinds. As fear becomes differentiated from startle after 6 months of age, it is manifested to more specific situations such as strangers at one year, or animals between 2 to 4 years. The general perceptual features which elicit fear in vertebrates were reviewed by Schneirla (1965) and discussed earlier.

The changing circumstances to which fear is shown depend upon maturational processes, perceptual growth and learning experiences. For these reasons fears often occur in children for little or no apparent reason, and die down as mysteriously, without further contact (Thompson, 1962; Thorndike, 1935). The rather constant ages at which some fears come and go have varying explanations. Where exposure is fairly constant, as with small animals and birds, fears of such objects are partly the consequence of changes within the child such as those due to maturation. Also, when children regress during illness forgotten fears may recrudesce until the child is well again, after which the fears disappear once more.

Phobias which develop with minimal or no traumatic exposure lead to the concept of sensitive or facilitatory periods of development during which the child is particularly responsive to certain stimuli. This is consonant with Sackett's (1966) demonstration of a critical period for the manifestation of fear to threat displays in rhesus monkeys reared in social isolation.

Yet other fears start at a given age simply because that is the age at which a child is first or most exposed to that situation. School phobias are a case in point. First exposure to a totally novel situation causes anxiety in young children, but they usually adapt rapidly, as Slater (1939) demonstrated in 40 children aged 2 to 3½ years (fig. 3.3). These

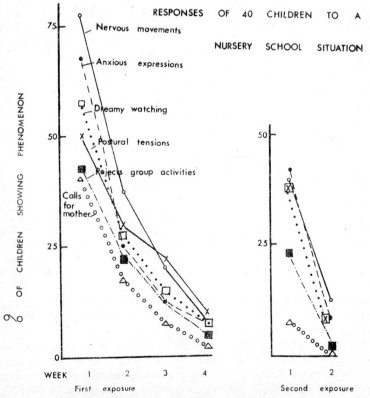

Fig. 3.3 Responses of 40 children to a school situation.

children attended nursery school initially for 4 to 6 weeks, and subsequently every 6 months they returned for additional observation over 2 weeks until they had reached kinder-garten age. Their responses to the novel nursery school situation were carefully studied. During the first period most of the children showed signs of uneasiness (fig. 3.3) but these declined steadily and disappeared in the great majority of children by the 4th week. During the second period of observation far fewer children showed signs of anxiety, and these disappeared rapidly within a week. The children had adapted far more quickly to the situation the 2nd time, presumably due to its greater familarity.

When a child develops a phobia of an object immediately after traumatic exposure to it or related events, then the causal mechanism is obvious. Conditioning of fear certainly occurs in many children. Watson and Rayner's case (1920) was a good example. However, as Thorndike (1935) noted, it is often difficult to condition new fears in children to certain stimuli, and one has to introduce the concept of stimulus prepotency—i.e. some stimuli can trigger phobias much more readily than others.

Trauma can result not only in specific fears of the traumatic situation but also in a general increase in fearfulness. In pre-school children who had experienced air raids the effects were still noticeable 6 months later in the form of an increase in ascertainable fears (John 1914). Another group of children who had had severe burns 2–5 years previously were contrasted with a control group of their siblings and a second control group of normal children (Woodward, 1959). Significantly more of the 198 burned children showed signs of emotional disturbance 2–5 years later (86%) than did either control group (7% and 14%). Of the disturbances, fears and anxieties were the commonest complaints.

Children can come to fear objects or situations they have never been exposed to. This occurs through social learning or modelling, the evidence for which was reviewed elsewhere. Many of the fears expressed by children in surveys appear to be cultural stereotypes which they have acquired.

School phobia (school refusal)

Refusal to go to school, also known as "school phobia" is a well-known problem for child psychiatrists, psychologists and teachers. However, as Rutter et al. (1968) point out, public concern over a problem is no measure of its frequency. Chazan (1962) noted that school refusal is quite uncommon even among children attending psychiatrists, amounting only to 1 to 3 % of all cases, while Graham (1964) found only 5 cases of school refusal in 172 cases referred to a local authority clinic. In the survey of the total population of 2139 children aged 10 and 11 on the Isle of Wight, Rutter et al. found but 3 cases of school refusal, which formed under 3 % of all those who had psychiatric disability. Although most children show anxiety about school at one time or another, these phenomena are generally short-lived and clear up with minimum or no treatment (Slater, 1939). Long-standing cases of school refusal present a more difficult problem (Hersov, 1960b.)

School refusal has been widely described, and we shall not attempt an exhaustive review of the problem, but will instead concentrate on the salient aspects. School refusal must be differentiated from truancy, in which the children do not refuse to go to school, but use many wily stratagems to stay away from school and wander alone or in the company of other truants, their whereabouts unknown to their parents, who first learn of the truancy from the school authorities. Truancy is often associated with other delinquent behaviour, with frequent change of school, with a history of parental absence in childhood, and with inconsistent discipline in the home (Hersov, 1960a). At school truants show a poor standard of work.

In contrast to truants, children with school phobias bluntly refuse to go to school, do not exhibit other delinquent behaviour, have no history of parental absence from home, and more often maintain a high standard of work and behaviour at school (Hersov, 1960a). School phobics also have significantly more somatic symptoms of anxiety than truants, especially disturbances of eating and sleeping, abdominal pain, nausea and vomiting (Hersov, 1960a).

Clinical features

The child will usually present simply with refusal to go to school. Young children may give no reason at all for their refusal, while older children will attribute their fears to various aspects of school life. The complaint may be of being bullied or teased, or self-consciousness about their appearance. They may be afraid of undressing in front of other children, or of taking a public bath or shower after games. Anxiety about poor performance at games or school work may be mentioned, or fear of a teacher. Thirty-six per cent of one sample experienced concern that harm would befall the mother while the child was at school (Hersov, 1960b). Overt anxiety about menstruation, puberty or masturbation may be revealed. Yet other reasons given for non-attendance include fears of vomiting or fainting during school assembly.

The child's fears are not only expressed directly but also in physical symptoms of anxiety which may appear particularly in the morning when he is encouraged to leave the house for school. These include nausea, vomiting, headache, diarrhoea, complaints of abdominal pain, sore throat and leg pains. Eating difficulties, sleep disturbance and various fears may be noted. The child's complaints may increase his parents' anxiety about him and lead sooner or later to open or covert agreement that he should stay at home. Once the child is assured he can stay at home the symptoms usually subside (Waldfogel et al. 1957). A typical picture is of a child who complains of nausea at breakfast and may vomit, and who resists all attempts at reassurance by his anxious—and ambivalent—mother, until a crisis is reached at which she gives in and allows him to stay at home. Then he feels better unless the pressure to go to school is resumed.

Mode of onset and precipitants

These and other features were described in detail by Hersov (1960b) in a sample of 50 cases seen in the children's Department of the Maudsley Hospital. All the cases had been out of school for at least 2 months. The features of this sample are in broad agreement with those in other series. Hersov's study has the additional and unusual merit of a control group which was contrasted with the school refusers.

In most cases the school refusal developed gradually with a period of increasing reluctance to attend culminating in outright refusal (64%). Outright refusal might be preceded by irritability, weepiness, restless sleep, nausea and abdominal pains at the time they were due to go to school, and pressure to get the child to school produced fear, pallor, tremulousness and sweating. A minority of cases began suddenly after a break in school-going (36%) on the Monday morning following a weekend, on the first day of a new term, or on the day of return to school following illness.

A common precipitant was a change to a new school at any level in the educational system (38%). Less commonly school refusal began after the death, departure or illness of a parent (18%). Nursten (1958) confirmed that change of school was a common trigger for the start of a school phobia.

Age and sex incidence

In the Maudsley sample the peak age of onset was 11 to 12 years, with a range from age 7 to 16 years. The peak age coincides with the period when most children move from a primary to a higher school in England. Sixty-two percent of Hersov's sample were boys, which agrees very closely with the composition of the sample described by Rodriguez et al. (1959). Intelligence was average in the Maudsley sample.

Family setting

Children with school refusal in Hersov's sample came from families which were of an average size, but which were unusually stable. When compared with controls, significantly fewer school phobics had experienced parental absence before age 5. However, a significant excess of the parents had a history of psychiatric disturbance, mainly of depression or anxiety.

Parental attitudes were also significantly unusual. Half the mothers were noted to be over-indulgent and to be dominated by their children, while a quarter went to the opposite extreme of being demanding, severe and controlling. More than half the fathers were assessed as being inadequate and passive in the home management of their children.

Hersov's description accords with others in the literature. Some mothers of school phobics develop unusually close dependence on and from their children as a compensation for their unsatisfactory marital or other relationships. The mothers themselves often have a history of an unhappy relationship with their own parents.

When there is excessive emotional interdependence between the mother and child, then both members of the dyad require treatment, for to treat the child alone may raise the mother's anxiety to a level which will lead her to terminate the child's treatment. Eisenberg (1958) pointed out that such mothers were reluctant to leave their children in the clinic playrooms, and would say in the child's presence "You won't be able to get him to leave me". The relationship between such mothers and children would become mutually constricting for both parties and soon became tinged with hostility.

Separation anxiety or fear of school?

It is often held that school phobia is a misnomer for school refusal, on the grounds that the condition is not a fear of school at all but is rather a fear of leaving mother. Separation anxiety undoubtedly plays a part in many cases, and there was evidence for it in 36% of Hersov's sample (1960b). However, to state as Waldfogel et al. (1957) did, that the condition is "invariably found to originate in the child's fear of being separated from the mother" is to take too one-sided a view. In 22% of the children in Hersov's study the fears were focused clearly on the school, not the mother.

Careful enquiry into the details of the places where the child shows fear can help to establish the relative importance of fears of school and fears of separation. It is to be emphasised that both factors are often present in the same case, and mature clinical judgment is needed to assess the situation. Psychodynamic interviews with the child must be supplemented by careful social assessment of the home and enquiry at the school by an educational psychologist. The latter point is borne out by Chazan's study (1962) of 24 children with school phobia, 5 of whom had some degree of backwardness which appeared to antedate the school phobia, rather than result from the child's irregular attendance. Cautious interpretation of the clinical evidence is necessary. Separation anxiety cannot be inferred simply from the fact that the child will go to school if his mother comes with him, even though he will go under no other circumstances. Any phobia is partly improved in the presence of a trusted companion, and a school phobia is no exception. Separation anxiety can be inferred with greater confidence when overt fears are expressed of leaving the mother rather than of going to school, together with fears that the mother may come to harm when out of sight of the child.

The importance of different factors may change with age. Dunsworth (1961) suggested that separation anxiety and neurosis in the mother is more important in pre-school children and those in their early years at school. In adolescents, phobias of school and college have been studied by Coolidge et al. (1960). This group represents a transition between school phobias and phobia of work situations in adolescents and young adults. Coolidge et al. reported that adolescents who refuse to go to school or college invariably have a history of school phobias in earlier years. The same type of family pathology was identified as in younger patients and there was the same occasional need to treat the whole family. Levenson (1961) studied a similar group of patients, all aged 16–20, and, in this case, all Jewish. They were free from anxiety once the pressure to return to college was removed. They were described as glib and articulate with an undercurrent of arrogance and hostility. They had been brought up to expect easy success but had little ability to tolerate frustration or to persist at tasks. Again, the father was found to be passive and dominated by the mother who was contemptuous of him and over-protective to the child. The parents were found, as others have done, to have such a close emotional involvement with the patient that they interfered with his treatment.

Chapter 4

TREATMENT OF PHOBIAS

Section I. **INTRODUCTION**
Prevention
Management immediately after trauma
Treatment of established phobias

Section II. **DESENSITISATION**
History
Technique. Difficulties during desensitisation
Results:
Controlled results in volunteer subjects:
Studies by Lang et al. with snake phobics
Studies by Paul with stage fright
Studies on role of reward and therapeutic expectations
The active components of desensitisation
Controlled results in patients:
Retrospective trial of inpatients and outpatients
Prospective trial of severely agoraphobic inpatients
Prospective comparison with insight psychotherapy in phobic outpatients
Crossover study in phobic outpatients
Prospective comparison with hypnosis in phobic outpatients
Physiological predictors of response to desensitisation
Retrospective study of modified leucotomy in severe agoraphobia
Summary of controlled studies in patients
Discussion of results in patients
Methods to facilitate desensitisation:
Group desensitisation
Automated desensitisation
Intravenous shortacting barbiturates
Standard vs. individually tailored hierarchies
Massed vs. spaced desensitisation

Desensitisation in imagination and in practice
    Transfer of improvement from imagined to
      real situations
Speed of change of different components of fear
Processes other than relaxation which inhibit fear
Desensitisation and insight
Elimination of nightmares by desensitisation of
    phobia

Section III.   **TECHNIQUES OTHER THAN DESENSITISATION**
    A. Experimental methods:
      Modelling
      Flooding (implosion)
      Paradoxical intention
      Cognitive manipulation
      Aversion relief
      Operant conditioning techniques

    B. Clinical methods:
      Relaxation techniques and hypnosis
        Meditation, faithhealing
      Psychotherapy (insight or analytically oriented)
        Psychoanalysis
      Drugs in phobic disorders
        Relief of phobic anxiety
        Relief of background anxiety
        Relief of panic attacks
        Relief of depression
        Acetylcholine
          Intravenous barbiturates
          Thiopentone
          Methohexitone
    Leucotomy

Section IV.   **THE PSYCHIATRIC MANAGEMENT OF PHOBIC
      PATIENTS**

Section V.   **TREATMENT OF PHOBIAS IN CHILDREN**
    Phobias in general
    School phobia
      Outcome of school phobia

Section I. INTRODUCTION

Nearly 2,000 years ago Celsus was probably the first person to use the word phobia in a medical context and to give a specific remedy for its treatment. Referring to hydrophobia, his term for rabies, he wrote:

". . . still there is just one remedy, to throw the patient unawares into a water tank which he has not seen beforehand. If he cannot swim, let him sink under and drink, then lift him out; if he can swim, push him under at intervals so that he drinks his fill of water even against his will; for so his thirst and dread of water are removed at the same time".

This drastic approach would be recommended today neither in the treatment of rabies nor of phobias proper. However, most other methods known to psychiatrists have been employed to alleviate genuine phobias. That many different techniques are currently in use is shown by the following passage which appeared in the newsletter of a phobic club whose members had answered a questionnaire (The Open Door, Nov. 1965). " HAVE YOU HAD ANY TREATMENT CONVENTIONAL OR OTHERWISE? Replies included: Drugs, Drugs and Drugs; Psychoanalysis; Narcoanalysis; Group therapy and other therapies including 'Heavy' Occupational Therapy (working in hospital kitchens and laundries!); Leucotomy; L.S.D.; Hypnosis; Autosuggestion; E.C.T. (Shock Treatment); Deep Relaxation; Yoga; Spiritual Healing; Acupuncture; Behaviour Therapy; Psychology correspondence course; Homeopathy; Naturopathy, etc."

To this impressive list of treatments for phobias one could add the methods of ridicule, disuse by avoidance, "willpower", forced retraining, graduated retraining, social imitation of fearless models, individual and group psychotherapy, autogenic training, paradoxical intention, habituation, desensitisation, deconditioning, counterconditioning, relearning, reciprocal inhibition and aversion relief. The reader might well feel confused by the bewildering array of techniques which have been employed in the treatment of phobias. Until recently no procedures had been subject to controlled trial, and it was consequently difficult to evaluate the merits of different methods. The recent surge of controlled studies enables us now to say with more confidence what some of the procedures can do.

We will discuss measures which are useful in the prevention of phobias and then will outline specific techniques for use in established phobias.

Prevention

Perhaps the most important measure to prevent the development of phobias is also the most difficult to put into practice. This measure is the provision of a milieu from infancy onwards in which the accepted mode of behaviour is that of readiness to face difficulties and overcome frightening situations. A courageous attitude is easier to nurture in a child of naturally brave disposition than in one who is born timid, and we have to accept the limitations imposed on this attribute by genetic endowment. Nevertheless it is desirable that a child's models show a consistent readiness to master frightening situations and to reward a similar attitude in the child himself. The model's example "of fearlessness is not so likely to succeed, however, if it involves the use of abilities and techniques that are beyond the child's capacities. Nor does an example of courage help if it merely strengthens the child's conviction or fear that he himself is a coward" (Jersild, 1950, p. 282).

When the child is sufficiently confident gentle encouragement should be given to enter mildly frightening situations until the child has lost all his fear. The child should not be ridiculed for being frightened, as shame reinforces fear. As a rule children should not be forced into frightening situations except under special circumstances where additional support is given until the fear has been overcome completely. Whatever happens the child should feel accepted and should not be rejected for appearing frightened, but praise and other rewards should be given freely for brave behaviour. This will be particularly necessary in a child who is naturally timid, whereas a tough child might require to be cautioned against excessive bravery when it amounts to fool-hardiness.

Children and adults are more likely to show fear when debilitated by illness, fatigue or depression. Attempts should not be made to face fear while in such a state as this may enhance rather than allay fear. Such attempts are best encouraged when the subject is feeling well.

Management immediately after trauma

Sudden trauma is often followed by a lag phase before a phobia develops. Animal experiments suggest that immediate re-exposure to the original situation during this phase protects against the development of fear to that environment (Willmuth and Peters, 1964). It is in fact common lore that subjects should re-experience a traumatic situation again immediately after the original trauma. For example, during World War II treatment of combat neuroses was advocated within the sights and sounds of battle; "the acute phase is the crucial period in which therapy should be instituted in order to head off the organisation of the neurosis" (Kardiner and Spiegel, 1947, pp. 76–7). Aeroplane pilots are encouraged to deliberately fly again as soon as possible after they have had a flying accident, and car drivers are recommended to drive once more as soon as they can after a car crash. It is sensible to help people face recently traumatic situations as soon as they can before the fear can be built into a phobia by the twin processes of first, repeated rehearsal of the trauma in the subject's mind and second, reinforcement by repeated avoidance.

While their phobias are still mild, patients can be helped to overcome their fear by warm reassurance and suggestion, and numerous strata-gems have been employed successfully in selected cases to encourage them to face the feared situation, e.g. Frazier and Carr (1967) cite a patient who was bet $1,000 by his doctor that he would not die of a heart attack should he venture forth from home, and promptly found himself able to go out alone for the first time in months. Prince (1898) described professional performers who were suddenly struck with stage fright, but who overcame this by constantly repeating aloud messages of reassurance written by the doctor on a piece of paper.

Treatment of established phobias

Once phobias are causing persistent avoidance of the phobic object then simple exhortations to bravery and willpower alone are not likely to help a patient. If anything they may aggravate his phobia by causing the patient to enter situations with which he cannot cope, he will get into a panic and escape from that situation, after which the phobia will increase. At this stage more specific techniques are necessary.

Many such techniques have been employed. In the past success has been claimed for a wide variety of techniques from faith healing and hypnosis to drugs and desensitisation. Most of these claims derive from isolated case reports or uncontrolled series of cases which are difficult to evaluate for two reasons. First, several kinds of phobias, especially those in children and in agoraphobics, fluctuate so much without treatment that improvement during administration of an uncontrolled technique might be due to this "spontaneous" change rather than to the technique itself. Next, many psychological techniques are complex assemblies of several procedures, so that even if they do produce change in phobics it is by no means clear which aspects of the technique were responsible.

In the last decade a rash of controlled trials of treatment for phobias has appeared, so that some order is gradually emerging about which treatments work, in which patients they work, and what the effective ingredients are in these treatments. Most controlled trials in phobics have contrasted desensitisation with another procedure, but recently other techniques have also been subjected to controlled scrutiny. The claims for these and some uncontrolled methods will be discussed, after which results of all the different methods will be integrated together. However, knowledge in this area is advancing so rapidly that present views may need considerable modification in a few years' time in the light of procedures which are currently being tested.

Section II.   DESENSITISATION

The procedure of desensitisation involves graduated exposure to phobic stimuli along a hierarchy while the patient simultaneously has a contrasting experience such as relaxation. Usually he is relaxed while he visualises a series of images of phobic situations, and later he also goes out to meet those situations in practice. Desensitisation is probably the commonest way in which phobias are treated today, and has been more thoroughly explored than any other technique. It is usually regarded as one of the many techniques which are called the behavioural psychotherapies.

History of desensitisation

The basic idea comes from common sense principles and was enunciated at least as early as 1644 by Sir Kenelm Digby: "Any aversion of the fantasy may be mastered not only by a more powerfull agent upon the present sense, but also by assuefaction, and by bringing into the fantasy with pleasing circumstances that object which before was displeasing and affrightfull to it". The term assuefaction was applied by Digby to the production of artificial responses by combining normally "frightfull objectes" with "pleasing circumstances" and vice versa.

Since the early years of this century many workers independently put forward the same idea. Jones (1924b) extinguished a 3-year-old boy's fear of a rat and rabbit by associating the rabbit with food which the child liked, while other children who were not afraid attended to foster social imitation. Herzberg (1941) described the treatment of phobias by the administration of graduated tasks, while Levine (1942, p. 132) actually used the term "desensitisation" in advocating methods to retrain phobias, giving as an example a child with a phobia of noise who might "be helped by an increased dosage of noise, starting with a minimal amount and increasing slowly. It may be done through a radio or phonograph, turned low at first, and gradually increased". It deserves mention that Levine also noted, in his discussion of psychotherapy, that "it may be possible to desensitise a patient (to psychologic material to which he is hypersensitive) by the presentation of the offending material, proceeding from a minimal dosage to a large dosage, so that better defences are prepared, and so that when the material comes up spontaneously, the individual's reaction to it may be less disturbed. In psychotherapy, this of course is done by discussion" (p. 123).

Discussing phobias in children Jersild (1950, p. 282) wrote that "apart from efforts to alleviate tensions and pressures in the situation that surrounds a child's fear, the most effective method of dealing with fear is to help him, by degrees, to come actively and directly to grips with the situation that scares him, to aid him in acquiring experience and acquaintanceship with it, to aid him in acquiring skills that are of value in coping with the feared event . . ." Jersild suggested that the feared stimulus be presented with an attractive or benign stimulus, this procedure being done in a larger setting which is reassuring.

The earliest psychoanalytic writings onwards emphasised the importance of facing the phobic situation, though they did not insist on the value of graduating the exposure. For example, Freud himself wrote in 1919:

"One can hardly ever master a phobia if one waits till the patient lets the analysis influence him to give it up . . . one succeeds only when one can induce them through the influence of the analysis to

... go about alone and to struggle with their anxiety while they make the attempt".

In a more recent review of psychotherapy in phobias Andrews (1966) described how many psychotherapists use their relationship with the patient to lever him into venturing out of safety into a direct confrontation of the phobic situation.

Finally, independent of these influences, other writers like Leonhard (1963) have also advocated the value of gradual retraining.

It is clear that the idea of desensitisation originated separately in several quarters. Jones' writings owed much to the influence of Watson and Rayner (1920), and Jersild was influenced by Jones. Herzberg Levine and Leonhard made their suggestions without acknowledgement of these ideas, and this was also true of Freud and Fenichel. In the last decade, however, desensitisation has been increasingly described in the language of learning theory, and it is now one of the accepted techniques of the behavioural psychotherapies. This is largely through the pioneering work of Wolpe (1954, 1958) and the writings of Meyer (1957), Rachman (1959) and of Eysenck (1960).

Technique of desensitisation

Desensitisation is usually carried out today in a manner derived from Wolpe (1958). Wolpe's method stemmed from his experiments in cats in which he found that the presentation of a pleasant stimulus like food could inhibit conditioned avoidance responses until they were gradually extinguished. He deduced that "if a response antagonistic to anxiety can be made to occur in the presence of anxiety-provoking stimuli so that it is accompanied by a complete or partial suppression of the anxiety responses, the bond between the stimuli and the anxiety responses will be weakened". Wolpe then devised a method of treatment whereby patients were first asked to prepare a hierarchy of their phobic situations from the least to the most frightening stimuli, then they were taught muscular relaxation, and finally while in this relaxed state they were asked to imagine the least frightening situation repeatedly until they could tolerate the image without anxiety. The patient was then asked to imagine a slightly more frightening situation and was relaxed repeatedly during the scene until this too could be tolerated, until finally all the phobic situations could be comfortably visualised in imagination. The patient practised entering those same situations in real life until the phobia was extinguished in practice as well as in imagination. Wolpe used the term "reciprocal inhibition" to describe the technique of coupling a pleasant with a frightening stimulus. Other terms which have also been employed to describe the same process are counterconditioning, deconditioning, relearning, habituation, and of course, desensitisation. The last named is now the commonest label for the procedure.

Most details of the technique have been elaborated by Rachman (1968). First a full history is essential to define the problems of the patient. The patient is then trained in progressive relaxation, the aim of which is to obtain a state of mental calm during subsequent presentation of phobic images. From 1 to 6 sessions may be needed to train the patient to the point where he can quickly achieve satisfactory relaxation. Jacobson's method is usually employed. This involves developing a "muscle sense", relaxing one muscle group (e.g. biceps) until a tingling sensation develops, relaxing consecutive muscle groups separately, relaxing various groups of muscles simultaneously.

Detailed instructions for this method of relaxation are given by Wolpe and Lazarus (1966, pp. 177–180) and appear in the appendix.

Various groups of muscles are flexed and then relaxed for up to 30 minutes, and the patient is also instructed to practise at home for two fifteen-minute sessions a day. It is usual to start with the arms and legs and then to move to the head and neck muscles. When the patient has successfully learned to relax each important group of muscles, an attempt is made to co-ordinate the relaxation of these disparate muscle groups. Final achievement of relaxation is indicated by bodily stillness, flaccid muscles, regular breathing and motionless eyelids.

An alternative method of relaxation is Schultz's authogenic training. The patient is asked to visualise one part of his body, to hold the image and to relax the corresponding part of his body, e.g. "get a clear picture of your right hand, see the outline of the fingers, the colour of the skin, the wrinkles on the knuckles. Now relax your right hand as you think about it, keeping the image in your mind all the time. Now try to see your right forearm in your mind's eye . . . etc." It is not important which mode of relaxation is employed provided the patient feels completely relaxed both muscularly and mentally after mastering the technique. Some therapists find it convenient simply to hypnotise the patient several times with suggestions of relaxation, though patients then cannot practise the hypnosis at home.

Constructing a phobic hierarchy involves grading those stimuli which frighten the patient from the least to the most frightening. Several hierarchies may be made where several phobias are involved. Information is used from the patient's history and from any questionnaires he may have answered. The therapist then isolates themes running through the phobic items and orders them into a graded and meaningful hierarchy, with equal increases of fear from one item to the next.

During desensitisation itself the patient is told which stimuli are to be presented in the sessions and is asked to indicate with each image whether that image was obtained and whether it aroused anxiety or could be tolerated calmly, e.g. "raise your left hand if you felt calm with the image, if it made you feel anxious raise your right hand". To facilitate ease of communication the patient can rate his feeling of anxiety during an image on a scale from 0—(absolutely calm) to 100— (a feeling of total panic). Mild fear might be rated as 20 and fairly intense fear as 70.

If mild anxiety occurs with an image, repetition of that image several times usually dissipates the anxiety, and the image should be presented several times more once the patient feels completely calm with it. However, if excessive anxiety occurs with an image, that image should be withdrawn and an item lower down on the hierarchy should be substituted.

At the start of treatment items lowest in the hierarchy (the least-disturbing ones) are introduced first, and the therapist proceeds slowly up the list depending upon the patient's reaction. Gradually it becomes possible for the patient to imagine formerly phobic stimuli without any anxiety. In this way a slowly increasing number of formerly phobic stimuli become tolerable in imagination by systematic desensitisation.

Once the phobic patient can tolerate a few phobic stimuli in imagination, he is asked to enter those situations in real life after the treatment session, having relaxed beforehand, and relaxing as much as possible while in contact with the phobic object. Usually the patient is able to manage this, though progress in real life often lags behind progress in imagination. This point will be discussed more fully later. The patient is asked to desist from encountering phobic situations which have not yet been dealt with in fantasy, since any experience of excessive anxiety with ensuing avoidance of that situation may enhance rather than improve the phobia.

Difficulties during desensitisation

Once the technique of desensitisation is given properly, the most important variable influencing results is the clinical status of the patient, how focal his problems are, how much anxiety there is at rest, how many compulsions and other neurotic symptoms there are. These will be reviewed. Even in suitable patients, however, progress in desensitisation can be hampered by many factors, most of which have been reviewed by Weinberg and Zaslove (1963), Wolpe and Lazarus (1966) and Rachman (1968). The problems are summarised in Table 4.1.

Problems during relaxation

First, progress can be slowed by difficulties during relaxation. During successful relaxation patients may feel sleepy and actually fall asleep. Other patients may show poor concentration not because of sleepiness but because they are distracted by upsetting occurrences outside treatment. To check these events it is necessary throughout desensitisation for the patient to signal that he is obtaining those images which are being presented.

Table 4.1
Difficulties during desensitisation

Difficulties during relaxation:
    Sleepiness
    Poor concentration
    Fear of losing control
    Muscular relaxation without mental relaxation
    Severe anxiety and depression

Problems of imagery:
    Inability to obtain images
    Dissociation of anxiety
    Dilution of image to more protective setting
    Intensification of image to panic proportions

Misleading hierarchies:
    Irrelevant hierarchies
    Fluctuating hierarchies

Relapse of desensitised phobias

Lack of cooperation

Life situation influences outside treatment

Patients may find it difficult to relax because they are afraid of losing control and may require reassurance that they have full control over the procedure at all times.

Some patients achieve excellent muscular relaxation yet complain that mentally they still feel tense There is much to suggest that the role of muscular relaxation in densensitisation is largely to induce a feeling of calmness, so its purpose is frustrated in such patients and desensitisation then becomes difficult.

The most serious obstacle to relaxation is the presence of general ("free floating") anxiety which causes patients to feel so tense that they are incapable of relaxing. Such patients may be helped by large doses of sedative drugs, but unfortunately desensitisation becomes less efficient the larger the dose of drugs, possibly because such drugs retard learning processes. Severe depression may also interfere seriously with relaxation, not only because it is frequently accompanied by anxiety, but also because depressed patients often have poor concentration and apathy, and so are incapable of adequate co-operation.

Problems of Imagery

Some people have great difficulty in producing any visual imagery for reasons unknown, and in desensitisation may be unable to conjure up any phobic image at all no matter how hard they try over several sessions. In such cases desensitisation in imagination is not feasible and desensitisation in practice has to be done instead if practicable.

A further problem during visualisation is dissociation, i.e. patients can visualise a phobic situation but feel no anxiety with it. As one subject remarked, " If that had really happened to me it would bother me, but the image is O.K.". In such cases desensitisation is likely to yield poor results since there is no anxiety to densensitise in imagination. Again desensitisation in practice will be required instead.

Yet another difficulty in the imaginal process is voluntary dilution of the phobic scene to a more protective setting, e.g. when a spider phobic had an image of a spider near her in the room the fantasy changed so that she promptly escaped by jumping out of the window. This is a form of avoidance response and suggests that the subject is not yet ready for desensitisation of that item.

The opposite may also happen in that the phobic scene may become involuntarily intensified instead of diluted, e.g. when a patient with a bird phobia imagined a small bird settling a few feet away from her the bird suddenly grew larger and flapped its wings violently, so that the patient startled out of her relaxed state. This phenomenon too is the result of too much anxiety in treatment. It can also occur if the patient is allowed to develop the scenes on his own instead of the therapist controlling the duration of presentation of a particular scene.

Misleading hierarchies

Hierarchies might be misleading because they may be irrelevant or fluctuating. Irrelevant hierarchies direct the therapeutic effort at the wrong source of fear and it is necessary to guard against these by constant check on the patient's reaction inside and outside treatment.

Fluctuating hierarchies can be a serious problem. On occasion items which were initially ranked as mildly disturbing may change inexplicably to become moderately or severely disturbing items. In these instances repeated checks are required in the structure and ordering of the hierarchy. This problem is particularly common in patients with diffuse phobias or with obsessive compulsive disorders.

Relapse of desensitised phobias

Fears which have been successfully desensitised often reappear to some extent at a later date. This partial reappearance of fear can often be managed by further desensitisation without subsequent relapse.

Motivational problems

Weinberg and Zaslove (1963) noted other problems in desensitisation which arise more indirectly. Such problems occur also in most other forms of psychiatric treatment. The patient may not carry out instructions, e.g. may fail to practise relaxation or to meet phobic situations in real life. The patient may be persistently late for treatment. He may suddenly announce that he is better and needn't come any more despite evidence to the contrary; this is an example of "flight into health".

Motivation is therefore important. Desensitisation may also be hampered by lack of motivation where there is frustration of motives prompting the volunteer, e.g. one student wanted to win out over her friends in being selected but grew dissatisfied as the non-competitive character of the research became clear.

Life situational problems intruding into desensitisation

Further problems may arise from life experiences outside treatment. In the students of Weinberg and Zaslove quarrels with parents and troubles with boy friends took precedence in their daily lives and invaded the desensitisation process. In their volunteers experiences with phobic stimuli were sparse and did not play a significant role in their current affairs. This latter point is less common in psychiatric patients with phobic disorders.

RESULTS OF DESENSITISATION

Wolpe claimed that his method markedly improved 90% of a series of 210 mixed neurotic patients at the end of treatment. This figure excluded patients who dropped out after fewer than 15 sessions of treatment. Of those who started treatment only 75% did well. Lazarus (1963), an associate of Wolpe's, used a similar treatment in a group of 126 mixed neurotic cases and noted that 62% improved. Unfortunately these claims could not be evaluated because firstly, different neurotic disorders have different prognoses (Cooper et al., 1965; Ernst, 1959) so that improvement rates for mixed groups of neurotics are not very informative about specific types of neurosis. Secondly, no control groups were available for comparison, so that it was impossible to say whether these cases improved because of desensitisation, because of other ingredients of treatment they received, or because of factors outside the treatment situation—so-called "spontaneous improvement".

From 1961 until the time of writing at least 18 controlled experiments have been made where groups of phobic subjects who were treated by desensitisation were contrasted with groups of subjects with similar problems treated by a control procedure. Because of these studies desensitisation is perhaps the only psychological technique for which we can give fairly complete answers to the questions whether it works, if so in whom, and which aspects of the procedure are responsible for the effects. The following account will only include those controlled studies of desensitisation which dealt with subjects who had focal fears. Controlled studies of subjects with other problems will be excluded. In this burgeoning field several more controlled trials will have appeared by the time these lines are read.

Controlled studies with volunteer phobic subjects

Most controlled investigations of desensitisation have dealt not with patients but with volunteer subjects who have been found on special enquiry to have circumscribed phobias but who were not sufficiently distressed by the phobias to seek psychiatric help for them. These investigations have been of undoubted value in determining the mechanisms by which desensitisation works, but their results have to be confirmed in a patient population because patients may differ from volunteers in important respects. Furthermore, at least a year's follow-up is essential to differentiate transient effects from more lasting changes. Fewer than 3% of psychiatric outpatients have phobic disorders and perhaps half of these complain of isolated phobias. Later we will enquire whether these psychiatric patients are helped by desensitisation.

Many of the studies with volunteers have had rather similar basic designs. Phobic subjects were usually obtained by questionnaire screening of a student population, after which subjects who reported intense fears were interviewed and subjected to an avoidance test in which they were required to approach the phobic object as close as they could, and to rate how much fear they felt during the test. Subjects who avoided the phobic object were selected for the experiment and filled in other measures of anxiety and personality. They were then assigned at random to treatment by desensitisation or by the control procedure, after which they had further avoidance tests, reported their fear during the test, and filled in other questionnaires. In some studies subjects were re-tested again after a period of follow-up.

Table 4.2 shows 13 studies with volunteers in which a group which received desensitisation was compared with a control group. All but three of the studies dealt with student volunteers, so the populations sampled have been rather homogeneous. Surprisingly few kinds of fear have been treated—8 studies dealt with snake phobias, 2 studies with stage fright. Several of the studies have had rather small numbers of desensitisation subjects, and follow-up has often been short, though a year's follow-up is usually regarded as a reasonable aim in clinical investigations.

Despite these imitations nearly all the investigations of volunteers show an impressive uniformity in their results. Each showed desensitisation to produce more change in the treated fear than did the corresponding control treatment, which included relaxation, graduated exposure, flooding, visualising non-phobic scenes, suggestion and hypnosis, insight psychotherapy, drug placebo and no treatment or a period on a waiting list (Table 4.3). It is true that significant differences were commonly found only in some of the measures cf fear which were employed, significance levels were often low, and the effects of desensitisation were not always significantly different from all the control groups employed in a given study. Nevertheless, there is an impressive overall trend in favour of desensitisation in volunteers with minor phobias. Further details of the studies in volunteers will appear in

Tables 4.4, 4.5 and 4.6. Meanwhile several of the best studies demand fuller attention.

Table 4.2

Controlled Studies of Desensitisation in Volunteers

Study	Fear treated	No. of subjects in des. group	Length of follow-up (months)
Lazarus (1961)	Acro, claustro.	16	9
Lang et al. (1966)	Snakes	23	8
Davison (1967)	,,	8	0
Lomont and Edwards (1967)	,,	11	0
Schubot (1966)	,,	15	0
Melamed and Lang (1968)	,,	7	7
Leitenberg et al. (1968)	,,	10	0
Ritter (1968)	,,	15	0
Bandura (1968)	,,	12	1
Rachman (1965)	Spiders	3	3
Paul and Shannon (1966)	Stage fright	20	24
Donner (1968)	Test anxiety	14	3
Kondas (1967)	,, ,,	12	5
	mean =	12·5	5

Table 4.3

Controlled Procedures Contrasted with Desensitisation in Volunteers

	No. of studies
Relaxation	4
Graduated exposure	5
Flooding	1
Visualising non-phobic scenes	2
Suggestion and hypnosis	1
Insight psychotherapy	2
Drug placebo	1
Modelling	1
No treatment or period on waiting list	11

Studies by Lang and his colleagues with snake phobias

Lang and his colleagues (Lang and Lazovik, 1963; Lang, Lazovik and Reynolds, 1965; Lang, 1969) pioneered a control design which was later adopted by many other workers. Their subjects were student volunteers with phobias of non-poisonous snakes. Desensitisation was contrasted with a relaxation-hypnosis procedure and with a no treatment control.

Subjects

There were 44 college student volunteers who were 1–2% of a normal class, selected by a questionnaire and subsequent interview. They were selected for inclusion in the trial if they rated fear of non-poisonous snakes as "intense" and this was confirmed in an interview. 80% of the volunteers were women. They systematically avoided snakes or places such as zoos or camping trips where they might be found. Subjects also showed anxiety to pictures of snakes and to the word "snake" itself. Subjects were excluded if they had physical disabilities or latent psychosis on psychotic scales of the MMPI or on interview.

Experimental Groups

Subjects were allocated at random into one of three groups:

1. **Desensitisation.** 23 subjects had a total of 16 sessions—5 of which were sessions of training in relaxation, and 11 sessions of systematic desensitisation in imagination along a 20-item hierarchy. Sessions lasted 45 minutes and were given 1–2 times weekly.

2. **Relaxation hypnosis (pseudotherapy).** 10 subjects had a total of 16 sessions—5 of which were sessions of relaxation training and 11 sessions of relaxation-hypnosis during which patients imagined pleasant scenes and then hierarchy items simply as starting points for discussion of snake-irrelevant material.

3. **No treatment.** 11 subjects were untreated controls.

Experimental measures. These were made before treatment, after training in relaxation, at the end of treatment and at 6 months follow-up.

1. An avoidance test in which the subject was invited to approach a live snake.

2. Self-rating of fear experienced during the avoidance test—the so-called "fear thermometer" (on a 10-point scale).

3. Fear Survey Schedule (FSS)—a list of 50 phobias, including 1 item covering snakes, rated on a 7-point scale.

4. Stanford Hypnotic Suggestibility Scale.

The experimenter who conducted the interview and administered the avoidance test participated in no other phase of the project.

Results (based on *change* scores)

1. Desensitisation subjects showed significantly less avoidance and less subjective fear after treatment than the groups which had relaxation-hypnosis or no treatment (Figure 4.1). Mean drop in subjective anxiety during the avoidance test on a 10-point scale was 2·4 for desensitisation, 1·3 for relaxation-hypnosis and 1·0 for untreated subjects. 10 out of 23 subjects who had desensitisation (45%) did not improve—they had completed less than 15 items of the 20 item hierarchy during desensitisation.

2. Successful desensitisation was relatively independent of suggestibility.

3. Improvement of the snake phobia was followed by improvement in other fears on the Fear Survey Schedule.

4. Among subjects who had desensitisation the improvement in the snake phobia corresponded to the number of hierarchy items

completed successfully during treatment. Subjects who completed less than 15 items during treatment were no better than untreated patients, suggesting that the therapeutic task must be well advanced before significant gains are made.

5. The intensity of the phobia at the start of treatment did not affect the subsequent outcome with desensitisation.

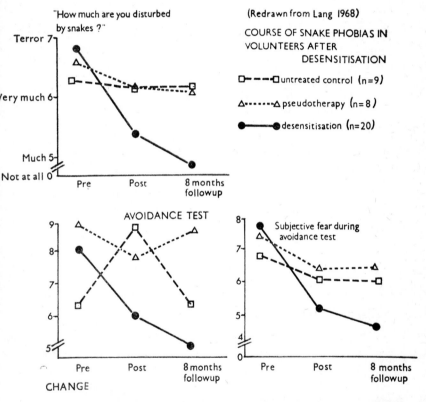

Fig. 4.1: Course of snake phobias in volunteers after desensitisation (Lang, 1968). From the chapter "The Mechanics of desensitisation and the laboratory of human fear", by Dr. P. J. Lang in Behaviour Therapy, edited by C. M. Franks. Used with permission of McGraw-Hill Book Co.

6. The total score on the Fear Survey Schedule, which correlates highly with the Taylor Manifest Anxiety Scale, correlated significantly negatively with improvement in desensitisation, suggesting that the presence of generalised anxiety adversely affected outcome.

7. Improvement in subjective reports of anxiety lagged behind that in overt avoidance behaviour. Avoidance scores differentiated between desensitised and untreated subjects immediately after

treatment, but it was not until the follow-up interview that the subjective scales yielded the same finding.

At follow-up eight months after desensitisation was completed the gains were maintained in the mean avoidance score, subjective anxiety rating and the snake item on the Fear Survey Schedule—in fact desensitisation subjects showed further improvement on the last two measures at follow-up (Lang, 1968. See Fig. 4.1).

Comment

The study by Lang and his colleagues provided the first adequate controlled evidence for the sustained efficacy of desensitisation in reducing phobias. It is important to note, however, that the snake phobias were usually reduced, not eliminated, and often much fear remained at the end of treatment while some subjects showed no improvement after desensitisation. Suggestion did not play a significant role in fear reduction, and generalised anxiety retarded the effect of desensitisation. In these studies, too, the complex nature of the fear response became evident, in that avoidance decreased significantly first, while improvement in subjective anxiety lagged behind. This finding was subsequently found also by Davison (1968).

Evidence from more recent work of this team suggests that the presence of a therapist during desensitisation is not essential for its efficacy (Melamed and Lang, 1968). This study contrasted 21 subjects with snake phobias who were randomly assigned into one of three groups: the first was a no treatment control. The second group of subjects were given desensitisation by a tape recorder on which they could control the speed of presentation of the stimuli. The third group of subjects were given live desensitisation individually by a therapist. In preliminary results both desensitisation groups showed greater reduction of avoidance than did controls (but p only $< \cdot 1$), and the automated group experienced greater decrease in subjective fear than the live desensitisation group (p $< \cdot 04$). An important qualification of this finding is that subjects who received automated desensitisation still expected to improve in their phobias, and saw a therapist before and after the automated series of sessions.

Studies by Paul

Paul (1966 & 1967) and Paul and Shannon (1966) studied the controlled effects of six procedures in male college volunteers on a speech course who had stage fright (fears of public speaking).

Subjects

96 men age 19–24 were selected from a college group of 710 students (14%) after completion of questionnaires about personality and anxiety. Selection was on the basis of indicated motivation for treatment, highest scores on performance anxiety scales and low falsification.

First study (Paul, 1965): *Experimental groups:* 96 subjects were allocated at random into 1 of 5 groups. Treatment was given over 5 weekly sessions.
1. *Individual Desensitisation:* (n = 15) Subjects were desensitised in imagination while completely relaxed, using a graded hierarchy.
2. *Insight psychotherapy:* (n = 15) Psychotherapy was focused on the area of public speaking. 3. *Attention placebo:* (n = 15) Subjects received a placebo capsule while doing a task in silence in the presence of the therapist. 4. *No treatment* (waiting list control): twenty-nine subjects were told that they would have to wait their turn before receiving treatment in the following semester, owing to the shortage of therapists.
5. *No contact:* Twenty-two subjects were not contacted at all.

Experimental measures
These were given before and after treatment for all treated groups. The "no treatment wait list" group was also assessed at the end of the waiting period. All groups had participated in the routine university tests of public speaking ability before treatment began and 6 weeks after treatment was completed. The measures were:

1. Anxiety scale questionnaire (self report)
2. Bendig's Extroversion-Introversion and Emotionality Scales (self report)
3. Interpersonal Anxiety scales in four stressful situations (self report)
4. Self-rating of confidence as a speaker
5. University test of public speaking ability—(objective behavioural assessment)
6. Pulse rate and palmar sweat index (physiological)

Results. Subjects who received individual desensitisation showed significantly more improvement than other groups on subjective reports of stage fright, the objective performance in a university test and in physiological measures (pulse rate and palmar sweat index and GSR) (see Fig. 4.2).

Second study (Paul and Shannon, 1966): Five groups of 10 subjects each were selected from the original larger groups used in the first study during the first university semester. Three groups—individual desensitisation, insight psychotherapy and attention placebo—had been treated during the first semester with concurrent enrolment in the speech course.

Ten subjects from the original "no treatment wait-list" group were now assigned to the 6th procedure—group desensitisation—during the second semester, after completion of the speech course. Each of five groups was matched for scores on all scales of the test battery for performance anxiety which had been obtained at original testing. The same measures were used as in the first study. The five groups were made up as follows:

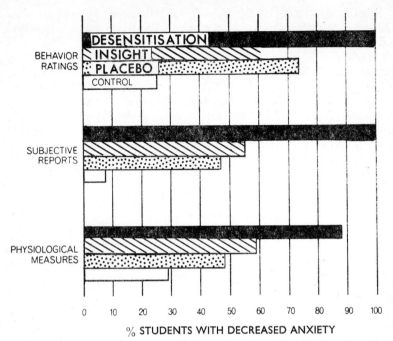

BEHAVIOR RATINGS
DESENSITISATION
INSIGHT
PLACEBO
CONTROL

SUBJECTIVE REPORTS

PHYSIOLOGICAL MEASURES

0   10   20   30   40   50   60   70   80   90   100

% STUDENTS WITH DECREASED ANXIETY

Fig. 4.2: Course of stage fright in volunteers after desensitisation (based on data from Paul, 1966).

1. *Group desensitisation:* 10 subjects who had spent three months on the waiting list for treatment. They were treated in 2 closed groups of 5 subjects each. They had 9 weekly sessions, 2 of which were spent in preliminary training in relaxation and 7 in systematic desensitisation in imagination along a 14–18 item hierarchy.

2. *Individual desensitisation:* 10 subjects, treated in the first study.
3. *"Insight psychotherapy":* 10 subjects, treated in the first study.
4. *Attention-placebo:* 10 subjects, treated in the first study.
5. *No contact:* 10 subjects, drawn by matching from the first study.

Results. Improvement with group desensitisation at least equalled individual desensitisation and both were significantly superior to results in the groups which had had insight psychotherapy, attention-placebo, simply a period on the waiting list, or no contact.

Treatment by group desensitisation resulted in significant reduction in stage-fright reported in a number of stressful situations, some reduction in other anxieties, and increased "extroversion" with decreased "emotionality". Objective performance in a university test also improved more than that in controls.

At follow-up 6 weeks after the end of desensitisation improvement was maintained.

Two years after treatment Paul (1967) followed up the subjects from the first study by posting questionnaires to them and obtained complete replies from all the tested subjects (n = 45) and from 70% of the controls (n = 31). As regards reduction in self report of stage fright (these scales were called "Speech Composite" by Paul), all three treatment groups showed significant improvement over controls, just as they had done at six weeks follow-up (Fig. 4.3). As at previous follow-up, the desensitisation group showed significantly more reduction in fear than the insight psychotherapy group (p < ·05). However, though desensitisation showed the same superiority to attention placebo as at six weeks follow-up, by two years follow-up this difference was no longer significant. The percentage significantly improved were 85% for desensitisation, 50% for insight psychotherapy and attention placebo, and 22% for untreated controls. A defect in this follow-up was the absence of any measure other than the subjects' self reports on various questionnaires.

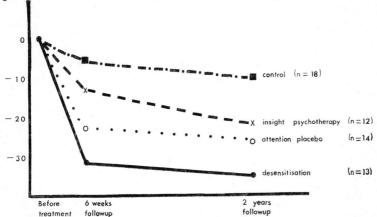

Fig. 4.3: Change in self report of stage fright over 2 years follow-up (Redrawn from Paul, 1967).

In general, therefore, the relative gains in focal treatment effects at 6 weeks follow-up were maintained over the subsequent 2 years. Though the attention placebo and insight psychotherapy groups improved significantly, the untreated control did not, the desensitisation group improved most, with no evidence of symptom substitution. The stability of improvement in all three groups is important and Paul (1967) suggested that no matter how change is brought about it is likely to be maintained in a supportive environment. In his subjects improvement from all three treatments was socially appropriate and was probably rewarded independent of the manner in which change initially came about. The lack of improvement in the untreated controls of Paul and of Lang is noteworthy in view of the myth of a two-thirds spontaneous improvement rate so frequently quoted for neurotic disorders.

A two year follow-up was also reported of subjects from the 2nd study (Paul, 1968) designed similarly to the previous assessment. Results again showed the desensitisation group to maintain its superior results on self-reports. In this investigation an objective measure was also reported—academic performance. Desensitisation subjects did significantly better than untreated controls in this regard.

Comment: This was a well designed and executed study whose results accord with those of other studies. Drawbacks were that 5 sessions are quite inadequate as a fair trial of the full potential of insight psychotherapy, and that the fear of public speaking was very mild in comparison with phobias seen clinically. This latter qualification will become important when we discuss implications of these results for psychiatric patients.

One other flaw is present in the design. One of the two long-term follow-ups was based solely upon questionnaire data sent through the post, so that no objective measure or independent witness was checked about validity of the self report.

Despite these flaws this series of studies is a good one with convincing results.

Study on the role of reward and therapeutic expectation

An important study by Leitenberg et al. (1968a) highlights the importance in desensitisation of verbal reinforcement of approach behaviour and the expectation of therapeutic benefit. They studied 27 female college students with snake phobias, and assigned them at random into one of three groups of 9 subjects each: 1. a control group which received treatment; 2. and 3. groups which both received 12 sessions of relaxation with desensitisation in imagination and in practice, but group 2 had desensitisation in the traditional manner, whereas subjects from group 3 had instructions designed to eliminate the expectation of improvement, and were simply told that their physiological responses would be measured while they visualised scenes. Furthermore, unlike the procedure in group 2, no praise was given when subjects from group 3 showed progress.

On testing at the end of treatment, decreased avoidance of snakes occurred in 9 subjects from group 2, in 6 subjects from group 3, and in 2 control subjects. Although both desensitisation groups improved significantly and the control group did not, improvement was significantly less in group 3. Leitenberg et al. concluded that therapeutically oriented instructions and selective positive reinforcement enhance the beneficial effects of systematic desensitisation. This might be because the patient receives constant feed-back from his own observations so that his behaviour can be changed in small steps to improvement.

Two flaws in this study do not affect the conclusions. There was only one measure of fear—the avoidance response, and no follow-up was reported.

Comparisons with the various control groups in different studies throw light on the mechanism by which desensitisation acts. This will be reviewed before the crucial question is raised about the effect of desensitisation in phobic patients as opposed to volunteers.

The Active components of Desensitisation

Granted that desensitisation is useful in phobic volunteers what ingredients of desensitisation are responsible for its effects? To answer this question studies in patients and in volunteers will be combined. The procedure of desensitisation involves graduated exposure to phobic stimuli along a hierarchy while the patient simultaneously has a contrasting experience such as relaxation. Usually he is relaxed and visualises a series of images of phobic situations, and later he also goes out to meet those situations in practice. Moreover, the patient expects to improve, is encouraged by the therapist at all stages, and develops a relationship with the therapist.

All these processes have been studied in desensitisation. Tables 4.4, 4.5 and 4.6 summarise the results for these and other variables which have been contrasted with the full desensitisation assembly of procedures. The full desensitisation procedure consistently gives better results than relaxation alone (otherwise known as extinction) (4·4B) or exposure to phobic stimuli without a hierarchy (otherwise known as flooding or implosion therapy) (4·4C). Desensitisation also gave better results than the visualisation of non-phobic scenes (4·4D).

Table 4.5 shows that desensitisation produced better results than suggestion under hypnosis (4·5E), than attention with a drug placebo (4·5F), or than an intense relationship with insight psychotherapy (4·5G). It deserves mention however, that significant improvement also occurred in some control groups which received hypnotic suggestions (Marks et al., 1968), attention with drug placebo (Paul, 1967), exposure (Schubot, 1966) or brief insight psychotherapy (Paul, 1967).

Studies which illuminate the role of the patient-therapist relationship in desensitisation are those which had psychotherapy controls, or where the therapist was absent during the desensitisation sessions, which were given instead by tape recorder, or where the quality of the relationship itself was manipulated.

In each of the three studies which had psychotherapy controls (Gelder et al., 1967; Lazarus, 1961; Paul, 1966) the desensitisation group did significantly better (Table 4.5G), even though the psychotherapy groups also showed improvement in two of the studies (Gelder et al., Paul). It follows that the benefit of desensitisation cannot be attributed solely to the relationship itself. This is borne out in two studies where the desensitisation was given by tape recorder with no therapist present during the procedure (Melamed and Lang, 1968; Donner, 1967). Desensitisation remained effective in the absence of the therapist, and his presence during the sessions did not produce consistent effects

Table 4.4. **Processes which have been compared with Desensitisation**
(Controlled trials in phobic subjects)

Process	Results	Type of fear	Population	n.	No. of sessions	Followup (months)	Study
A. Relaxation	Desen. better	Snakes	Students	8	9	0	Davison (1967)
	”	Spiders	”	3	11	3	Rachman (1965)
	”	Test anxiety	Students & children	10	12	5	Kondas (1967)
	”	Snakes	Students	8	9	3	Davison (1967)
B. Exposure i.e. Visualisation of phobic scenes along a hierarchy	”	Spiders	”	3	11	0	Rachman (1965)
	”	Snakes	”	11	11	0	Lomont & Edwards (1967)
C. Flooding (exposure without hierarchy; implosion)	” (but exposure group also improved)	Test anxiety	Students & children	5	12	5	Kondas (1967)
	”	Snakes	Students	15	9	0	Schubot (1966)
	”	Spiders	”	3	10	3	Rachman (1965)
D. Visualisation of non-phobic scenes	”	Snakes	”	8	9	0	Davison (1967)
	”	”	”	10	16	8	Lang et al. (1965)

Table 4.5. **Processes which have been compared with Desensitisation**
(Controlled trials in phobic subjects)

Process	Results	Type of fear	Population	n.	No. of sessions	Follow up (months)	Study
E. Suggestion and hypnosis	Desen. better (but hypnosis group also improved)	Mixed phobias	Psychiatric outpts.	14	12	9	Marks et al. (1968)
F. Attention-placebo.	”	Snakes	Students	10	16	8	Lang et al. (1965)
	” (but attention-placebo group also improved)	Stage fright	”	10	6	24	Paul & Shannon (1966)
G. Relationship to therapist 1. Intense psychotherapy	”	Agoraphobia Acro-claustrophobia	Psychiatric outpts.	26	60	12	Gelder et al. (1967)
	”		Volunteers	14	22	9	Lazarus (1961)
	” (but psychotherapy group also improved)	Stage fright	Students	10	6	24	Paul & Shannon (1966) Paul (1967)
2. Therapist absent, tape-recorder used	Des. works without therapist { bit better with therapist / bit worse with therapist	Test anxiety	”	14	8	<3	Donner (1968)
	”	Snakes	”	7	12	7	Melamed & Lang (1967)

Table 4.6. **Processes which have been compared with Desensitisation**
(Controlled trials in phobic subjects)

Process	Results	Type of fear	Population	n.	No. of sessions	Follow up (months)	Study
H. *Verbal reinforcement* (expectation of improvement)	*Des. signif. worse without reinforce-ment or expectation of improvement*	Snakes	Students	10	12	0	Leitenberg et al. (1968a)
I. *Conventional hospital care*	*No significant difference*	Agoraphobia	Psychiatric inpts.	10	60	12	Gelder & Marks (1966)
J. *Live modelling with exposure*	*Live modelling + exposure better (but des. group also improved)*	Snakes	Volunteers	12	7	1	Bandura (1968)
K. *Passage of time* (no treatment controls)	No significant improvement in any study. Desensitisation significantly better	,,	Children	14	—	8	Ritter (1968)
		,,	Students	11	—		Lang et al. (1965)
		,,	,,	10	—	0	Leitenberg et al. (1968a)
		,,	,,	4	—	0	Davison (1968)
		,,	,,	3	—	3	Rachman (1965)
		,,	,,	7	—	0	Melamed & Lang (1967)
		Stage fright	,,	10	—	0	Paul & Shannon (1966)
		Test anxiety	,,	14	—	3	Donner (1968)
		,,	Students & children	9	—	5	Kondas (1967)

(Table 4.5G).   Nevertheless, it may be important that the subjects expected to improve and saw the therapist before and after the desensitisation procedure, so that the subjects may have had subtle reinforcements apart from the tape recorder.

In the only study so far which has examined the role of praise of progress and expectation of improvement (Table 4.6 H), the effect of desensitisation was significantly impaired when these elements were removed from the treatment situation (Leitenberg et al., 1968a). Students in this study were simply told that it was an experiment about fear, and they were not praised when they reported a decrease in their fears during the sessions.   Since desensitisation produced greater benefit than the control methods reviewed in table 4.4, 4.5 and 4.6 despite the fact that all groups expected to improve, the greater value of desensitisation cannot simply be the result of the expectation of improvement.   From the study of Leitenberg et al., one concludes that it is not the mere fact of a relationship which is important but *what is done with that relationship*. Where the relationship is used to praise the subject when he progresses, this enhances results because he receives constant feed-back that his behaviour can be changed in small steps to improvement.   This can also be construed as a process of operant conditioning.   However, even without this element desensitisation still produced more improvement than no treatment at all, so that the counter-conditioning procedure itself remains an integral part of the effective procedure.   The term counter-conditioning is used purely descriptively to denote the way a subject is brought into graduated contact with the phobic situation during a contrasting state such as relaxation.

Desensitisation conferred no significant advantage in agoraphobic in-patients (Table 4.6 I). This was not because conventional hospital care is such an effective treatment but because severe agoraphobics are resistant to any treatment.   The nature of one's clinical material is one crucial factor which determines results, a point which will be expanded later.

Desensitisation consistently gives significantly better results than simple observation of subjects over a period of time—so-called "spontaneous improvement" (Table 4.6 K).   All these studies involved focal phobias in volunteers, not patients, and specific phobias are rather more stable in the absence of treatment than diffuse phobic states (Marks and Gelder, 1966).   Untreated control groups of patients with diffuse phobias have not yet been compared with desensitisation groups.

Only one procedure has been superior to desensitisation viz., live modelling with exposure along a hierarchy (Table 4.6 K).   In this study the subjects were volunteers with fears of snakes, and it will be of interest to see how far these findings can be repeated in patients.

Summarising these results, desensitisation has produced better results than relaxation alone, exposure alone along a hierarchy, exposure without a hierarchy, visualisation of non-phobic scenes, suggestion under hypnosis, drug placebo, psychotherapy, or no treatment. Though desensitisation is effective in the absence of a therapist, its effect is significantly impaired when subjects do not expect to improve and do not receive verbal reinforcement for reports of calmness.

It is true that some improvement was occasionally obtained with simple exposure to phobic images, suggestion-hypnosis, insight psychotherapy or attention with a drug placebo, but this was never as great as with the full desensitisation procedure. Desensitisation is thus an assembly of techniques several of which may contribute to improvement when used alone, but which produce the maximum effect when combined together.

That relaxation alone and exposure to phobic images alone are less effective than the two together supports the view that a process of counter-conditioning is involved. However there is very little evidence that a new response takes the place of the earlier phobic one. After successful treatment patients rarely state that when they think of phobic images they experience relaxation instead of tension. That repeated exposure to phobic images alone is not enough suggests that extinction or habituation is only one aspect of the mechanism of improvement. That verbal reinforcement significantly improves the results argues that operant conditioning plays an important part in the method. As the patient constantly monitors small changes in his affect during treatment and his reports of calmness are repeatedly reinforced by approval, so his fear is gradually diminished and he beomes more willing to meet the phobic situation. Many autonomic responses are subject to operant or instrumental control (Miller, 1966, 1968) and fear seems no exception to this rule.

Studies of Desensitisation in Patients

For the psychiatrist it is crucial to know whether results obtained in volunteers are also applicable to patients in the clinic, because patients usually have much more distressing phobias and other problems than volunteers. So far the only investigations of desensitisation to include control groups of patients have been published from the Maudsley Hospital (Table 4.7). Since results in patients are the acid test of the clinical value of desensitisation, these studies require description in some detail.

Retrospective trial of phobic in-patients and out-patients
(Cooper, Gelder and Marks, 1965; Marks and Gelder, 1965.)

The first study was a preliminary retrospective assessment of results in all patients who had had desensitisation and other behavioural techniques at the Maudsley Hospital by that time (1964). It was hoped to identify those patients who did well and then to do prospective studies of desensitisation in such patients. The study was necessarily

Table 4.7

Controlled Studies of Desensitisation: Phobic Patients

Study	Fear treated	No. of pts. in des. group	Length of follow-up (months)	Control procedure
Cooper et al. (1965)	Mixed phobias	41	12	Mixed treatment without des.
Marks and Gelder (1965)	,, ,,	31	12	Mixed treatment without des.
Gelder and Marks (1966)	Agoraphobia	10	12	Hospitalisation
Gelder et al. (1967)	Mixed phobias	16	12	Insight psychotherapy
Marks et al. (1968)	,, ,,	14	9	Hypnotic suggestion

retrospective, and rater bias had to be controlled by the use of "blind" assessors who rated behavioural patients and matched controls without knowing which group they belonged to. Because the study was retrospective, reliable information was only available about outcome and not about details of the treatment process itself.

In all, 77 patients were found who had had behaviour therapy until that time. These were matched with control patients with similar type, duration and severity of symptom, and similar age and sex. All available information about patients' symptoms and activities before and after treatment was then extracted from the case notes of the behavioural and control groups. Progress of patients at the end of treatment and over 12 months follow-up was rated blindly by two assessors working independently.

Of the 77 patients, 29 had severe agoraphobia, 12 had other more circumscribed phobias, while 10 had obsessive rituals and fears. The remaining patients had a variety of other neurotic omplaints. Patients with obsessive disorders did no better with behavioural treatments than with control methods, severe agoraphobics did slightly but not significantly better with graded retraining, while in the more focal phobias desensitisation in practice produced a useful improvement which diminished with time. Results for most of the agoraphobics and the milder phobias are shown in fig. 4.4.

Among the agoraphobics, percentage much improved at the end of treatment was 45% for desensitisation and 25% for the control group. Among the other phobics the percentage much improved at the end of treatment was 55% for desensitisation and 20% for controls. In the severe agoraphobics, most of them in-patients, desensitisation in practice had been carried out for a mean of 66 sessions, compared with 27 sessions for control treatments. Furthermore, these patients were not only retrained but also received skilled clinical casework for their personality and social problems. By comparison, in studies of desensitisation with volunteers which were reviewed earlier, treatment lasted on average only

12 sessions and problems other than the phobias were not usually dealt with.

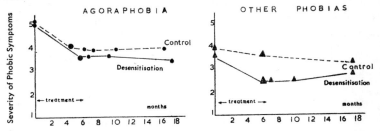

Fig. 4.4: Retrospective study of Marks and Gelder (1965): Course of phobias in severe agoraphobia and in milder phobias.   Score 5 = maximum disturbance.

Despite the vigour and enthusiam with which the patients had been treated in hospital, the results did not justify expenditure of such effort to re-train in-patient agoraphobics. However desensitisation in practicd did seem to be a useful procedure in patients with more circumscribee phobias, though these patients on average had 29 sessions of treatment. Another conclusion was that the nature of the clinical material was of great importance in affecting prognosis.   The commonly reported figure of a two-thirds improvement rate in mixed groups of neurotic patients is misleading in that it conceals marked differences in improvement rates from 0 to 100% in the course of different clinical syndromes depending upon the timing and degree of improvement under consideration.

These findings were then extended in four prospective studies. In these four studies the patient's progress was rated independently by the patient, by 2 doctors and by a psychiatric social worker. Relatives were interviewed to check reports by patients. For the crucial ratings in these studies—those of phobias—ratings of the 2 doctors correlated 0·81 with one another, while ratings of patients correlated 0·76 with those of the doctors. Ratings were made of 6 symptoms—the main phobias, other phobias, general anxiety, depression, depersonalisation and obsessions: of 5 areas of social adjustment—work, leisure, sex, family relationships, other relationships, and the patient filled in questionnaires about personality and symptoms—sections G,I,J, and L to R of the Cornell Medical Index (Brodman et al. 1949) the Eysenck Personality Inventory (Eysenck and Eysenck, 1964) and social and phobic check lists from the Tavistock Self-Assessment Inventory. (Dixon et al. 1957a & b).

Prospective study of severely agoraphobic in-patients
(Gelder and Marks 1966)
In the first prospective study 20 patients with severe agoraphobia were allocated at random to desensitisation or to a control group on admission as an in-patient or to a day hospital. Patients were included if

they presented with a main complaint of agoraphobia; severely depressed patients primarily requiring antidepressant treatment were excluded. These patients with agoraphobia complained of intense fears of going out alone into open spaces, into streets, shops, crowds, trains etc. All were severely handicapped by their symptoms which had been present for a mean of 7 years, their mean age at treatment was 34 years and 75% were women. Three-quarters were unable to leave the house un-accompanied, and their symptoms made it very difficult for them to work, shop, take their children to school, or enjoy their leisure. In addition to their phobias, patients in both groups presented other symptoms, such as fluctuating depressive mood, obsessions and minor degrees of depersonalisation; however, these were always less severe than their phobias. Sexual difficulties, mainly frigidity, were present in $\frac{3}{4}$ of the patients. All but 4 were married and had children. The desensitisation and the control groups were well-matched on several clinical variables.

Patients were treated by desensitisation in imagination and in practice while control patients had supportive psychotherapy. All patients were treated 3 times weekly over 5 to 6 months (a total of 60 to 70 sessions). Patients were rated every 2 weeks during treatment and every 3 months during a year's follow-up after treatment.

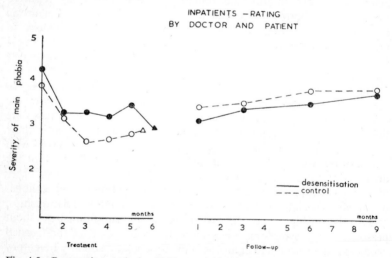

Fig. 4.5: Prospective study by Gelder and Marks (1966): Course of phobias in severely agoraphobic inpatients. Score 5 = maximum disturbance.

Results for the main phobias were disappointing and are seen in Fig. 4.5. Desensitisation and control treatments did not differ significantly in their effects. Both groups improved slightly in their main phobia, but were left with much residual social disability. The percentage of patients rated much improved at the end of treatment was 40% for desensitisation and 20% for controls. Patients did best who had few symptoms other than phobias. Attacks of panic and anxiety were one reason for the poor results. Patients who had recently overcome their fears sometimes reported that a single panic attack might undo the effects of weeks of treatment, and if less severe attacks of anxiety were repeated the fear might also be re-learnt. It was often extremely difficult to treat such attacks. The same conclusion emerged from this prospective study as from the previous retrospective one viz., that desensitisation can produce only limited changes in severe agoraphobia, although sometimes these can be worthwhile, e.g. in reducing a patient's fear of travelling to work, despite his retention of multiple other phobias.

When the poor results of desensitisation in severe agoraphobia were first published, 2 criticisms were levelled against them. The first was that the therapists were "novices" inexperienced in desensitisation. (Wolpe, 1965; Eysenck, 1965). The second asserted that desensitisation was used alone without regard for the complex nature of the patients' problems. (Lazarus 1966).

The first criticism overlooked the fact that Wolpe, Lazarus and most other workers in the field were themselves fairly new to desensitisation when they undertook their first studies. Most therapists in the retrospective study of Marks and Gelder (1965) were lecturers and senior lecturers in a University Department of Psychology who were well acquainted with the principles of desensitisation. Therapists in the prospective study (Gelder and Marks, 1966) were psychiatrists or psychiatrists in training, all supervised by a therapist with special experience of desensitisation. The therapists were at least as skilled in clinical techniques as the average clinician in a psychiatric teaching hospital. The aim of the studies was to answer the practical question "How valuable is desensitisation under routine hospital conditions?" For desensitisation to be of general value it has to be a technique which is learned fairly readily by most clinicians. This in fact occurred. Clinicians quickly mastered the technique of desensitisation and in suitable patients with focal phobias they obtained useful results with the method. The clinicians only failed to achieve success when they applied desensitisation to a different kind of patient. The fault lay not in the therapists but in the unsuitability of the technique itself for problems like severe agoraphobia.

The second criticism claimed that desensitisation had been applied too narrowly in severely agoraphobic patients, and that problems apart from the presenting phobias were not dealt with. In fact in both studies not only were patients desensitised, but they also received broad spectrum treatment in the form of skilled clinical casework, relatives were interviewed to unravel family problems, and sedative and antidressant drugs were given when required. Control groups received similar management, but without desensitisation. In both desensitisation groups the patients received 3 times more treatment than milder phobics in the retrospective and a later prospective study (Gelder et al. 1967) yet desensitisation only yielded superior results in the milder phobics who were treated much less vigorously. The evidence pointed over-whelmingly to the nature of the clinical material being the main reason for the failure of desensitisation in severe agoraphobia.

Close examination of uncontrolled work of Wolpe (1958) and Lazarus (1961) reveals that the clinical material determined their results just as it did in the later controlled studies. Their subjects were not in-patients, unlike the severe agoraphobics, and only required an average of 22 sessions of desensitisation, which is similar to the amount of desensitisa-tion required for milder phobics in the controlled studies. Yet when Wolpe (1964) treated a case with obsessive phobias, more than 100 sessions of desensitisation in imagination yielded very little result, and many more sessions of desensitisation in practice were required before any gains were obtained.

The main point is that every treatment has certain indications and contra-indications. Of course skill is important, but the most skilful therapist will obtain poor results with unsuitable patients. The practi-cal question is to delineate those conditions which can be successfully treated by therapists of moderate experience. The controlled studies did this to some extent.

Prospective study of phobic out-patients (Gelder, Marks and Wolff, 1967)
The second prospective trial examined a series of 42 less severely ill out-patients with a main complaint of one or more phobias. About half the patients had agoraphobia to a milder degree than the agoraphobics from the in-patient trial or the retrospective trial; for example, all could make the journey to out-patients with a companion, many could come alone, and associated symptoms of depression, anxiety and obses-sions were also less intense than in the in-patient series. About half the patients had other more circumscribed phobias like those included in the retrospective trial—these included phobias of animals and of social situations. Variables significantly differentiating out-patients from in-patients are seen in table 4.8. Mean age at treatment was 31 years, and mean duration of symptoms was 9 years. 67% of the patients were women.

Patients were allocated at random into 3 matched groups: 16 received desensitisation in imagination and in practice, 16 had group psycho-therapy, and 10 had individual psychotherapy. The 3 groups were well-matched on clinical variables. Treatment was carried out once a week in all groups, and lasted on average 6 months for desensitisation (25 sessions), 12 months for individual psychotherapy (50 sessions), and 18 months for group psychotherapy (75 sessions). Psychotherapy was analytically oriented, and was given by psychotherapists or by training psychiatrists under supervision of a psychotherapist.

Table 4.8

Comparison of inpatient and outpatient phobics: Mean scores at start of treatment

	Inpatients (Gelder and Marks, 1966)	Outpatients (Gelder et al., 1967)	
	Severe agoraphobics (n = 20)	Agoraphobics (n = 22)	Other phobics (n = 20)
Other phobias	3·8	3·2	2·9
General anxiety	3·0	2·6	2·2
Work adjustment	3·9	3·0	2·0
Cornell check list	35	26	22
Social anxiety list	17	12	13
Phobic list	13	10	7
Neuroticism—E.P.I.	33	30	26

Higher scores indicate greater disturbance.

Inpatients were significantly more disturbed than outpatients on every variable shown. Within the outpatients agoraphobics were more disturbed than other phobics, but less disturbed than the inpatient agoraphobics.

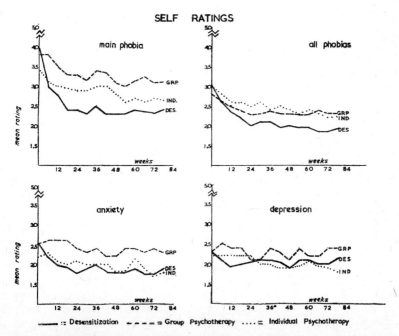

Fig. 4.6: Prospective study by Gelder, Marks and Wolff (1967): Course of phobias and other symptoms in mixed phobic outpatients: self ratings.

Patients were rated every 6 weeks over 18 months during treatment and follow-up, and were rated again 2 years after starting treatment.

Results are seen in Figs. 4.6 and 4.7. All raters agreed that of the 3 treatments, desensitisation produced greater and faster improvement in the main phobia than did other treatments. The difference became significant after 6 months but diminished later, as patients in psychotherapy went on improving slowly. At the end of follow-up desensitisation patients still showed the most improvement, though the difference

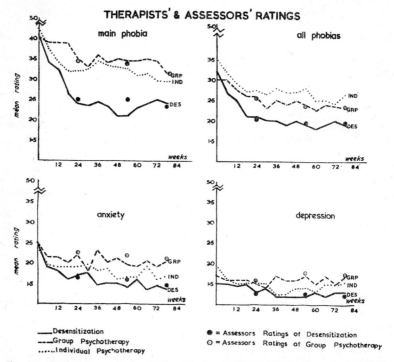

Fig. 4.7: Prospective study by Gelder, Marks and Wolff (1967): Course of phobias and other symptoms in mixed phobic outpatients: The 2 doctors' ratings.

was then no longer significant. Only 2 patients lost their symptoms, both with desensitisation. The percentage of patients whose phobias were rated much improved by 2 of 3 raters at the final rating were desensitisation 56%; group psychotherapy 13%; individual psychotherapy 30%. Figs. 4.6 and 4.7 show that desensitisation patients also improved more in all their phobias, and that they did not show any increase in their general anxiety or depression during treatment. There was no evidence that symptom substitution accompanied improvement. Ratings of social adjustment were less sensitive and reliable than symptom ratings. However, significantly greater and more rapid improvement occurred in leisure adjustment with desensitisation. These patients also improved significantly in work adjustment (fig. 4.8). No group of patients relapsed significantly after the end of treatment.

Patients who did badly with treatment tended to be agoraphobic, to be older at treatment, and to have more severe obsessive and other neurotic symptoms. Patients who did badly with desensitisation

Course of phobic outpatients

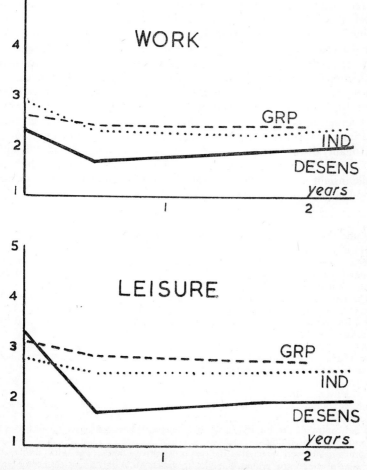

Fig. 4.8: Prospective study by Gelder, Marks and Wolff (1967): Course of work and leisure adjustment: The 2 doctors' ratings.

resembled the larger sample, but agoraphobia and high initial anxiety were relatively more important and age at treatment was unimportant. Neither the intensity nor the duration of a particular phobia was an important determinant of response to desensitisation; the important consideration was the extent of the disturbance in terms of number of phobias and other symptoms such as anxiety and depression.

Results of this study agreed with those of Marks and Gelder (1965) that milder phobias responded usefully to desensitisation. Patients whose phobias improved with desensitisation also improved in work and leisure adjustment. Although patients in psychotherapy did not improve much in their phobias, a few sometimes showed improvement in interpersonal relations, even though they did not improve in their phobias, and the change in interpersonal adjustment appeared related to events in psychotherapy. Though the different raters shared this impression, the rating scales for interpersonal adjustment were unsatisfactory and could not detect this change, so that the point requires further testing. It was concluded that desensitisation and insight psychotherapy can each contribute in different ways to the treatment of phobic patients. Where patients have a circumscribed phobia and good interpersonal adjustment, then desensitisation alone was indicated. However, psychotherapy could be offered as well to those patients whose phobias had improved with desensitisation but who were left with troublesome personality disturbances. In other words the 2 techniques had different indications. Desensitisation was indicated for relief of focal phobias while insight psychotherapy was not helpful for phobias, but might be useful in alleviating interpersonal difficulties.†

---

† **Criticisms of the clinical studies reviewed so far**

The clinical investigations discussed until now were stringently criticised by Paul 1968a). Since they have been widely read the criticisms require detailed correction. Some of the criticisms showed misunderstanding of the purpose and design of the work, while others were factually incorrect.

The retrospective study was a preliminary assessment of results of behaviour therapy in all patients treated in the past until 1964 at the Maudsley Hospital. This was a necessary survey before more definitive prospective studies were undertaken. Paul asked what the controls were controlling for. The anwer is for the effect of traditional hospital treatment. The problem was a practical one: phobic patients will always have a mixture of problems and so will need a variety of treatment procedures in the course of hospital treatment; does the addition of desensitisation confer any advantage over traditional treatments alone? Paul claimed that the controls were selected from a different population in terms of age, sex ratio and duration of disability; but this statement is incorrect, as was the suggestion that there were more experienced clinicians in the control group. Finally, it was claimed that rater bias was not controlled for, but in fact the two independent assessors had no idea which patients they were rating.

Similar sallies were directed at the two prospective studies. The critic dismissed the value of the control groups, implying mistakenly that only a no-treatment group is a valid control. The control group which is relevant depends of course upon one's question. The prospective studies were designed to answer the same question as the

Cross-over study of phobic outpatients (Gelder and Marks, 1968)

A third prospective study was a cross-over design in which desensitisation was given to those phobic patients who had not improved with group psychotherapy in the trial of Gelder et al. (1967). Of the 16 phobic patients who had had group psychotherapy for 18 months, 7 had not improved 6 months after treatment ended. These patients were then desensitised. Ratings and raters were the same as before.

Raters agreed that on average phobic patients improved about 3 times as much in the 4 months of desensitisation as they had done in the previous 2 years (Fig. 4.9). Changes in other symptoms were less

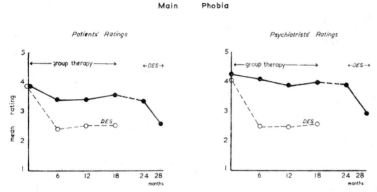

Fig. 4.9: Crossover study of Gelder and Marks (1968): Changes in mean rating of main phobia during group therapy and subsequent desensitisation. (Changes in original desensitisation group shown for comparison).
●———● = crossover patients (n = 7). o————o = original desensitisation group (n = 16).

striking. This confirmed the original findings that most change occurred in that area on which desensitisation focused. The treated phobias changed more than the untreated phobias, while general anxiety

---

retrospective study viz. does traditional treatment plus desensitisation do better than traditional psychiatric treatment alone? It was erroneously claimed that the second medical assessor based ratings upon therapists' interviews or case notes, but in fact they were based upon independent interviews by the assessor.

Paul was correct in pointing out that the assessors were not "blind", but this was impossible to arrange since any extensive interview gave passing clues about the treatment involved. To minimise this problem patterns of change were looked for across every set of raters. Paul quoted the misleading correlation of ·67 for all symptom ratings combined, when in fact the ratings of main importance for the study—those of the phobias—had a mean reliability of ·77.

Also criticised was the inexperience of the therapists, but they were all trained in desensitisation in the same way as those employed in his own studies. Similar inaccuracies marred Paul's account of the outpatient study, where he discovered "lack of reliability between ratings" without evidence and contrary to the figures reported in the paper.

and depression changed least. It was particularly striking that changes occurred in a few months in those patients who had resisted so much earlier treatment by group psychotherapy.

Desensitisation lasted only 4 months on average in the cross-over patients, whereas patients who were desensitised from the start needed about 6 months treatment. This finding resembles that of Lazarus (1961) with volunteer subjects who had isolated phobias: he too found that subjects who had had group psychotherapy (for 22 sessions) improved faster than when desensitised from the start. It may be that desensitisation takes place more speedily after group psychotherapy because the latter resolves some social and personality problems, leaving the phobias as a more isolated disorder and thus more amenable to desensitisation.

The crossover report also described one patient who received both group psychotherapy and desensitisation over the same period of time. Detailed assessment showed the role of each treatment. Group psychotherapy had very little immediate effect on the phobias, whereas desensitisation was followed by an immediate improvement in those phobias which had been treated during the session. This improvement was significantly greater than that produced by group psychotherapy. Much of this improvement which was found immediately after desensitisation was lost by the end of the week, but even so, desensitised phobias retained twice as much improvement as untreated phobias. No other symptom showed this consistent improvement which accumulated week by week until eventually the effect was seen in the patient's extending her range of daily activities.

This study added to previous evidence that desensitisation has a specific effect on phobic symptoms in psychiatric patients.

Phobic outpatients: Prospective comparison of desensitisation with hypnosis (Marks, Gelder and Edwards, 1968)

In this prospective trial, desensitisation was compared with hypnotic suggestion in phobic patients who were similar to those in the previous outpatients study. Mean age at treatment was 32 years, mean symptom duration was 11 years, and 64% of the patients were women. 43% of the patients were agoraphobics.

Twenty-eight patients were originally allocated at random into 2 equal groups of 14 which received either desensitisation or suggestions of improvement under hypnosis. Patients were treated individually, and were rated before and after 12 weekly sessions of treatment. After a delay patients who were unimproved then had 12 sessions of the alternative procedure in a crossover design. 23 patients finally had desensitisation (14 + 9) while 18 patients finally had hypnosis (14 + 4).

Ratings and raters were the same as in the previous prospective studies. All patients were rated before, during and after treatment, and a year after treatment first began.

Both desensitisation and hypnosis produced significant improvement in phobias. All raters agreed that desensitisation produced rather more improvement in phobias than did hypnosis, but only one set of ratings differed significantly. Most patients were left with some residual disability at the end of each treatment. No prognostic variables could be identified to predict improvement with desensitisation within this sample of patients.

Changes in this study were very similar to those observed in the previous investigation of phobic outpatients (Gelder et al. 1967) and in phobic volunteers (Lang et al., 1965). Thus for the main phobia on a 5-point scale, in this study patients improved 1·0 and 0·7 points for desensitisation and hypnosis respectively. In the previous outpatients study improvement for the main phobia after 12 weeks' treatment was respectively 1·1, 0·6 and 0·2 points for desensitisation, individual and group psychotherapy. In the volunteers improvement was respectively 1·1 and 0·6 points for desensitisation and hypnosis subjects after 16 sessions of treatment (correcting for differences in scaling procedures).

Why then did this study generally not yield significant differences between the two treatments? The consistency of trend among all raters makes it rather unlikely that the difference was simply due to chance. Closer inspection showed that short duration of treatment in a variable patient population was probably an important factor. In the outpatient study of Gelder et al. (1967) the difference between desensitisation and psychotherapy, though similar to the present study at 12 weeks, only became significant at 24 weeks; in the retrospective study of Marks and Gelder (1965) the significant difference between graded retraining and a control treatment was obtained after a mean of 29 sessions of treatment.

One cannot ignore the similarity of decrement in main phobia achieved in these 3 separate studies of desensitisation. It suggests that the same general process was at work. How much benefit a patient derives from a certain decrement in the main phobia will of course depend upon the extent of his phobias relative to his other difficulties. The more focal the phobia and the fewer the other problems the less is the amount of desensitisation required to benefit the patient. In this context it is worth repeating that although in volunteers desensitisation produced significantly more improvement than control methods after a mean of only 12 sessions, in those phobic patients where it was useful significant differences were only obvious after 24 sessions of desensitisation.

How did hypnosis produce improvement? Both relaxation and suggestion might have placed a part. Suggestion could act by counteracting the anticipatory anxiety which phobic patients experience before they enter a feared situation. If the effects of suggestion are long lived, they will see the patient through a number of new situations without anticipatory anxiety, so that a form of desensitisation will occur.

Physiological predictors of response to desensitisation
(Lader, Gelder & Marks, 1967)

Patients who were desensitised in the 5 trials just described were tested to see whether physiological correlates of prognosis could be obtained. All underwent a standardised laboratory procedure. Their palmar skin conductance was recorded during 20 pure-tone auditory stimuli, each of 100 dB intensity and 1 second duration applied automatically at intervals ranging from 45 to 80 seconds. Measures derived included the rate of habituation of the GSR's and the number of spontaneous fluctuations in skin conductance.

Thirty-six patients were treated—11 agoraphobics, 8 social phobics and 17 animal phobics. Animal phobics habituated more rapidly and had fewer fluctuations than the other 2 groups of patients and in these respects resembled normals. This group also showed the best response to desensitisation.

Rapid habituation and few spontaneous fluctuations correlated significantly with clinical improvement and with low overt anxiety (see Table 4.9). A discriminant function analysis employing these physiological variables discriminated well between patients who had a good and a bad social outcome (Fig. 4.10). This analysis omitted 6 patients who had no social disability to begin with.

Table 4.9

Palmar skin conductance and clinical correlates
(Lader, Gelder and Marks, 1967)

	Improvement with des.	Overt anxiety	Spontaneous fluctuations
Habituation rate	·49	— ·36	— ·58
Spontaneous fluctuations	— ·42	·61	
Overt anxiety	— ·52		

If correlation > ·33, p < ·05
  „ „   > ·42, p < ·01
  „ „   > ·53, p < ·001

Interpretation of these findings are necessarily complex. One might regard the physiological measures as concomitants of anxiety and therefore the patients with good outcome would be those with the lowest levels of anxiety. Other studies suggested (Gelder and Marks, 1966; Lazarus, 1963) that the presence of anxiety tends to interfere with progress of treatment by desensitisation in two ways, first by encouraging partial relapse between treatment sessions, and second by interfering with the progress of desensitisation. Findings from this study support the second suggestion, that anxiety may impair response to the desensitisation procedure itself, since the habituation procedure to individual auditory stimuli in the laboratory resembles the desensitisation technique with anxiety-evoking stimuli in treatment. Patients who do not habituate readily to auditory stimuli probably do not habituate well with desensitisation and so have a poorer prognosis. This poor habituation is accompanied by subjective anxiety and panic attacks at rests. These features are the hallmark of severe agoraphobia rather than of other kinds of phobia.

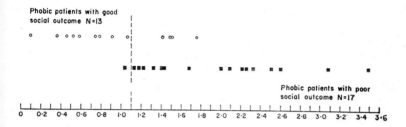

Fig. 4.10: Discriminant function score of autonomic activity as a predictor of social disability after treatment (Lader, Gelder and Marks, 1967). The discriminant function score for each patient is obtained by substitution of the patients' values in the equation: Discriminant score $= -0{\cdot}03488$ (habituation rate) $+ 0{\cdot}02035$ (spontaneous fluctuations) $+ 1{\cdot}81975$ ("habituator"). 6 patients were omitted from this sample because they had no social disability.

The other reason for the poorer prognosis of anxious phobics is the fact that even after their phobias have been desensitised they are liable to sudden panic attacks in the course of which phobias are regenerated, usually of the agoraphobic variety. These patients have much anxiety at rest, and this is reflected by the high level of physiological arousal, as testified by their spontaneous fluctuations. Lader and Wing (1966) suggested this may trigger off episodes of positive feedback which are seen clinically as panic attacks.

Severe agoraphobia: Retrospective study of modified leucotomy
(Marks, Birley and Gelder, 1966)

Further light on the role of anxiety in the treatment of agoraphobia comes indirectly from a serial retrospective study of modified leucotomy. This operation damages far less nervous tissue than the standard leucotomy of earlier times and so carries less risk of producing serious personality change.

Twenty-two patients were studied who had had a modified leucotomy in the past for severe phobias and general anxiety. They were more severely disturbed than the phobic patients in the studies described earlier, and had had extensive treatments of many kinds without lasting benefit. Cases were excluded in which the phobias were part of a depressive or paranoid illness. Thirteen patients were from one hospital (Series A) and 9 were from a second hospital (series B). The two series were matched separately with control patients who had similar type, duration and severity of symptom, and similar age and sex. As only 16 fully suitable controls were available there was some overlap across the series. Both series and their controls corresponded closely on all matching variables. Mean age at treatment was 39 years, mean symptom duration was 16 years. 82% of the patients were women.

Methods of rating followed those of the earlier retrospective study (Cooper et al., 1965; Marks and Gelder, 1965). All available information about patients' symptoms and activities before and after treatment was extracted from the case notes. Progress of patients at the end of treatment and over 5-years follow-up was rated blindly by 2 independent assessors; these reached good agreement about changes in phobias, anxiety and depression.

Results were similar in Series A and B, and are seen in Fig. 4.11. Through 5 years follow-up leucotomy patients did significantly better than controls with respect to phobias and general anxiety; depression remained mild; work adjustment improved markedly. At 3 years follow-up phobias were rated much improved in 64% of leucotomy patients and 31% of controls. Personality changes after operation were mild and not related to outcome.

Maximum improvement of general anxiety occurred within the first three months, whereas phobias continued to improve until 3 years' follow-up (Fig. 4.11).

Poorer outcome was associated with an anxious, shy, premorbid personality with prominent depression before operation.

It was concluded that modified leucotomy had a useful part to play in highly selected patients with long-standing severe agoraphobia and anxiety.

How did modified leucotomy produce improvement? The operation aims to cut thalamo-frontal fibres thought to play a part in maintaining anxiety (Falconer and Schurr, 1959). The dramatic fall of anxiety, which was maximal soon after operation in both series A and C, points to a direct effect of the operation.

By contrast, phobias in both series improved more gradually, which suggests that gradual relearning played some part in the improvement of phobias after operation had reduced the general anxiety. The course of several cases illustrates this. One patient had had 3 months' intensive desensitisation in practice before leucotomy without lasting benefit; several weeks after leucotomy she had a further 3 months of desensitisation; this time she made good progress, until at one year she was almost symptom-free—her anxiety had been reduced immediately after operation, thus allowing retraining to proceed successfully. A second patient lost much of her anxiety immediately after operation, but did not lose her phobias until many months later, when in an emergency she ran alone into the street for the first time and found that she did not feel anxious; thereafter she gradually went out further. Thus it appears that leucotomy reduced anxiety directly; once anxiety diminished, phobias improved gradually, at least partly through relearning. Phobias changed less in patients who were depressed or had anxious personalities perhaps partly because they were less inclined to go out and so met

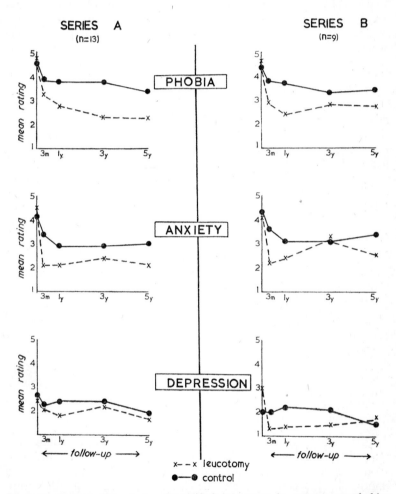

Fig. 4.11: Retrospective study of modified leucotomy in severe agoraphobia: (Marks, Birley and Gelder, 1966). Mean ratings for Series A and B throughout 5 years follow-up. Initial ratings on admission; subsequent ratings date from time of operation (or discharge from admission for controls). Ratings of 5 and 1 indicate maximum and no disturbance respectively.

fewer opportunities for relearning, whilst active sociable patients met more opportunities for learning to reduce their phobias.

It was mentioned earlier that severe agoraphobics often begin to improve with desensitisation and then have a sudden unexpected attack of panic, in, say a crowded shop, after which the patient will not venture out again into the shop for fear that the panic attack will recur there. Once severe general anxiety has occurred it is attached secondarily to its setting and a phobia has developed. In patients with such general anxiety, desensitisation becomes a sisyphean task because of the repeated regeneration of phobias. In the leucotomy series, as soon as the operation had reduced anxiety this obstacle was removed, and desensitisation could then be applied usefully, as in the case described.

Summary of controlled studies in patients

Table 4.10 and Fig. 4.12 summarise the results of four of the studies described above. In two separate groups of severe agoraphobics desensitisation conferred no significant advantage over other forms of treatment, whilst in two separate groups of patients with more focal phobias including mild agoraphobia desensitisation did produce significantly more improvement than did the control procedures. The type of patient being treated was clearly a crucial variable, patients with circumscribed phobias and few other symptoms improving most with desensitisation.

Table 4.10
Percentage of patients who were much improved after treatment

	Percentage	
	Desensitisation	Control
Specific phobias: Retrospective Study		
(Marks and Gelder, 1965)	55	20
Mixed phobias: Prospective study		
(Gelder *et al.*, 1967)	56	19
Severe agoraphobia: Retrospective study		
(Marks and Gelder, 1965)	45	25
Severe agoraphobia: Prospective study		
(Gelder *et al.*, 1967)	40	20
	Leucotomy	Control
Severe agoraphobia: Retrospective study		
(Marks *et al.*, 1966)		
(figures at 3 years follow-up)	64	31

Milder phobias which did not improve during group psychotherapy improved after a crossover design in which they received desensitisation. In another study both desensitisation and hypnosis produced significant improvement in milder phobics, desensitisation producing rather more improvement, but not significantly so.

Once phobias improved fresh symptoms did not develop, i.e. there was no symptom substitution. On the contrary, improvement in phobias allowed patients to improve in other aspects like work and leisure adjustment.

Predictors of a poor response to desensitisation were the presence **of** agoraphobia, severe obsessive and other neurotic symptoms, high general ("free floating") anxiety, and physiological correlates of anxiety such as slowed habituation of the galvanic skin response and increased spontaneous fluctuations of palmar skin conductance.

Poorer results in severe agoraphobics were largely due to their general anxiety. Once this anxiety was relieved by modified leucotomy then phobias could usefully be unlearned or desensitised.

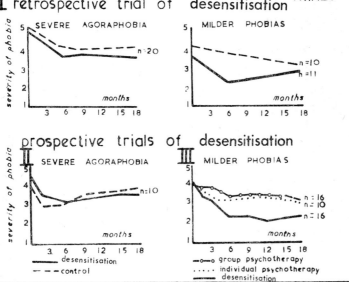

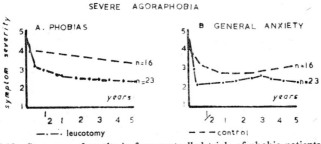

Fig. 4.12: Summary of results in four controlled trials of phobic patients: Mean ratings of phobias.

I   = study of Marks and Gelder (1965)
II = study of Gelder and Marks (1966)
III = study of Gelder, Marks and Wolff (1967)
IV = study of Marks, Birley and Gelder (1966)

Discussion of results in patients

The findings point to an important limitation to the value of desensitisation in psychiatric patients, since few patients require treatment for focal phobias without general background anxiety. The best results with desensitisation are obtained where patients closely resemble the volunteers used in the studies cited earlier. Unfortunately this similarity is found in only a small minority of psychiatric patients. In this minority, however, desensitisation is a useful treatment. In patients with more extensive phobias desensitisation can still occasionally be of limited value, e.g. in reducing an agoraphobic's fear of travelling to work despite his retention of multiple other phobias.

After desensitisation very few patients lose all their phobias, and most are left with some residual disability. However, there is little tendency to relapse except in anxious agoraphobics or during periods of depression, so that any improvement is useful even though it does not amount to a cure.

An advantage of desensitisation is the ease with which clinicians can learn the technique and obtain good results with it in suitable patients. However, desensitisation is often a lengthy treatment. About 20 sessions are the average to achieve definite gains. Furthermore, desensitisation can be intensely boring for the therapist. This is a real drawback since many therapists will be reluctant to embark on a protracted and tedious procedure to achieve rather limited goals.

The cost-effectiveness of a treatment is an important consideration in deciding whether or not to use it. Unfortunately, desensitisation is often costly in time and limited in effectiveness. If a patient has a very mild focal phobia of an object which he does not encounter much in everyday life, e.g. snakes in Britain, there is little point in embarking on desensitisation when the busy clinician has many distressed patients who require treatment for urgent problems. Equally, desensitisation is not economical in an anxious agoraphobic with multiple fears, with whom hundreds of therapeutic hours will be required for slender gains which are liable to be lost at any moment. On the other hand, if a patient with a bird phobia cannot get to work for fear of birds which are prevalent in the streets around her, then a lot of time spent in desensitisation may well be justified. Similarly, desensitisation might be valuable to help an agoraphobic woman simply take her child to and from school even if one leaves her many other fears untouched. In any given case the cost-effectiveness of desensitisation has to be weighed up.

In psychiatric patients desensitisation is simply one tool in the total context of psychiatric management. Clinical skill is required to assess the detailed handicaps of each patient, and many techniques additional to desensitisation may be necessary for other problems which are found so frequently in phobic patients. Measures such as drugs, rehabilitation training, family counselling and insight psychotherapy may all be required in selected patients. Desensitisation inevitably has to be part of a broad therapeutic approach, and its aims and importance will differ from one patient to the next.

Methods to facilitate desensitisation

Several methods have been tried to apply desensitisation more economically. One way is to save the therapist's time through group desensitisation or by automated desensitisation. Another possible method is to speed up the desensitisation process itself by the use of drugs or other manoeuvres.

1. Group desensitisation

This is the administration of desensitisation to several subjects simultaneously. At least 5 controlled trials of desensitisation have employed this method and shown it to be significantly superior to techniques without desensitisation (Donner, 1968; Kondas, 1967; Paul and Shannon, 1966; Lazarus, 1961; Ritter, 1968). Paul and Shannon (1966) showed that results with group desensitisation at least equal those with individual desensitisation.

Group desensitisation is particularly suited to groups of subjects who share the same stereotyped phobia. This has often been the case in experiments with volunteers. However, the phobias of psychiatric patients are far less stereotyped and show much individual variability in the details of their phobic stimuli. Furthermore, patients progress in desensitisation at widely varying speeds which are not readily catered for in a group situation. Group desensitisation is therefore less practicable for most psychiatric patients. It might, however, be useful for teaching groups of patients to relax before desensitising them individually afterwards, thus saving some time for the therapist.

2. Automated desensitisation

At least 2 controlled studies have reported that desensitisation was successful when administered by a tape recorder (Melamed and Lang, 1968; Donner, 1968). Subjects were volunteers who expected to derive therapeutic benefit, and saw the therapist before and after desensitisation, so that there was some therapist contact, albeit an attenuated one. Migler and Wolpe (1967) reported an uncontrolled case of successful automated desensitisation.

Automated desensitisation holds some promise in volunteers. No studies in patients have yet been reported. A potential snag in patients is the variability of their phobic stimuli and the uneven speed of their progress. It is also possible that the time involved in preparing a tape recording suitably tailored to each patient's needs may equal that involved in routine desensitisation. Nevertheless, this method deserves further exploration.

3. Drugs to speed up desensitisation

D. Friedman (1966a) suggested that desensitisation was speeded up if given while patients were under the influence of small doses of a short-acting barbiturate such as methohexitone.   This drug is rapidly meta-bolised and excreted so that its effects have almost disappeared 20 minutes after intravenous injection. In Friedman's technique the patient first prepares a hierarchy in the usual way. A 2·5% solution of methohexitone is then prepared by adding 20 mls. of distilled water to 500 mgs. of methohexitone. With the patient in a reclining position the drug is injected slowly into a vein in the antecubital fossa until he feels calm and relaxed. More is injected as necessary to maintain this state, and the needle is kept in the vein throughout treatment. 25–50 mgs. methohexitone is usually just sufficient to induce relaxation with no cognitive impairment. Desensitisation is administered in the usual way while the patient is relaxed under the influence of methohexitone instead of by the traditional muscular technique of relaxation. Recovery from the drug occurs 3–4 minutes after withdrawal of the needle and the patient may drive himself home after the session.

Friedman and Silverstone (1967) claimed encouraging results in an uncontrolled series of 20 phobic patients. Early controlled trials of the method have not had particularly encouraging results (Yorkston et al., 1968; Mawson, unpublished).

The use of other drugs in phobic disorders will be discussed later.

4. Massed versus spaced desensitisation

Learning in general occurs better under conditions of spaced (distributed) practice rather than massed practice. Since desensitisation can in some ways be construed as a learning situation, a potentially important variable is the rate of presentation of phobic stimuli during desensitisation.

Ramsay et al. (1966) examined this variable in 20 students with fears of animals and insects. During spaced desensitisation subjects imagined fear situations 20 times during each 20 minute session given once daily over 4 days. During spaced practice subjects imagined fear situations 40 times during each of two 40 minute sessions given on day 1 and 4. Subjects were thus balanced for time spent in treatment, number of images seen and times between testing. Both groups showed signifi-cantly reduced subjective fear, but spaced desensitisation yielded significantly greater reduction than did massed desensitisation. No avoidance test was given and there was no follow-up.

In an agoraphobic patient Sergeant (1965) compared the effects of spaced desensitisation given at the rate of 6 stimuli a minute with massed desensitisation given at the rate of 12 stimuli a minute. Improve-ment between sessions was significantly better for spaced than for massed desensitisation. In fact, massed desensitisation made the patient rather worse.

Evidence suggests, therefore, that desensitisation produces better results when done more slowly. It is not clear, however, what the optimum rate should be.

5. Standard versus individually tailored hierarchies in desensitisation

During group or automated desensitisation for subjects with stereotyped phobias it is possible that time need not be spent drawing up fresh hierarchies for each subject, but that a standard hierarchy for that fear would suffice. In students with examination anxiety Emery and Krumboltz (1968) compared the effects of standard versus individually-tailored hierarchies, and found that subjects improved equally with either type of hierarchy, desensitisation with both types producing significantly more reduction in subjective fear than occurred in controls with no treatment.

In psychiatric patients use of a standardised hierarchy is not generally desirable since patients vary greatly in the details of stimuli which trigger their phobias and important stimuli may easily be missed. In any case hierarchy construction does not take long, so little is to be gained by using a standard hierarchy.

Desensitisation in imagination and in practice

Wolpe's main contribution to psychiatry was his technique of desensitisation in imagination. The technique allowed treatment of a far wider range of situations than was possible by desensitisation in practice alone. Clearly it is much easier and quicker for patients to imagine travelling by train or being in a thunderstorm than having to go through those experiences in real life. Most desensitisation today combines both desensitisation in imagination and in practice, i.e. the patient is first accustomed to the phobic situation in fantasy and is then asked gradually to enter it in real life outside the treatment situation.

How effective is desensitisation in imagination compared to desensitisation in practice? These two modes of desensitisation have been contrasted in 2 studies in volunteers. In students with fears of rats Cooke (1966) noted that desensitisation in practice and in imagination produced similar reduction in avoidance. In students with snake phobias Garfield et al. (1967) found that desensitisation in imagination alone produced less improvement than desensitisation combined both in fantasy and in practice.

In a related problem Ritter (1968) contrasted vicarious desensitisation alone with vicarious desensitisation plus desensitisation in practice. 44 children with fears of snakes were assigned to one of three treatment conditions: (1) Vicarious desensitisation—children observed models engage in gradually bolder inter-actions with a tame snake over 2 sessions; (2) Contact desensitisation—children not only observed those models but themselves were brought into gradual physical contact with the snake itself; (3) Control children who had no treatment.

In the results both desensitisation groups showed significantly less avoidance than untreated controls, but contact desensitisation yielded significantly greater reduction of avoidance than vicarious desensitisation alone. Percentages completing the terminal task of the avoidance test were 80% for contact desensitisation, 53% for vicarious desensitisation and 0% for controls.

In an elegant study of a similar problem Bandura (1968) assigned 48 adult volunteers with snake phobias to one of four treatment conditions: (1) symbolic desensitisation—subjects were desensitised in the usual way; (2) self-regulated symbolic modelling—subjects watched a film of models engaging in gradually bolder inter-actions with a tame snake, were taught to relax throughout the procedure, and also controlled the rate of presentation of the film sequence (vicarious desensitisation by film alone); (3) live modelling with contact desensitisation

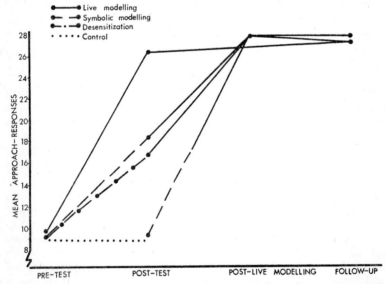

Fig. 4.13: Treatment of snake phobic volunteers by 1) desensitisation 2) symbolic modelling 3) live modelling with practical retraining. (Bandura, 1968; Bandura, Blanchard and Ritter, 1968). All 3 groups improved more than untreated controls, but the live modelling group did best. In a crossover design the desensitisation and symbolic modelling groups then had live modelling with practical retraining and improved to the level of the original group which had had live modelling.

(vicarious desensitisation plus desensitisation in practice). These subjects watched models engaging in gradually bolder inter-action with a snake in real life instead of in a film, and then were brought into gradual physical contact with the actual snake itself; (4) no treatment control. At the end of treatment and 1 month follow-up all the 3 treated groups avoided significantly less than the untreated controls (Fig. 4.13). However, the group which had live modelling with desensitisation in practice (group 3) did significantly best with regard to decreased avoidance and change in attitude and subjective fear during the avoidance test. The group which had self-regulated symbolic modelling (group 2) did next best, and the group which only had desensitisation in imagination (group 1) did only third best. When groups 1 and 2 subsequently had live modelling in a cross-over design they improved further to the same extent as the original live modelling group (Fig. 4.13).

It appears therefore that the more the subject is allowed to engage in graduated contact with the real life situation itself as opposed simply to the fantasy alone, the better he does. This fact is recognised in the current practice of usually combining desensitisation in imagination and in practice whenever possible. Clearly desensitisation in practice is not always feasible e.g., in fears of thunderstorms and lightning these cannot be produced at will and films and tape recordings of these events may not suffice. Similarly, in phobias of sexual situations our present culture will permit desensitisation in imagination but will baulk at guided desensitisation in practice.

Transfer of improvement from imagined to real situations

Clinical impression suggests that when fears have been reduced in patients' fantasies during desensitisation the patient is usually more willing to face them in the real life situation and indeed this is confirmed by the improvement noted in controlled trials which were reviewed earlier in this chapter. However, there is great individual variability in the amount of transfer. In 3 students with spider phobias Rachman (1966b) found that adequate exposure to the imaginary stimulus usually produced an immediate reduction in fear responses to the real object. However, these immediate reductions in fear were not always stable. During the succeeding hours and days reduction in fear was partially lost in 38% of instances, though in 48% further decrease in fear did not occur.

Agras (1967) studied the transfer of improvement from imagined to real situations during the desensitisation of 5 agoraphobic patients. Improved performance in the feared situation lagged well behind progress during desensitisation in all but one subject, though gradual improvement did eventually appear in real life. Diminution of the galvanic skin responses to images of phobic scenes accompanied progress in desensitisation of fantasies, but individuals varied in this.

Patients find it easier to transfer improvement outside treatment if shortly after the end of a treatment session they can enter a phobic situation similar to the one just treated. This is often not feasible either because their phobic object is rare, or more commonly because in real life the degree of exposure to a phobic situation is not so easily controlled as it is in treatment, and the patient is afraid of excessive exposure which will enhance rather than reduce fear.

Certain phobic patients find that though they are clearly able to visualise their phobic situations in treatment they feel perfectly calm during the fantasy and are unable to experience any anxiety. Yet as soon as they encounter the identical situation outside treatment they experience anxiety once more. This phenomenon may be termed "dissociation" and constitutes a real drawback to treatment, since such patients do not produce any anxiety to be desensitised in imagination.

Occasionally with repetition of the fantasy in increasing detail the patient learns to experience the anxiety, but some patients never manage to do so. In such cases the technique of desensitisation in imagination is inappropriate and little transfer of training can be expected from fantasy to real life. Lang (1968) noted some evidence that improvement occurs mainly where phobic images were accompanied by mild anxiety (as opposed to panic or no anxiety) but systematic study of the importance of anxiety with the images remains to be done.

Speed of change of different components of fear

"Fear is not some hard phenomenal lump that lives inside people that we may palpate more or less successfully. On the contrary, . . . fear is a loosely woven fabric of responses, with many edges where an unravelling process may be initiated" (Lang, 1968). Fear consists of internal subjective feelings, multiple autonomic components and behavioural responses. Measures of these often correlate lowly with one another, and in monkeys Brady et al. (1968) has shown how behavioural and cardiovascular changes in emotion can be parallel but independently conditioned effects of the same stimulus events. It would thus be surprising if in humans the different components of fear did not sometimes change at different speeds relative to one another. The development of an effective instrument to reduce fear, viz. desensitisation—highlights this phenomenon in man.

Many studies of desensitisation do not report on separate components of fear, and not all measures are comparable. Nevertheless, where these are reported and comparable, no consistent relationship emerges in the order or speed with which each component of fear is reduced during desensitisation. In studies of desensitisation in volunteers with snake phobias, 3 workers found significant changes only in avoidance behaviour, while changes in subjective estimates of fear were either not obtained or came later (Lang et al., 1965; Davidson, 1968; Ritter, 1968), but in 4 other studies both avoidance and subjective fear changed together either significantly or nearly so (Schubot, 1966; Lomont and Edwards, 1967; Melamed and Lang, 1967; Bandura, 1968).

The fragmented evidence to date supports the view that

" the organisation of fear responses and the order of their change is idiosyncratic to the subject" (Lang, 1968). Lang went on further to suggest that " this has implications for the acquisition as well as the reduction of fear. Thus, disrupting autonomic responses may be evoked in the presence of specific discriminative stimuli. The organism may learn to avoid these stimuli. Subsequently, the fact of co-incident avoidance and somatic arousal may be remarked, and the unit self-labelled as fear. However, such a process could as well start with the verbal or overt behavioural components and it need not necessarily involve all the organism's potentially expressive systems or sub-systems. It seems very unlikely that most fears are initiated by the traumatic conditioning of the total behavioural output of the organism. Fears may develop piecemeal . . ."

Lang then pointed out the potential importance of the operant conditioning of fear. " If responses innervated by the autonomic nervous system can be shaped by the environment, we can more easily understand the slow development of fear via social learning, and the frequent absence of traumatic experience with the phobic object in the reports of very fearful subjects.

The systems of behaviour . . . undoubtedly influence each other, such that events in one system become initiating cues and terminating responses for other systems. Thus, peripheral vaso-constriction, alterations in stomach motility or acid secretions, may prompt avoidance behaviour which terminates the autonomic sequence. However, positive feedback loops also can develop in which awareness of autonomic events preciptitates avoidance which is a cue for further autonomic and verbal distress responses. Thus, the important therapeutic changes depend on training pro-grammes designed to eliminate specific response components, and interrupt mutually augmenting feedback between response systems".

This concept of the specificity of different components of fear and the necessity for treating them separately is useful, but it would be premature to overstate it at this early stage before all the evidence is in.

Processes other than relaxation which inhibit fear

The essence of desensitisation is that the patient is gradually brought into contact with the phobic situation while simultaneously undergoing a contrasting experience such as relaxation which inhibits the anxiety. Under certain conditions relaxation may not be feasible, e.g. in children, and then different settings are required to inhibit fear.

In children eating may reduce fear and sweets or food may be given each time the phobic stimulus is presented. Sometimes the mere presence of a loved or trusted companion is itself sufficient to counteract anxiety during desensitisation. At other times "emotive imagery" may be used in children (Lazarus and Abramovitz, 1962). In this method instead of relaxation, imagery capable of arousing positive feelings is used to block the occurrence of anxiety. A hierarchy of the child's phobias is drawn up, and he is then asked to describe his fantasy heroes and wish-fulfilments. The child is asked to imagine a scene containing both his hero and himself, and then as part of the narrative the therapist introduces the lowest item in the phobic hierarchy. If the child gets anxious the therapist withdraws the phobic item from the narrative and again evokes the scenes of the hero.

Rachman (1968) has described the use of self-assertion in the inhibition of social anxieties. The patient is encouraged to express his spontaneously-felt emotions in a clear and forthright manner. It is claimed that repeated self-assertion eventually results in conditioned inhibition of social anxiety. A closely related technique is the "behavioural rehearsal" of Wolpe and Lazarus (1966). This consists of assertive training combined with real-life rehearsals of anticipated social situations which are expected to give rise to anxiety. The patient and the therapist exchange roles in practice situations until the patient is capable of behaving appropriately and without anxiety.

Sexual stimulation can be used to inhibit fear, but its scope is rather limited for obvious reasons. As an example of its effect, a patient with a phobia of trains began to feel anxious when he imagined himself in a railway carriage, but relaxed with a beatific smile on his face when the therapist suggested that a beautiful woman entered the train and sat down opposite him. Patients with sexual fears or with complaints of impotence are instructed not to attempt any sexual activity unless they feel intense sexual arousal, under which condition they may engage in immediate sexual activity (Wolpe and Lazarus, 1966). This method was anticipated by John Hunter in 1786 when he described the rationale for successful treatment of a case of impotence.

"A complete action (in the parts of generation) cannot take place without a perfect harmony of body and of mind; that is, there must be both a power of body, and disposition of mind; for the mind is subject to a thousand caprices which affect the actions of these parts.

Copulation is an act of the body, the spring of which is in the mind; but it is not volition; and according to the state of the mind so is the act performed. To perform this act well, the body should be in health, and the mind should be perfectly confident of the powers of the body; the mind should be in a state entirely disengaged from everything else; it should have no difficulties, no fears, no apprehensions; not even an anxiety to perform the act well.

So trifling often is the circumstance which shall produce (impotence) depending on the mind, that the very desire to please shall have that effect, as in making the woman the sole object to be gratified ... A gentleman told me, that he had lost his powers in this way ... he had at unnecessary times strong erections, which showed that he had naturally this power; that the erections were accompanied with desire, which are all the natural powers wanted; but that there was still a defect somewhere ... some women he could have connection with, as well as ever ... there was but one woman that produced this inability, it arose from a desire to perform the act with this woman well which desire produced in the mind a doubt, on fear of the want of success, which was the cause of the inability of performing the act ... I told him that he might be cured, if he could perfectly rely on his own power of self-denial ... He was to go to bed to this woman, but first promise to himself, that he would not have any connection with her, for six nights, let his inclinations and powers be what they would; which he engaged to do ... About a fortnight after he told me that this resolution had produced such a total alteration in the state of his mind, that the power soon took place, for instead of going to bed with the fear of inability, he went with fears that he should be possessed with too much desire, too much power, so as to become uneasy to him, which really happened . . . ."

Desensitisation and insight

In psychotherapy it is commonly assumed that "insight" by a patient into the mechanism of a symptom leads to its alleviation. In a perceptive paper Cautela (1965) described 3 subjects who gave "insightful" statements as their phobias improved during desensitisation, in the course of which there had been no discussion of aetiology or dynamics of the phobia. This phenomenon touches crucial issues about the interaction between cognitive and emotional variables, and little is known about it. Since clear observations about this are so rarely documented, especially in the literature of phobias, Cautela's report merits detailed description.

In Cautela's first case the "insight" which developed was essentially a change in attitude of the same kind which occurs in patients recovering from other psychiatric disorders, e.g. paranoid or depressive illnesses in which the delusional content undergoes steady change and dilution as improvement occurs. The patient was a 35 year-old truck driver with a fear of driving his truck. He improved after 9 sessions of desensitisation and remained well at 3 weeks follow-up:

At the start of the 4th session he said he was feeling a little better in traffic. He realised most people were probably alright. There were just a few fanatics out to get truck drivers. Still, there were enough of these fanatics to make driving dangerous for a truck driver.

In the 7th session he said most drivers were conscientious working people like himself and there was probably no group of fanatics out to especially get truck drivers. He did feel, though, that truck drivers got more than their share of bad luck.

In the 9th session he wondered where he got the "crazy ideas" about truck drivers and accidents. Accidents were bound to happen and truck drivers just got their share. "That's the breaks of the game".

In Cautela's third case the insight which developed was about the origin of the phobias, knowledge which is often called insight into the dynamics of the disorder. The case was a 29 year-old woman with a phobia that her hands would tremble in social situations:

At the beginning of the 5th session she said : "You know, I've been thinking. Do you think the trembling has anything to do with the fact that my parents have been separated since I was 12? You know my mother deserted me and my father then".

At the beginning of the 6th session she said she was afraid people might think she had an emotional problem because she came from a broken home. She heard a lot about broken homes in her psychiatric training as a nurse.

In the 7th session she said that 2 years earlier her boy friend broke the engagement because he felt she was emotionally immature. Right after this her fear of trembling developed. She now realised she was afraid people would think she was emotionally unstable because she came from a broken home. She feared people would see her tremble and guess the truth about her family situation. "That's really all silly; to think that people have nothing better to do than watch me all the time. Besides, so what if they knew. What did that prove? Some people adjust well even if their parents are separated".

In both these cases insightful remarks followed progress, and did not precede it. Improvement through desensitisation released a change in attitude and self-knowledge, and not the reverse. In controlled trials of psychotherapy phobias have not shown impressive change despite discussion of and working through the origins of the phobias. However, occasional cases are documented (pp. 87–88) in which during treatment or chance events the patients recalled the original trauma which triggered the phobia, and this recall heralded disappearance of the phobia. It appears, therefore, that insight follows improvement in some cases, and precedes it in others. Yet other patients improve without insight ever developing into the origin of their phobias. Be it said that in many instances the origin of the phobia remains a mystery for the therapist as well.

Elimination of nightmares by desensitisation of phobias

Some recurrent nightmares are direct expressions of chronic fears and can be attenuated by desensitisation of the fear-producing stimuli. Geer and Silverman (1967) described the treatment of a long-standing frequently occurring nightmare by systematic desensitisation. The content of the nightmare (that the sleeper was awakened by an unknown intruder brandishing a knife) suggested a chronic fear which could be manipulated in the same manner as fears experienced in the waking state, even though the subject did not consciously experience a fear of being accosted in his sleep.

Silverman and Geer (1968) then applied desensitisation to a recurrent nightmare in another case, in which the subject experienced a phobia of the same content as the nightmare, and the nightmare disappeared as the phobia was successfully treated. The subject was a 19-year old female student with frequent nightmares of 4 years duration. The nightmare occurred in 3 variants, all containing the fear of falling from a bridge. The subject had a conscious phobia of bridges as long as she could remember, and also was afraid of heights. The patient lost her fear of bridges after 7 sessions of desensitisation, during the course of which her nightmares ceased. Towards the end of treatment she instead experienced 2 pleasant dreams about bridges. At follow-up 6 months later the patient reported no recurrence of the nightmare of the phobia, and no other problems of a psychological nature.

The process by which chronic fears become manifest in recurrent nightmares is obscure. Related phenomena are the recurrent nightmares of soldiers depicting a trauma of the battlefield, and counter-phobic behaviour in the waking state which involves the repeated arousal and confrontation of fear-producing stimuli e.g. the tendency of children to repeat frightening games. Such phenomena were labelled repetition compulsions by Freud (cf. Jones 1953, vol. 3. 289–90) who considered them to be attempts to master the unpleasant experiences (p. 269).

Section III. PROCESSES OTHER THAN DESENSITISATION WHICH IMPROVE PHOBIAS

Although desensitisation is at present the most widely used method in the treatment of phobias, and has been studied more carefully than any other technique, many other procedures have also been employed. Some of these are experimental techniques which have been subject to controlled scrutiny, but which have not yet been applied clinically very much. Others are more traditional clinical methods, only some of which have been studied in controlled fashion.

A. Experimental Methods

These are procedures which reduce fear in an experimental setting, but whose role in psychiatric treatment is not yet clear.

Modelling (vicarious conditioning)

It is well-known that fears can often be allayed by the sight of fearlessness in others. At least 8 controlled studies have shown the value of fearless models in the reduction of avoidance responses in volunteers with fears of snakes and dogs (Table 4.11A). Four of the studies were in children and 4 in adults. Bandura et al. (1967) studied 48 children aged 3–5 who had fears of dogs and found that observation of models who gradually approached dogs over 8 sessions reduced avoidance behaviour in the children at one month follow-up significantly more than mere observation of dogs without a model, and more than the pleasant experience of a party. Observation of models yielded equal effects regardless of whether it occurred in a neutral context or in the context of a pleasant party atmosphere.

Bandura and Menlove (1968) tested the value of diversity of modelling stimuli, and the importance of observers' susceptibility to emotional arousal. Of 48 children aged 3–5 who had fears of dogs, one group observed a graduated series of films in which the model displayed progressively more intimate inter-actions with a single dog. A second group of children observed a similar set of graded films depicting a variety of models interacting non-anxiously with numerous dogs varying in size and fearsomeness, while a control group was shown movies containing no animals. Both the single model and multiple model groups displayed significantly more decrease in avoidance than controls up to one month follow-up, but only the multiple model group lost their fears sufficiently to approach dogs very closely.

Among the multiple model group those children who had not only fears of dogs but also fears of interpersonal and inanimate situations showed less improvement than children who were less "emotionally prone". This finding parallels that of Gelder et al. (1967) and Lang et al. (1965), whose phobic patients and subjects did less well if they had multiple symptoms and fears.

Table 4.11. **Processes other than Desensitisation which reduce fear**
(Controlled trials in phobic subjects)

Process	Results	Type of fear	Population	n.	No. of sessions	Follow up (months)	Study
A. *Modelling*	Signif. decreased avoidance	Dogs	Children (3–5 yrs.)	24	8	1	Bandura et al. (1966)
	,, ,,	,,	,,	32	8	1	Bandura & Menlove (1968)
	,, ,,	,, Snakes	Volunteers	9	1	0	Hill et al. (1968)
	,, ,,	,,	Children(5–11 yrs.)	12	7	7	Bandura (1968)
	,, ,,	,,	Students	30	2	0	Ritter (1968)
	,, ,,	,,		20	1	0	Geer & Turteltaub (1967)
	,, ,,	,,	,,	9	1	0	Hart (1966)
	,, ,,	,, Rats	,,	10	1	0	Spiegler et al. (1968)
		Rats	,,	16	1	0	Kirchner & Hogan (1966)
B. *Flooding* (implosion)	(therapist absent: tape-recorded instructions)	,,	,,	21	1	0	Hogan & Kirchner (1967)
	,, ,, (therapist present)	Snakes	,,	10	1	0	,, ,, (1968)
	Signif. decreased avoidance	,,	Psychiatric inpts.	2	5	1	Wolpin & Raines (1966)
C. *Cognitive Manipulation*	No improvement	Spiders	Students	?	?	?	Larsen (1965)
	,, ,,	Snakes	?	3	10	3	Rachman (1966)
	Signif. decreased avoidance	,,	,,	51	2	0	Valins (1968)
	,, ,, ,,	,,	,,	9	1	0	Hart (1966)

Studies by Ritter (1968) and Bandura (1968) extended these findings by showing that modelling is even more effective when subjects are in addition exposed to the phobic object along a hierarchy as occurs in desensitisation in practice. Fuller details were reviewed on p. 226. In fact in Bandura's study which was carried out in adults, one experimental treatment was as good and another was superior to desensitisation in imagination alone. One of these treatments was symbolic modelling, where subjects watched models on film at a pace the subjects could regulate themselves while feeling relaxed, and the other treatment was live modelling with graded exposure, where subjects watched live models and were then themselves under guidance brought into gradual contact with the phobic object (desensitisation in practice). 92% of the original group which observed live models and then had desensitisation in practice managed terminal behaviour in the avoidance test at one month follow-up. In a cross-over design those subjects who had not improved with the other treatments then observed a live model and were desensitised in practice. All of these managed to handle a snake as the terminal task in the avoidance test. In fact this study is the only one so far to yield a method which emerged superior in a controlled comparison with desensitisation alone.

The extent of improvement obtained in Bandura's study greatly exceeds that reported in any other controlled study of the treatment of phobias. In nearly all studies of desensitisation most subjects or patients were left with residual disability, but the great majority of subjects in Bandura's study completed the stringent terminal task at the end of treatment and at a month's follow-up. Though the follow-up was short the study suggests that the addition of modelling to desensitisation requires investigation in psychiatric patients to ascertain how much it can improve the rather slow and limited effects usually obtained with desensitisation alone. The technique may be applicable to patients with fears of concrete situations like animals or heights. It remains to be seen how far it will be useful in conditions like severe agoraphobia which are the hardest of all phobic disorders to treat.

One might wonder at the good results obtained by modelling combined with desensitisation in practice, since many phobic patients observe other people encountering the phobic situation without fear, yet the patients are not improved by this, and may actually feel worse because they then feel cowards. However, few real life opportunities for modelling occur in *finely graduated* fashion. We often see a parent ineffectually trying to urge a terrified child to follow his own example of patting an enormous dog which towers above the child. This is not outstandingly successful because the child is being asked to do too much at once. The essence of Bandura's study was that the modelling and the contact was gradual.

One final point requires emphasis. Whatever the final role of modelling becomes in the treatment of phobias, results will not necessarily shed light on the origin of phobias. As a general rule for any treatment, its efficacy does not necessarily tell us much about the aetiology of the condition being treated.

Flooding (implosion therapy)

Results of this method are particularly interesting, since it is almost the opposite of desensitisation. Flooding aims at the patient experiencing the phobic stimulus as vividly and as long as possible until finally the patient is unable to feel fear any longer. "The patient is helped to break the phobic cycle by having him make a deliberate effort to feel and to experience fully his fear without trying to escape from it" (Malleson, 1959). This process has also been termed "implosion", which implies a bursting from within, and depicts the onslaught of phobic cues and the subsequent intense anxiety reaction which is reputedly followed by collapse of the symptoms because of extinction of the anxiety which supports them (Hogan and Kirchner, 1967).

Experimental analogues of flooding in animals were reviewed in Chapter 2. In these experiments extinction of avoidance responses was obtained when animals were prevented from making an avoidance response in the presence of the feared stimuli. In the clinical situation the patient is asked to experience his fear fully without avoiding it. The report of Malleson (1959) is one of the few to concern patients, and gives a good idea of the technique.

Treatment of an examination phobia by flooding

The patient was an Indian student with examination panic 48 hours before an examination. He had already failed a previous examination because of a similar attack of panic. "He was made to sit up in bed, and to try to feel his fear. He was asked to tell of the awful consequences that he felt would follow his failure—derision from his colleagues in India, disappointment from his family—financial loss . . . at first, as he followed the instructions, his sobbings increased. But soon his trembling ceased. As the effort needed to maintain a vivid imagination increased, the emotion he could summon began to ebb. Within half an hour he was calm". He was instructed to repeatedly experience his fears. " Everytime he felt a little wave of spontaneous alarm he was not to push it aside, but was to enhance it, to augment it, to try to experience it . . . more vividly". The patient was intelligent and assiduous, practiced his exercises methodically, and became almost unable to feel frightened. He passed his examination without difficulty.

Several controlled trials of flooding have been completed on volunteers who had fears of animals and insects (Table 4.11B). All except one found that flooding reduced avoidance behaviour more than control procedures. The exception was Rachman's study, which also differed from the others in that his subjects only visualised the phobic images for a maximum of 2 minutes, whereas in the other experiments the frightening experiences went on for much longer. Duration of exposure may well be a crucial variable, and premature termination of exposure may actually increase rather than decrease fear.

The best studies of flooding or implosion so far are those of Kirchner and Hogan (1966) and Hogan and Kirchner (1967). Kirchner and Hogan studied the effect of one session of flooding in female student volunteers who had intense fears of rats. The subjects were told that listening to tapes might help them unlearn their fears, and were assigned at random to one of two groups. 19 subjects underwent a control procedure of sitting in a booth and listening through earphones to tape-recorded instructions to imagine pleasant scenes while listening to music. The other 16 subjects sat in a booth listening through earphones to tape-recorded instructions eliciting imagery with high anxiety connected with fears of rats. Early imagery stressed both the approach of a rat toward the subject and the necessity for experiencing as much feeling and emotion as possible. Initial scenes suggested a sewer rat slowly approaching the subject and snapping at an outstretched finger. At this point all subjects jumped back in their seats in a single movement. Later scenes suggested rats biting and ripping the flesh of the subject. Towards the end subjects were asked to imagine the rat attacking them as they reached to pick it up. Throughout the session subjects moved and grimaced. All subjects were free to stop the taped material at any time. Each subject had an avoidance test with a rat before and after the experiment. In the test before the experiment no subject picked up the rat. In the test after the experiment 26% of controls and 62% of the subjects who had flooding picked up the rat (p $< \cdot$ 03).

Flooding thus significantly reduced avoidance behaviour even when the procedure was given by tape recorder without a therapist being present. Both control and experimental groups expected to improve, so this factor would not account for the difference between the two groups. Defects in the design were the absence of any follow-up and the absence of measures of fear other than avoidance.

Hogan and Kirchner (1967) again studied the effect of one session of flooding on volunteers with fears of rats, but this time treatment was given by a therapist, not by a tape recorder. 22 students underwent a control procedure in which they were asked to imagine neutral or relaxing scenes. 23 subjects were flooded or "imploded": they were asked to imagine touching a rat, having a rat nibbling at their fingers, running across their hand and body, devouring their eyes, jumping into their mouth and being swallowed, after which the rat destroyed various internal organs of their bodies. Subjects imagined themselves locked in a room full of rats. Each subject was given those scenes which he feared most.

On average the treatment session lasted 30 minutes for controls and 39 minutes for subjects who were flooded. During the sessions pulse rates were monitored on a physiograph. Pulse rates increased significantly more in the flooded groups than in the controls.

Before treatment all subjects failed to pick up a rat in an avoidance test. After treatment 9% of controls and 67% of flooded subjects picked up the rat (p < ·001). Unfortunately again there was no follow-up, nor were any measures of fear employed other than avoidance. Nevertheless, these results substantiated the authors previous work that one session of flooding or "implosion" significantly reduced avoidance behaviour in phobic subjects. Similar results were obtained again by the same workers in a third controlled study, this time with snake phobias in volunteers (Hogan and Kirchner, 1968).

Other studies which showed the effect of flooding applied rather less systematically were those of Larsen (1965) and Wolpin and Raines (1966). In these studies other procedures like hypnosis with or without relaxation achieved similar effects, unlike a no-treatment control group. Folkins et al. (1968) studied volunteers who watched a stressful film and noted that, compared with a control procedure, the imagining of frightening scenes reduced anxiety to the same extent as listening to taped instructions to relax, or undergoing an analogue desensitisation procedure. Subjects in this study were not phobic, and there were no pre-test measures.

The results of flooding in volunteers warrant controlled trials being done in patients. Until such studies have been completed one can only say that the technique holds promise and deserves further investigation. Such intense phobic anxiety as occurs in flooding has hitherto been regarded as harmful rather than beneficial. Flooding or implosion procedures may also throw light on broader issues than the treatment of fear alone, e.g. why some patients in psychotherapy improve after an abreaction which may be a reliving of past experiences or may be non-specific.

Paradoxical intention ("logotherapy")

This is a clinical method which has certain similarities to flooding. The technique was publicised by Frankl (1960). The patient is asked to cease fleeing or fighting his symptoms, and instead is asked to exaggerate them, after which he is no longer haunted by the symptoms. The technique depends upon observations that anticipatory anxiety brings about precisely what the patient had feared, while excessive intention or self-observation of one's own functioning may make this functioning impossible. Anxiety or compulsions may be increased by the endeavour to avoid or fight them.

Gerz (1962) illustrated the use of paradoxical intention in a man afraid that he might die of a heart attack:

"when I asked the patient in my office to 'try as hard as possible' to make his heart beat fast and die of a heart attack 'right on the

spot' he laughed and replied 'Doc, I'm trying hard, but I can't do it.'
Following Frankl's technique I instructed him to 'go ahead and try
to die from a heart attack' each time his anticipatory anxiety troub-
bled him. As the patient started laughing about his neurotic symptoms, humour helped him to put distance between himself and his
neurosis. The patient . . . (was) instructed to 'die at least 3 times
a day of a heart attack, and instead of trying hard to go to sleep,
try hard to remain awake' . . . In the moment he started laughing at
his symptoms and when he became willing to produce them
(paradoxically) intentionally, he changed his attitude towards his
symptoms . . . With this change in attitude, he . . . interrupted the
vicious cycle and strangled the feed-back mechanism".

It is possible that in very selected patients paradoxical intention may
have certain uses, though the extent of its applicability is by no means
clear at the moment.

The rationale and method of paradoxical intention and of flooding
have certain resemblances to one another. As the rationale for use of a
flooding procedure Malleson (1959) suggested that "fear or panic is
always integrally bound up with the wish to escape. So long as that
wish persists, reciprocally the fear persists". This suggestion is reminiscent of John Hunter's rationale for his treatment of impotence—as
long as the patient was afraid of failing with his mistress he failed mis-
erably. As soon as he was told not to engage in intercourse his potency
returned (Hunter, 1786).

Paradoxical intention and flooding also have elements in common
with *Morita therapy* as practised in Japan. Kora (1964) described the
treatment of patients with severe anxiety and fear of death:

"The patient will always entertain a premonitory fear that the
seizure (of anxiety) might attack him any moment and his sphere of
activity is usually very much limited because of this anxiety.
. . . he should be told that it is important not to upset the regular
pace of his life even if he had a premonitory fear that the seizure
might attack him, by accepting such fear as it is calmly and passively.
When he does not have the fit, the patient should be made to go
out all by himself even if he has an anticipatory fear or is suffering
from anxiety. He should ride the bus or the street car if that is
necessary and should attempt to enlarge his sphere of activity in
any way possible. If he takes advantage of his disease and leads a
life like that of a patient by capitalising on his condition, he will
never be cured."

Similarly, in the treatment of intrusive thoughts "the only
solution is to accept the desultory thoughts as something inevitable
and to keep on reading without repelling them, but tolerating them
as they are. If this stage of self-resignation is achieved, there will no
longer be any antagonistic ideas . . ."

Finally, the meditative techniques of Zen buddhism include principles reminiscent of paradoxical intention and flooding. Describing the stages of training Maupin wrote (1962): "There is an initial phase in which concentration, difficult at first, eventually becomes more successful. Relaxation and a kind of pleasant 'self-immersion' begin to follow. At this point internal distractions, often of an anxiety-arousing kind, come to the fore . . . the only way to render this disturbance inoperative is to 'look at it equably and at last grow weary of looking' ".

Cognitive Manipulation

Since cognitive cues partly determine how a subject will label emotions he is feeling at a given moment (Schachter & Singer, 1962), it is to be expected that manipulation of these cues can modify emotional feeling. Two controlled studies of students with snake phobias have shown that cognitive manipulation can effectively decrease avoidance of a phobic stimulus (Table 4.11C). Subjects of Valins and Ray (1967) were given false auditory feedback of their heart sounds while watching slides of snakes. They were led to believe that their heart rate did not increase on seeing the snakes. This procedure led to significantly decreased avoidance of snakes. Hart's (1966) subjects were simply asked to prepare a tape recording supposedly to help teach other students with snake phobias to overcome their fears. This procedure of cognitive rehearsal alone reduced their avoidance of snakes compared to control procedures. There was no follow-up in either of these studies of cognitive manipulation. Nevertheless, they confirm the work of Leitenberg et al. (1968a) that cognitive processes may be quite important in the treatment of phobias. Though these methods have little direct clinical application at the moment they open up important areas of research which may broaden our understanding of psychotherapeutic processes.

Operant conditioning techniques

These have already been touched on in the section on desensitisation, where the work of Leitenberg et al. (1968a) was described. These workers showed that expectation and praise of progress (i.e. social reinforcement) significantly improved the effects of desensitisation in a group of snake phobic volunteers. Other preliminary studies by the same group of workers confirmed that operant methods can improve patients, but the clinical value of this approach is not yet clear, as little follow-up and no controlled studies of groups of patients are yet available.

Barlow et al. (1968) treated an agoraphobic woman by arranging for a nurse to ask the patient to go out twice daily and see how far she could walk by herself. Each session was timed with a stop watch. After a baseline was established social reinforcement was made contingent on increasing the time she spent away from the starting point (Fig. 4.14). Each time the patient attained a given criterion she was praised by being told "that's fine" or "very good" i.e. by social reinforcement. Although the instruction did not explicitly mention time the patient consistently increased her time away on a walk. When social reinforcement was withdrawn (extinction) no further improvement was noted (Fig. 4.14). When reinforcement for time was reinstated the patient increased her time away. During this period her distance away remained relatively stable. Subsequently praise was switched from time to distance with the result that distance away increased more than time. Praise was withdrawn once more (extinction), and after an "extinction burst" (Fig. 4.14) performance declined sharply. Reintroduction of social

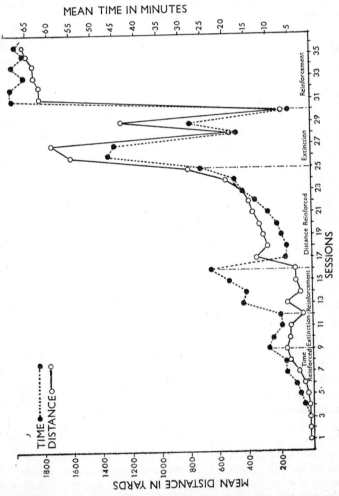

Fig. 4.14: Effect of social reinforcement: Time away and distance away from the starting point in a case of agoraphobia (Barlow et al., 1967).

reinforcement was again followed by rapid improvement to the maximum performance possible within the design. Unfortunately there was no follow-up and subjective anxiety was not reported. Similar findings were repeated in 2 other agoraphobic patients.

Patients found the periods of extinction to be particularly trying. They expressed anger at the programme, insisted it would not work, and were often tearful. They usually blamed themselves for their deterioration in performance during extinction, and indeed after reinforcement was removed one patient even apologised for doing so poorly the previous week.

In another experiment the same group of workers (Leitenberg et al., 1968b) showed that a claustrophobic patient became able to sit increasingly longer in a small enclosed room simply by sitting for repeated trials in the room and being told how long each trial lasted, i.e. by obtaining feed-back about her progress. After withdrawal of this feed-back performance remained stationary, but restoration of feed-back was followed by resumption of improvement in performance which generalised to situations outside treatment. Improvement remained at 3 months follow-up. Similar results were obtained in a patient with depression and an obsessive phobia of knives who was asked to practise looking at a knife repeatedly. Feed-back about the time spent improved her ability to look at knives. Adding praise to the feed-back did not further improve her performance. Withdrawal of this praise did not impair performance, but when this was followed by withdrawal of feed-back as well, performance then deteriorated, i.e. extinction began. With restoration of feed-back performance improved once more. The patient now became able to use sharp knives in the ward for the first time, but had to have special treatment for her depression.

Both social reinforcement (e.g. praise) and feed-back may act as repeated reminders of the specific objectives of treatment, and thus facilitate patients' efforts to attain those aims. Presumably where a patient is motivated to change, feed-back alone will help to modify his behaviour, but in the absence of motivation social reinforcement can instigate change in the desired direction, especially if the patient is in a state of relative social deprivation.

Further evidence that social reinforcement can improve fearful behaviour was provided by Wagner and Cauthern (1968) in 3 snake phobic volunteers.

If operant techniques or feed-back prove to be as successful as desensitisation they would offer hope of cutting down the time spent by doctors and psychologists in treatment, since nurses can be easily trained to praise patients or provide feed-back in the right manner. Praise takes a few minutes at most, unlike the half to one hour of a desensitisation session. This issue can only be settled by controlled trials in patients.

Operant methods can in fact be construed as a subtle form of desensitisation, since patients entering the phobic situation may have their anxiety allayed by the expectation of praise for their daring. Conversely, an important aspect of desensitisation is praise of the patient for his progress up the hierarchy, and this can be seen in part as operant conditioning. Indeed, at some point the procedures of desensitisation and operant conditioning are hard to tell apart.

It is obvious that operant conditioning applies systematically what most clinicians do routinely when they praise patients for their efforts at recovery. Done systematically, however, it may achieve more than the haphazard encouragement which is usually all that is possible in busy routine conditions.

Aversion relief

Recently a few phobic patients have been treated by the unusual method of aversion relief (Solyom and Miller, 1967), an idea which was originally used by Thorpe et al. (1964). Though it is much too early to know whether this method will eventually have a definitive place in the treatment of phobias, it is worth detailed description.

The technique involves the presentation of phobic stimuli to the patient as he presses a button to terminate an aversive electric shock. Solyom and Miller seated the patient in an armchair and presented a tape-recorded narrative of the phobia through earphones. The text was interrupted by periods of silence averaging 30 seconds in duration. These pauses were followed immediately by an electric shock to the patient's finger which the patient could terminate by pressing a button which restarted the taped narrative of the phobia. Similarly, slides of phobic stimuli selected by the patient were paired with aversion relief after the cessation of electric shock. The intensity of the shock was "midway between ... shock-perception and shock-tolerance thresholds". Sessions lasted about half an hour.

Several tapes were used depicting the same phobia in different situations, and each tape was presented repeatedly until the patient reported improvement in that phobic situation, after which this tape was used less frequently. If the patient anticipated a phobic situation in the near future a tape recording of his anticipated phobic reaction was prepared and presented.

When a tape was played for the first time each 30 second period of silence was followed by shock. On subsequent occasions the shock was omitted after some of the pauses to provide a partial reinforcement schedule. Patients reported that the periods of silence evoked anxiety even in the absence of shock.

The phobic stimuli were thus selected by the patient in the form of pictures or were expressed in the patient's own words. These were presented in the context of a total experience. The expression of phobic anxiety itself was not punished by shock.

By this method Solyom and Miller treated 7 female phobic patients. Six of these patients were much improved after treatment, and this was maintained over follow-up to 10 months or more. During treatment changes in the galvanic skin response reflected clinical changes. One patient discontinued treatment after 12 sessions—she was a house-bound phobic anxious patient with social fears. Two of the patients had desensitisation as well as aversion relief—these required only 6–10 sessions of aversion relief. The four patients who were treated successfully solely by aversion relief had an average of 21 sessions of treatment. This is very similar to the usual length of treatment required for successful desensitisation of phobic patients.

Solyom and Miller's technique requires a fair amount of technical preparation before treatment. Whether aversion relief shortens treatment time or can be extended to phobias which don't respond to other methods of treatment such as desensitisation is a matter for future controlled investigation. To be acceptable clinically an unpleasant method such as aversion relief must have a clear advantage over other forms of treatment.

B. Clinical Methods

These procedures have a tradition of use in some psychiatric clinics. Though most of them have had limited study in a systematic controlled manner, a rough evaluation of their clinical value is possible.

Relaxation Techniques and Hypnosis

Relaxation exercises are an integral part of the usual desensitisation procedure and contribute to its effectiveness. However, relaxation by itself usually produces but slight if any lasting improvement in phobias, and cannot be regarded as a definitive technique for their treatment. The role of relaxation in desensitisation is not clear. It is obvious that muscular relaxation does not of itself produce mental relaxation, since total muscular relaxation under curare can be accompanied by intense fear in conscious subjects. Furthermore, conditioned avoidance responses in animals can be readily acquired in dogs whose muscles are totally paralysed by curare (Solomon and Turner, 1962). It appears that muscular relaxation is a useful method of inducing a state of mental calmness in most patients, and that the latter is the state which is important. Following relaxation exercises the mental calmness is accompanied by a significant decrease in spontaneous fluctuations of skin conductance (Mathews and Gelder, 1969). Lowered activity of skin conductance is associated with faster habituation during procedures like desensitisation (Lader et al., 1967). Many patients find it helpful to listen periodically to a tape recording of relaxation instructions which they can play at home whenever necessary.

A state of mental calmness can equally well be obtained by a hypnotic induction procedure. Treatment of phobic disorders by **hypnosis** is difficult to evaluate since so few controlled trials have been done. Table 4.5E on p. 200 shows two studies in which hypnosis was compared with desensitisation.   Hypnosis emerged in both as less effective. Nevertheless, hypnosis did produce significant improvement in phobias in the psychiatric out-patients who had mixed phobias (Marks et al., 1968).   This work was described earlier.   Another controlled study in which hypnosis significantly reduced avoidance behaviour was that of Larsen (1965) in volunteers with snake phobias.

Over the last 80 years occasional claims have also been made for the efficacy of hypnosis in phobias on the basis of uncontrolled work (e.g. Moll, 1891; Schilder, 1921; Schneck, 1954).   Cautela (1966) reviewed some of these and pointed out that hypnosis often involves relaxation and repeated visualisation of the phobic situation, rather as in desensitisation.   Cautela argued that this might be responsible for occasional cases of improvement under hypnosis.

Suggestion may also be important.   This can be given without hypnotic induction if suitable task-motivating instructions are used, as Barber (1962) has shown.   Edwards (1965) has demonstrated that the effect of suggestions given during hypnosis can last weeks or even months in some patients, while in others they are short-lived. Suggestion might act by counteracting the anticipatory anxiety which phobic patients experience before they enter a feared situation. If the effects of suggestions are long lived, they will see the patient through a number of new situations, so that he will enter each without anticipatory anxiety and a form of desensitisation will occur. Hypnotic suggestions may thus act partly by facilitating relearning, but this leaves unexplained the psychological mechanism of suggestion.

Improvement of phobias under hypnosis also rarely follows abreaction under hypnosis (e.g. Gill and Brenman, 1943) or by other methods such as ether administration (Little, 1964), with reliving of a trauma which may have originally triggered the phobia. The mechanism of relief from abreaction is by no means clear.

Hypnosis may thus effect some improvement in various patients with phobic disorders. However, the effect is uncertain and does not compare particularly well with desensitisation. Hypnosis is therefore not one of the definitive techniques in the treatment of phobias.

Another way of achieving mental relaxation is by techniques of **meditation.** There are many such techniques, and unfortunately none have yet been tested systematically in phobic patients, so that the extent of their usefulness is unknown.

Autogenic training

(Schultz and Luth, 1959). This is a further technique for obtaining mental relaxation, and was described earlier in this chapter. Claims have been made for its value in phobias. Though autogenic training is a useful way to produce relaxation as a preliminary to desensitisation, by itself, as with relaxation exercises alone, there is little evidence that it has a lasting effect in improving phobic disorders".

Faith healing

About one-sixth of agoraphobics in Britain have consulted a spiritual healer at some stage of their disorder (Marks and Herst 1969). Obviously data about outcome is not very likely to be available. It is possible that faith healing could help in certain cases by suggestion in a manner similar to that in hypnosis.

Psychotherapy (Insight or Analytically Oriented)

Until desensitisation came into vogue about five years ago insight psychotherapy was probably the commonest mode of treatment for phobic disorders. It is particularly difficult to assess the value of psychotherapy as nearly all reports of its use are uncontrolled.

Most methods of psychotherapy assume the psychoanalytic idea that phobias are a façade which is symbolic of other fears or conflicts, and that the task of psychotherapy is to uncover these, upon which the phobias will resolve. This formulation is extremely difficult to test adequately in the absence of clear criteria for symbolism, as was discussed earlier on p. 94–100.

Many reports of success with psychotherapy demonstrate how relief follows the patient's understanding of meaningful connections or symbolism of the phobic symptom, as in the case of Lief (1955) described on p. 000 and in a case described by Moss (1960). This factor may be useful in selected cases, but limited evidence from the few controlled trials available (Table 4.5G, p. 200) suggests that as a rule this procedure is not particularly helpful for phobias themselves, though it may benefit patients in other ways. For example, Gelder et al. (1967) showed that desensitisation produced significantly quicker and better results than psychotherapy in relieving phobias, but in some patients psychotherapy did seem to produce improvement in interpersonal adjustment, though this could not be measured in the absence of sensitive scales. Interpersonal adjustment appeared to improve despite the fact that phobias had not improved. The two different techniques of desensitisation and psychotherapy each seemed to produce its own pattern of change, desensitisation improving phobias and psychotherapy improving interpersonal adjustment. However, this effect of psychotherapy is by no means a hard finding and still requires definitive demonstration.

That group psychotherapy may facilitate subsequent desensitisation is suggested in the studies of Lazarus (1961) and Gelder and Marks (1968). In both studies the time necessary for desensitisation to effect improvement in phobias was shorter in patients who had already been treated by group psychotherapy than in patients who had desensitisation without any previous treatment. This suggests that amelioration of problems of adjustment in patients may make their phobias more amenable to change by desensitisation.

Although most psychotherapists aim at improving a patient's phobias by resolution of his personality problems, many psychotherapists in fact use the therapeutic relationship as a lever to urge the patient to enter the phobic situation, often along an informal gradient of fearfulness (Andrews, 1966, and see p. 183). Some psychotherapists thus employ a rudimentary form of desensitisation, though they do not usually call it this. It is important to differentiate improvement through this procedure from improvement due to resolution of personality conflicts. If desensitisation is the mechanism by which some psychotherapists effect improvement in phobias, then analysis of personality conflicts is a wasteful way of trying to apply desensitisation, and it is surely more sensible in such instances to give desensitisation systematically rather than indirectly.

This is not to say, however, that psychotherapy has no value in phobic disorders. Phobic patients commonly have personality problems and difficulties in relating to their spouses, parents or friends, and these difficulties can require treatment in their own right as well as prevent successful desensitisation. Clinical impression suggests, though definitive proof is lacking, that psychotherapy is useful for these interpersonal difficulties.

Some patients present for treatment of a phobia but in the course of treatment it becomes apparent that they are more incapacitated by their personality problems than by the phobia, or that improvement in their phobias will bring them into contact with situations they cannot cope with—that is, their phobias bring them secondary gain. In such cases it may be worth leaving the phobia untreated for a while and deal first with the personality difficulties by psychotherapy. Once these are less distressful for the patient, then desensitisation can be given for the phobia.

Occasionally it appears that the phobia was only the pretext for seeking help when the patient tacitly wanted treatment for other problems, for some of which psychotherapy is appropriate. Mechanic and Volkart (1961) have shown how patients are more likely to seek treatment for a variety of complaints when they are feeling lonely and need support. Lonely or depressed patients may use a minor phobia, a trivial wart or slight indigestion as the face-saving excuse to visit and talk to their doctor, perhaps in the hope of revealing some of their less obvious but more important problems if he proves to be sympathetic and helpful. As Mechanic (1962) suggested, "interpersonal stress is a significant factor affecting who will seek medical care and when. Aside from clear emergencies and acute illnesses, which scarcely permit alternatives, the maintenance of a doctor-patient relationship involves an interaction between certain services the physician offers and certain needs of the patient which may go beyond "traditional medicine" in its usual connotation".

Psychotherapy is also required in phobic patients in whom in the course of desensitisation it appears that improvement in the phobia is upsetting a dynamic equilibrium in the patient's environment. Husbands and wives may have adjusted to or even thrived while the patient was handicapped by phobias. A frigid wife may prefer her husband to be impotent because of his sexual fears, and will not be pleased if he gains sexual potency. A spouse or parent may prefer the patient in the passive-dependent role which results from a crippling phobia, and may find it threatening when the patient achieves more independence after the shackles of the phobia are loosened. Strain then ensues in the marital or parental relationship, and further attempts to improve the phobia may be thwarted by subtle strategies of the relatives or of the patient himself. In this event the patient requires psychotherapy, sometimes alone, sometimes in a series of joint interviews with the chief relative concerned.

Desensitisation and insight psychotherapy can thus be complementary procedures in certain cases and are not mutually exclusive. However, there are many phobic patients without severe maladjustment in whom desensitisation alone is required and insight psychotherapy is quite unnecessary. The relationship between behavioural and insight methods of psychotherapy has been detailed elsewhere (Marks and Gelder, 1966). Desensitisation itself is very different in procedure from traditional psychotherapy, but the more "broad-spectrum behaviour therapy" described by Lazarus (1966) and others is almost indistinguishable from the more active forms of insight psychotherapy.

Indications for insight psychotherapy in phobic patients may be summarised as follows:

1. When the patient presents with a phobic disorder but is found also to have troublesome problems of personal maladjustment. This may be obvious when the patient is first seen or come to light only after he has been in treatment for some time.

2. When in the course of definitive treatment of the phobia by desensitisation or other means it becomes clear that removal of the phobia is causing loss of secondary gains which are so important to the patient that further progress is prevented.

3. When improvement of the phobia through desensitisation or other means upsets the dynamic equilibrium of the patient's relationships to an extent which causes serious difficulties. Psychotherapy of the patient, and if need be of the family, may then be necessary.

Psychoanalysis

This technique is considered by some to be simply a form of intensive psychotherapy, whilst others hold that it is different in kind. Though reports have been made of improvement in phobias during psychoanalysis (e.g. Sterba, 1935; Schmideberg, 1951; Rangell, 1952; Ruddick, 1961), most of these are of single cases, and no study was controlled. There is no indication from these reports that psychoanalysis achieved any more than psychotherapy. The treatment is expensive and time consuming, and cannot be regarded as a definitive technique in the treatment of phobic disorders, though it may be helpful for personality problems in the few patients who can afford it.

THE USE OF DRUGS IN PHOBIC DISORDERS

The use of appropriate drugs may afford considerable relief to phobic patients who have several kinds of distress. These drugs have particular indications and are not intended for all patients who have phobias.

Relief of the phobic anxiety itself. Phobic patients usually find it much easier to enter the phobic situation while under the influence of sedative drugs or alcohol. Relief of the phobia lasts only as long as the action of that drug or alcohol, and the patient does not find it any easier to face subsequent phobic situations without these aids. The effect of sedative drugs or alcohol is thus palliative and not curative. They are a valuable help to the patient who is particularly handicapped in his everyday activities, but need to be taken each time he anticipates facing the phobic stimulus, since such drugs when ingested orally take up to 30 minutes to be absorbed and exert their effect. It is of little value for a patient who is phobic of trains to get on the train, wait to see if he is frightened, and then take a sedative, since 30 minutes of acute fear may elapse before he feels better. In patients who encounter their phobic object several times a day the only way to make life tolerable might be to give them several doses of sedative every day.

A variety of sedative drugs are in common use, and many have been subjected to controlled trial in anxiety states, but not in phobic disorders. A concise review of the subject appears in Wittenborn (1966). Several classes of drug are available.

1. **Barbiturates:** Barbiturates have long been used in the control of anxiety and related symptoms, but Wittenborn included them in his review primarily for historical reasons. Not all controlled trials have shown barbiturates to be significantly superior to placebo in reducing anxiety. Barbiturates used for phobic anxiety are given half an hour before the patient anticipates entering a phobic situation, or up to 3 times daily if the phobic effect is met with daily. Among the commonest barbiturates used are amylobarbitone sodium 50–100 mgs., and pheno-barbitone 15–50 mgs. up to 3 times daily. Higher doses tend to cause sleepiness, and allergic reactions occur occasionally with pheno-barbitone. Addiction is sometimes a complication.

2. **Benzodiazepine derivatives** (chlordiazepoxide, diazepam, oxaze-pam). These drugs have all been shown in repeated controlled trials to reduce anxiety more than placebo and sometimes more than bar-biturates. Usual doses of the drugs, given up to 3 times daily, are

10–20 mgs., for chlordiazepoxide, 5–10 mgs. for diazepam and 10 mgs. for oxazepam. All 3 drugs may produce drowsiness in higher doses.

3. **Meprobamate:** This drug has been used rather more in North America than in Britain. Usual dose is 400 mgs. up to 4 times daily. Side effects are said to be less common than in barbiturates.

4. **Phenothiazines:** Because these drugs often have troublesome side effects there is a tendency to reserve them only for severe anxiety, and even then they have no clear advantage over the drugs mentioned above in the reduction of anxiety.

Patients who are on these drugs require warning that the drugs potentiate the effect of alcohol. When drugs have been given in high doses for a long period withdrawal needs to be slow, as convulsions may follow abrupt withdrawal of drugs such as barbiturates.

Since drugs afford but transient relief of a phobia, whenever possible a more definitive method of reducing the phobia permanently should be tried e.g. by desensitisation. Clinical impression suggests that the phobia returns as soon as the drug effect has worn off, whether drugs are withdrawn rapidly or very slowly. There have been no controlled trials examining this in patients, although there is slight evidence that gradual withdrawal of sedatives may facilitate improvement in fear motivated behaviour (Sherman, 1967).

Drug dependence and addiction

Danger of addiction exists in patients with severe chronic phobias. Terhune (1949) found no cases of drug or alcohol addiction in 86 phobic patients, but Sim (1968) noted that 21% of 191 patients in a psychiatric department developed dependence on drugs and/or alcohol which was either unable to contain their anxiety or had become sufficiently severe to warrant treatment in its own right. Addiction can be treated by withdrawal of the drug while the patient receives chlopromazine to minimise withdrawal effects. Despite their addiction 45% of these patients improved markedly during treatment, so that phobic anxiety complicated by severe addiction can still have a reasonably good prognosis.

Relief of background ("free-floating") anxiety

Many phobic patients have in addition to their fear in the phobic situation, continued anxiety at rest even in the absence of the phobic object. This is true particularly of patients with severe agoraphobia (phobic anxiety state), and this background of anxiety may be more distressing than the phobias themselves. When this occurs patients require relief by sedative drugs of the same kind and in similar doses as those given for anxiety in the phobic situation. *Chlordiazepoxide* and *diazepam* are probably the most frequently used. The drugs will need to be given several times a day. The danger of addiction or alcoholism in patients with severe anxiety is a real one, since large amounts of drugs are often needed, and tolerance may develop after a while. Sometimes tolerance can be countered by switching from one drug to another at intervals.

Relief of panic attacks

In addition to a continuous background of anxiety regardless of his environment, phobic patients also may have crippling phasic panic attacks. These come on suddenly, are accompanied by signs of extreme anxiety such as palpitations, rapid breathing, unsteadiness, weakness and a feeling of impending death, and subside as rapidly as they began. Such panic attacks are particularly common in patients with severe agoraphobia who have a background of marked constant tension, and are also often accompanied by depressive episodes. Panic attacks are the most distressing experience complained of by phobic patients.

Panic attacks can be improved by sedative drugs such as *chlordiaze-poxide* and *diazepam*. In addition, claims have been made for the value of "anti-depressant" drugs in this problem. There are two main classes of these drugs.

1. **Monoamine oxidase inhibitors** (e.g. iproniazid, phenelzine, tranyl-cypromine). These drugs have not been subjected to controlled study in phobic anxious patients, though claims have been made for their value (e.g. King, 1962; Sargant and Dally, 1962). This class of drug has two important drawbacks. First, several have been responsible for rare cases of fatal hepatitis. Second, patients on these drugs who eat foods with a high content of tyramine, e.g. cheese, yeast and meat extracts, occasionally develop hypertensive crises with severe headache and even subarachnoid or intracerebral haemorrhage with fatal results. These side effects naturally make many doctors wary of prescribing this class of drugs.

2. **Iminodibenzyl derivatives** (e.g. imipramine, amitriptyline, nortrip-tyline): Both imipramine and amitriptyline have been shown in controlled trials to be superior to placebos in relieving depression, and are to be preferred to the monoamine oxidase inhibitors since they have fewer serious toxic effects. *Imipramine* has also been shown to be superior to placebo in the reduction of panic attacks in severe agoraphobia (Klein, 1964). Imipramine might therefore be prescribed for panic attacks in doses of 25–75 mgs. up to 3 times daily. *Amitriptyline* is a similar compound and could probably be used equally well in the same dosage. Unlike sedative drugs, which exert their action as soon as they are absorbed, imipramine and amitriptyline may not have a beneficial effect until the patient has been on the drug for several days or weeks. Treatment may need to continue for many months, or even a year or more until the tendency to have panic attacks disappears. A trial of slow withdrawal will indicate whether this has happened.

Side effects are dryness of the mouth, blurred vision, constipation, and postural hypotension, and sleepiness with amitriptyline. Very rarely blood dyscrasias have occurred in patients on these drugs.

Relief of depression

Patients with severe agoraphobia often have episodes of depression, usually together with increased background anxiety and panic attacks. Use of anti-depressants may help such patients considerably. Iminodibenzyl derivatives such as *amitriptyline* or *imipramine* are the most preferable drugs for depression. Mode of administration of these is the same in depression as for panic attacks. Many phobic patients find that their phobias increase during a depressive phase, and resolution of the depression is usually accompanied by improvement of the phobias to the state obtaining before the depression began.

Acetylcholine. Sim and Houghton (1966) treated 191 phobic patients (mainly agoraphobic) in a psychiatric department by intravenous injections of acetylcholine 2 to 3 times weekly to a total of 30–45 injections. Rationale for the drug was that its peripheral action counteracts an over-secretion of adrenaline. Acetylcholine is destroyed extremely rapidly in the blood stream by anti-cholinesterase action, but the authors hoped that "through frequent repetition the patient is able to gain a new mastery over the tendency to sympathetic over-stimulation". Sim and Houghton claimed that 89% of 141 patients who were followed up to 2 to 10 years later by their general practitioners were "materially improved". Unfortunately criteria for improvement were not stated, and there was no control group, so that it is impossible to assess this claim. Furthermore, patients not only had injections of acetylcholine but were also given graduated tasks to perform with an escort in a manner indistinguishable from desensitisation in practice. In the absence of controls one cannot assess how much improvement was due to this desensitisation, how much to the acetylcholine, and how much to other factors in treatment. The authors themselves recognised that their findings were not conclusive.

Unless further evidence comes to light, there is no good reason at the present time to recommend injections of acetylcholine for the relief of phobic disorders.

Intravenous barbiturates: Thiopentone: Use of this drug was described in a preliminary report by King and Little (1959). The rationale was based on Roth's observations that a series of 10–12 injections of thiopentone administered 3 times weekly produced cumulative relief in tension in phobic anxious patients, even when no abreaction had taken place. King and Little injected a 2·5% solution intravenously at a rate sufficient to induce sleep in about 15 minutes. Injections were given on alternative days. Forty-four patients with phobic anxiety and depersonalisation were treated in a controlled design: patients were allocated at random so that 50% received thiopentone, 25% had placebo injections and 25% had psychotherapy. The patient assessed her overall change, and progress was also rated by a doctor unaware which treatment the patient had had.

At one month follow-up the doctor rated improvement in 80% of thiopentone and 50% of control patients (p not significant), while patients rated themselves improved in 90% and 70% of cases respectively. At 3 months follow-up the doctor and patient rated improvement in 85% of thiopentone and 50% of control patients (p < ·05). Only one case achieved complete recovery.

No follow-up was reported after 3 months and unfortunately no subsequent report was published with fuller details, so that adequate assessment of the method is not possible. It does seem unlikely that intravenous barbiturates would confer any long term advantage over oral barbiturates, and justification for the procedure would require more definitive assessment than was described in the preliminary report of King and Little.

Methohexitone: Claims have been made that intravenous injections of this short-acting drug facilitate desensitisation. Controlled evidence does not yet support this claim. The subject has already been dealt with earlier.

In summary, drugs may be of considerable value as a palliative for various kinds of distress in phobic patients. Anxiety in the phobic situation as well as background anxiety away from it can be relieved by drugs such as chlordiazepoxide or diazepam, but anxiety returns as the effect of the drug wears off. In patients with severe phobias and much general anxiety there is some danger of drug dependence or addiction. Panic attacks and depressive episodes in phobic patients can be relieved by the administration of imipramine or amitriptyline, but these may need to be continued for a year or more.

Leucotomy

Leucotomy has been recommended in the past as a useful treatment for chronic tension states. A drawback to the standard leucotomy of earlier years was the marked personality change which often ensued. The later modified leucotomy was a more anterior cut which damaged much less brain tissue than the earlier operation and produced less change in personality. A controlled retrospective study of this modified leucotomy in severe agoraphobics (Marks et al., 1966) was reviewed on p. 217 and results were shown in fig. 4.11. Results showed that leucotomy patients did significantly better than controls with respect to phobias and general anxiety, and work adjustment improved markedly. Personality-changes after operation were mild and not related to outcome. The conclusion emerged that in long-standing cases of severe agoraphobia with prominent anxiety, modified leucotomy produced more useful sustained improvement than other

forms of treatment.   Leucotomy also facilitated desensitisation by
reducing anxiety.

Doctors are naturally extremely cautious in recommending such an
operation even in suitable cases.   Fewer than 2% of patients with
phobic disorders were treated by leucotomy in the Maudsley Hospital.
The need for careful selection is evident, based on long duration of
illness, severe chronic anxiety, and a sociable previous personality.
Reluctance to recommend leucotomy would be even greater in patients
who engage in intellectual or responsible pursuits like university
academics or top professionals.   Modified leucotomy is thus an occasional but useful last resort for the severest phobic anxious patients
who have not responded to other forms of treatment over many years.

Section IV.   TREATMENT OF PHOBIAS IN CHILDREN
(M. G. Gelder and I. M. Marks)

Phobias in general

Views about treatment of these conditions in children are divided as
they are when the symptoms occur in adults.   The assessment of treatment results is even more difficult than in adults because fears and
phobias tend to disappear without treatment as the child grows older.

What accounts for the gradual diminution of children's fears? The
acquisition of fears depends to an important extent on the child's
experience in the family: children who see that their mothers have many
fears become fearful themselves.   Similarly, the decline in fears depends
to an important degree in the way the mother responds to her fear and
tends to help him over them.   For this reason it is important to know
what measures mothers adopt.   Jersild (1950) and Hagman (1932)
report that parents most often attempt rational explanation. However,
Hagman (1932) found that explanation was most effective when
combined with gradual exposure to the source of fear. Jersild (1950)
reported that the three most effective methods were (a) imitation of
adults or other children who show no fear in the presence of the
object (b) "reconditioning" (c) gradual experience in dealing with
the feared object or situation.

Rutter et al. (1968) noted how readily children's fears respond to
sensible handling. In their survey of the Isle of Wight they found several
examples of children with school phobia in which the phobia had never
reached the point of significant handicap or had been handicapping
only for a short while. In these cases the parents had a good relationship
with the child, were unflustered by the situation and dealt with the child's
fears calmly and confidently.

Many children are treated by a variety of approaches and others are
given support in the expectation of spontaneous improvement.

There are a number of reports of psychoanalytic treatment of individual cases, beginning with Freud's famous description of the therapy of Little Hans (Freud, 1909). Little Hans was, of course, not treated directly but through his father; subsequent reports deal with direct analysis of the child. Sterba (1935) treated a dog phobia in a $7\frac{1}{2}$ year old girl; Schnurmann (1949) described the analysis of a dog phobia in a child of $2\frac{1}{2}$. The phobia was interpreted as a manifestation of castration anxiety. The method of treatment adopted in the cases followed the familiar methods of psychoanalysis in children and will not be set out in detail here. The results are impossible to assess, because they are presented as uncontrolled single case studies.

At the other extreme lie supportive methods which attempt no more than the methods traditionally used by sensible parents. Jersild (1950) surveyed these. The most commonly used method was rational reassurance and explanation, but it was not the most effective method; indeed it seemed to have little value unless supplemented by another technique. Other methods identified by Jersild were: imitation of adults or peers; gradual passive-re-exposure; and active acquisition of skills in handling the feared situation. Hagman (1932) found that mothers reported that a combination of explanation and gradual re-exposure produced the best effect.

More recent developments in behavioural techniques arise from these traditional methods but have refined them and increased their efficiency. Systematic desensitisation either in practice or imagination is the usual method and it follows the same essential lines which were described with adults. Somewhat different means of inhibiting anxiety must be found in younger children, who do not easily learn the methods of relaxation which are used extensively in adults. The reassuring presence of an adult therapist can inhibit anxiety, and so can feeding. Younger children also find difficulty in calling up imagery in the precise way that is required in the desensitisation methods used in adults. Lazarus and Abramowitz (1962) have shown how games, stories and emotive imagery can serve the same purpose of exposing the child to carefully controlled and graded items in a hierarchy of anxiety provoking stimuli.

Unfortunately the results of desensitisation in children are as hard to assess as those of psychotherapy and for the same reason: reports are usually of single cases, or of very small series, and adequate control procedures are not included. In view of the high remission rates of fears and phobias in childhood, this latter precaution is essential. At present it is only possible to say that deconditioning methods, like psychoanalysis, can sometimes produce dramatic cures. How far the observed changes are related to the specific techniques which are used, is quite uncertain. This is a field where further research is urgently needed.

School phobias

It is not our purpose to enter into details of treatment in child psychiatry. Nevertheless some comments are required about the broad therapeutic lines which are to be followed. Several problems arise. Should the child be returned to school as early as possible? Should treatment focus on his professed fears of school, or are these rather displacements of fears which originate in the family and which can only be approached indirectly? How far should treatment be concerned with the child and how far with the parents?

Many authorities emphasise the need for prompt intervention and early return to school. Rodriguez et al. (1959) stressed this and could find no evidence that their policy of early return to school led to any other functional disturbance replacing the school phobia when psychiatric treatment was provided for the child and family. The same finding was reported by Waldfogel et al. (1959) and Glaser (1959). In the sample of Waldfogel et al. (1959) children treated by early return did much better than those who weren't. Rodriguez et al. even indicated the occasional need for legal action to overcome the parents' own problems in allowing the child's early return. Kahn (1958) points out that punishment alone nearly always fails as it increases the tension between parents and child and makes the child feel even more insecure.

On the other hand, Johnson et al. (1941) have suggested that all pressure to return to school should be removed until insight has been gained.

Eisenberg (1958) set out the contrary argument, namely that school is a very important part of the child's life. To keep the child away cuts him off from normal experience and further retards his psychological development.

This is one of the situations where no single rule will fit every case. Phobias which are not severe may respond well to immediate return to school, but if they are severe forced return to school can lead to increasing anxiety. A gradual exposure to school is more desirable. This can be arranged in milder cases simply by letting the mother accompany the child to school, first being with him in the classroom all the time, then going into a room nearby while the child remains in the classroom, and gradually increasing her distance and time away from the child until normal separation is effected. Enlightened schools encourage a policy along these lines and rapid resolution of the phobia can follow.

In more severe cases a therapist may need to participate in the treatment. The child may first be shown pictures of school, then taken by the therapist, then gradually spend longer and longer periods there himself. In this way he can return early, and keep the benefits of school life, without being exposed suddenly to overwhelming fear which provokes further insecurity and hostility to the therapist.

Of course, this programme of gradual re-exposure had been used by therapists on purely empirical grounds with no particular regard for learning theories. Talbot (1951) treated 24 children; social workers carried out a graduated programme even though their orientation was a psycho-dynamic one. A series of temporary plans were worked through on the same principle as a hierarchy in desensitisation.

Treatment of the child along these lines may need to be accompanied by social work or psychotherapy with the parents, usually with the mother. School phobia can in some instances be a family disorder, in which case treatment must be directed to the whole family if it is to succeed.

Outcome of school phobia

Assessment of results is difficult because no controlled studies have been made. Those reports which are available claim good results with a policy of early return to school. Few reports described the outcome of these cases in later life, but there are several follow-up studies a few years after treatment. Warren (1961) reported 16 patients (7 boys and 9 girls) who had been admitted to an adolescent unit after out-patient treatment had failed. They were followed up about 6 years later. Four were still handicapped by phobias, 3 were living lives limited by phobias and 3 more had shown other kinds of neurotic symptoms since discharge but were improving at the time of follow-up. Less than half (6) were well. The outcome was worse if school phobia was accompanied by additional phobias or other symptoms.

Rodriguez et al. (1959) followed 41 children (14 females and 27 males). The children's ages ranged from 5–13 with a mean age of 9·3 years. The cases were followed after an average of 3 years by telephone or by letter to parents and by studying school attendance records, but the children were not seen. Outcome depended partly upon the age of the children.   89% of those under 11 at the time of treatment were attending school regularly at the time of follow-up, but only 36% (14 children) of those who were over 11 when treated had returned to school by the time of follow-up. In those who returned to school there was no evidence that other obvious disturbances had replaced the phobias. Dunsworth (1961) also noted that prognosis was better in younger children.

Waldfogel et al. (1959) followed up 36 children with school phobia 6 to 18 months after treatment. Of the 20 who were treated by returning to school, 18 continued to attend school at follow-up without showing symptoms and 2 were at school with mild anxiety. The parents of another 7 patients had refused to allow the children to return to school at the time of treatment and in 4 cases treatment was not available. Of these 11 patients only 3 were attending school at the time of follow-up.

Glaser (1959) saw 38 cases of school refusal 1–2 years after treatment with emphasis on early return to school. Of these, 36 cases were in regular school attendance at follow-up, only 3 of whom had major persisting symptoms.

The prognosis of school phobia thus seems quite good for return to school, especially where treatment emphasises the importance of early return. It is not known whether these children are prone to other fears or disturbances when they become adults.

Section V. THE PSYCHIATRIC MANAGEMENT OF PHOBIC PATIENTS

In the community at large there are many phobics who do not require treatment because their phobias do not interfere with their lives or the phobias respond to simple measures. By the time a phobic reaches the psychiatrist, however, he is "already a highly selected, resistant patient. His friends, his environment and the patient himself will all have tried to cure him, and failed.   This is a patient who does not respond to 'easy' forms of therapy.   There may be many agoraphobic patients who benefit from such wild measures as a slap on the back or a kick in the pants, but these do not reach the doctor's office". (Miller, 1968b).

The psychiatric management of phobic patients presents special problems. Patients who seek help from psychiatrists for phobic complaints are not usually treated by any one technique alone, since they commonly have many problems which require a variety of approaches together. Skilled clinical assessment is necessary to evaluate the main problems and their management.

Phobias, like other neurotic symptoms, occur in a variety of clinical conditions. When a patient first presents with a phobic complaint a full psychiatric history and examination is essential to check whether the phobia is indeed the main problem, or whether it is a small aspect of another psychiatric disorder which requires treatment in its own right. For example phobias are often aggravated or begin de novo during depressive illnesses. It is common clinical practice to give antidepressant drugs to those patients whose phobias start abruptly in a depressive setting, and this often improves both the phobias and the depression. In such cases it is assumed that the phobias have a depressive basis, and the practice of giving antidepressant drugs is justifiable before embarking on a protracted course of desensitisation. The procedure is less warranted in phobic patients with lifelong personality disorder, insidious onset or prolonged course.

Paranoid schizophrenics may have marked fears of being watched by other people, together with delusions and hallucinations. Treatment of the schizophrenia alone, e.g. by administration of phenothiazine drugs, can alleviate all these problems together. It is possible that phobic symptoms in schizophrenia might be amenable to treatment in their own right, though attempts to do this have not been strikingly successful (Cowden and Ford, 1962). Multiple phobias are often found as part of an anxiety state, in which case the latter requires treatment. Minor phobias are frequently an incidental complaint in abnormal personalities, and treatment of the personality problem by psychotherapy may be more important than treatment of the phobic symptom.

In all cases the relative importance of the phobic problem has to be determined. If after full examination the phobic state appears to be the dominant handicap of the patient then it will require treatment in its own right. This section will outline the general principles. Particular techniques were discussed in detail earlier.

At the moment desensitisation is the most definitive technique for the reduction of phobias. Desensitisation is usually given both in imagination and in practice. The patient is asked to practise outside treatment that which he has learned to cope with easily inside treatment, and the therapist must actively support and encourage him in this at all times. The patient can keep a diary in which he is asked to enter a daily record of his activities. Limited targets are set which the patient feels can realistically be achieved without experiencing exhausting fear. The patient is instructed not to enter any situation which he feels will precipitate a panic attack. Sedative drugs may be necessary if the patient cannot avoid such situations in his everyday life—benzodiazepine derivatives such as chlordiazepoxide or diazepam are the commonest preparations used for this.

Focal phobias

When the phobia is a focal circumscribed problem in the absence of other complaints, then treatment presents little difficulty since the phobia should respond to desensitisation, though 20 or more sessions are usually necessary for worthwhile improvement to occur. In such cases one can hope realistically to eliminate most of the phobic problem.

Less circumscribed phobias

Unfortunately, most psychiatric patients are less straightforward, since their phobias are rarely monosymptomatic. The commonest variety of phobias seen clinically is that cluster of phobias known as the agoraphobic syndrome or phobic anxiety state. Here there are several phobias, often with a varying degree of other symptoms as well such as anxiety at rest, mild depression and obsessive-compulsive phenomena. When such patients have relatively few phobias and other problems, they are more likely to respond to desensitisation, and it is usually well worth while giving desensitisation to agoraphobics of this kind. However, the therapeutic aims will be less ambitious, and most patients will have some residual symptoms at the end of treatment. Treatment will have been rewarding if it helps patients back into their everyday activities with minimal avoidance despite occasional feelings of fear. A longer course of desensitisation will be necessary than in the most focal phobics, progress is likely to be more uneven, and retreatment may be necessary for occasional relapse. Patients may experience difficulty in achieving relaxation, and find it helpful to listen to a tape-recording or record of relaxation exercises at home every day. When background anxiety is a problem, sedative drugs in small doses may be valuable.

Depressive episodes may occur during or after treatment and produce setbacks in the improvement which was achieved by the hard work of desensitisation. During such periods it is wise to postpone further desensitisation until the depression has been relieved by antidepressant drugs, the iminodibenzyl derivatives (e.g. imipramine or amitriptyline) having the most to commend them. Depression may take up to a month to clear on appropriate medication, and desensitisation can then be resumed.

Agoraphobic patients often have minor setbacks after breaks in their activities due to enforced immobilisation. After a week in bed with flu, or a month in hospital with a broken leg, patients may find it more difficult to enter situations they were able to cope with previously. Desensitisation will need to be intensified at such times, and the patient will need active encouragement to overcome this setback and return to his previous capabilities.

Diffuse phobias

Patients who have diffuse phobias and much anxiety at rest usually have a severe form of the agoraphobic syndrome or phobic anxiety state. They are difficult to treat and may need intensive support over several years. Desensitisation is only useful in such patients to achieve very limited goals, e.g. in a severely agoraphobic man who has had to give up his job because he cannot face the bus journey from home to work, it would be sensible to spend much time simply desensitising him to the route to work, and so enabling him to resume employment, even though one leaves his many other fears and symptoms untouched. Apart from these restricted goals, the cost-effectiveness of desensitisation in such patients is so low as not to make it worthwhile. The therapist faces an endless sisyphean task in which hundreds of therapeutic hours may be wasted achieving modest results which are repeatedly lost because of relapse through fresh upsurges of anxiety which condition new phobias. However, after some years many of these patients lose their acute anxiety and panic attacks, and at that stage of "burnt out agoraphobia" desensitisation might be applied with great profit to the patient, whereas in the earlier acute phase it would not have been useful.

In patients with diffuse phobias, severe chronic anxiety is common and sedative drugs are necessary to control these, though there is a risk of addiction. Alcoholism occasionally complicates the picture when patients use alcohol to control their tension, and it may be necessary to admit the patient into hospital and protect him from stress until he has been "dried out". Panic attacks and depressive episodes can be improved by use of antidepressant drugs, and if these fail electroconvulsive shock treatment (ECT) may occasionally prove helpful. In patients whose tension and depression are severe a brief spell in the sheltered environment of hospital may be required.

A small number of such patients are handicapped for many years without any reduction in their chronic tension and phobias despite every form of intensive treatment. In such cases modified leucotomy has been beneficial, though such action would only be recommended as a last resort in the severest of cases.

Whether patients have diffuse or focal phobias, traditional psychotherapy has limited indications which were summarised earlier. These are a) when the patient presents with a phobia but is found to have troublesome interpersonal difficulties; b) when improvement of the phobia during treatment reveals secondary gains which prevent further progress; or c) when improvement of the phobia seriously upsets a dynamic equilibrium in the patient's relationship with others, in which case psychotherapy may be needed not only for the patient but also occasionally for the family, either together or separately, depending on the circumstances.

General supportive measures

Apart from specific therapeutic techniques, there are many other ways to help patients with phobic disorders. Each patient needs to be closely questioned on all factors which aggravate or improve his phobias, and to plan his treatment schedule accordingly. It is important at all times to maintain an attitude of support, and to encourage any efforts of the patient to gradually face phobic situations with confidence, if need be initially with sedative drugs. Patients are reassured if allowed to carry a small supply of such drugs around with them just in case a panic attack occurs unexpectedly. However, an exhibition of willpower alone is not a sufficient treatment régime. The patient should not be pushed too far into doing things for which he is not yet ready, since panic which results in avoidance will retard his progress. A fine balance needs to be struck of general encouragement of his initiative without straining him beyond his capacities. Friedman (1959) summarised the desirable attitude in a short verse:

> "Which Epitaph Shall be Mine?"
> She couldn't try
> For fear she'd die;
> She never tried
> And so she died

> or

> She couldn't try
> For Fear she'd die;
> But once she tried
> Her fears—they died.

At the same time regular practice of relaxation exercises at home is desirable and these are easier if the patient can play a record or tape recording of relaxation instructions whenever required. This may be in the therapist's voice or the patient can prepare his own version from a written script.

Patients usually find it easier first to enter phobic situations in the presence of a reassuring person, and then to do it alone. Agoraphobics find various simple stratagems of great benefit. They feel more confident while pushing a perambulator or a shopping basket on wheels, or if they walk around with a dog on a leash. Frequently it is easier for them to enter new situations outside at night rather than in the day, and to do it at a time when crowds of people are not expected. If they wish to practise going on a bus or train it is better to avoid rush-hour travel at the start, and to choose trains or buses which stop frequently so that they feel free to get out whenever they wish. In a cinema, theatre or church for the first few times they will be more relaxed sitting on an aisle seat near an exit, and as they get accustomed to it can allow themselves to sit in more central positions from which it is less easy to escape with speed and dignity. Some patients also find it easier to go out when it is raining, if they wear dark glasses, or if they chew gum or suck sweets during their ventures.

The majority of agoraphobics feel much safer in a car, and being able to drive a car themselves is a great boon which immediately enables them to extend the range of their activities and become more self-sufficient. If an agoraphobic can afford a car and learn to drive this should be encouraged enthusiastically, since this measure alone reduces their handicap considerably.

The telephone is another useful device for some agoraphobics. Women with severe agoraphobia may be afraid to be left alone at home, and their husbands may have been forced to remain at home for periods simply to keep their wives company. Such women feel safer when they have a telephone with which to call somebody if they are feeling particularly distressed. It also enables them to maintain contact with friends and relatives and so reduce their social isolation.

Agoraphobics often have a fear of heights and prefer to live on ground floor accommodation. The nearer their home is to shops, friends and helpful relatives, the easier their lives will be. They may need help in taking their children to and from school, or in getting to and from work if they are employed outside their home. Agoraphobics would benefit from a community service which gave them lifts to and from work, but this does not exist at present.

Special community services for patients with phobic disorders are rather limited at the moment. Phobic patients can obviously utilise existing services provided by general practitioners, psychiatric outpatient and inpatient departments, and day hospitals. They can also attend day centres if they cannot be left alone at home and need to be in a sheltered environment during the day. If the patient needs to find work suitable for his own particular disability help can be obtained through various employment agencies and personnel in the community, including the local labour exchange, disablement resettlement officer and industrial rehabilitation units and training centres. A patient may be able to work, for example, if the place of employment is a short walk or bus ride away from home, but fail to manage if he has to cross a crowded main road or change buses in order to get there. He may find it easier to work at his own place in a quiet room with a few other workers present rather than as part of a chain of workers or a busy assembly line which requires split second efficiency.

In Britain and Australia phobic patients have formed clubs in a few areas which arrange social activities and enable members to help one another. An extensive correspondence club has also been formed in Britain called The Open Door. This is a nationwide non-medical organisation which distributes a monthly newssheet and puts phobic subjects in touch with one another so that they can be of mutual help. Some members were referred by their medical advisers, but the majority joined in response to radio and television broadcasts and articles in newspapers and women's magazines which described typical agoraphobic symptoms in some detail. Membership in 1967 was 2,000, of whom 90% were women.

Prognosis

Before discussing the prognosis in phobic disorders it is necessary to dispel a myth which is prevalent about the prognosis of neuroses. This myth holds that about two-thirds of neuroses recover or improve markedly regardless of the treatment they undergo (Eysenck, 1952): The magic figure of two-thirds has often been seized on as a rough baseline which any new treatment ought to exceed to prove its worth. This misconception is unfortunate as the improvement rate of neuroses varies tremendously with the amount of improvement under consideration, the time when the improvement was measured and the clinical syndrome which is being discussed. In Eysenck's paper itself, for example, a paper by Denker is cited as finding that 45% of a series of psychoneuroses had recovered by 1 year, 27% by 2 years, 82% by 3 years, 87% by 4 years and 91% by 5 years follow-up. Eysenck arbitrarily selected the figure of 72% at 2 years as the "most suitable". A further 19 studies in his paper were cited as giving improvement rates varying from 41% to 77% with a mean of 64%. Unfortunately these percentages included not only "cured or much improved" but also the category "improved", which is much broader than Denker's criterion of "recovery", and is therefore not comparable. Furthermore, the time when improvement was measured was not stated for any of the papers other than that of Denker, nor was the clinical composition of the different series. The figures cited are therefore no guide to the clinician about prognosis. These points were further emphasised by Cooper et al. (1965), who found improvement rates in neurotic syndromes which varied from 0 to 100% depending upon the time and degree of improvement and the clinical syndrome concerned. The two-thirds improvement myth can thus be disregarded in any discussion of prognosis of phobic disorders, which form a small proportion of all neuroses.

Comparisons of various figures reported in the literature for the outcome of phobic disorders are not always meaningful. Most reports combine several varieties of phobias of unequal severity together, and use differing criteria of improvement with different forms of treatment and varying periods of follow-up. These variables significantly influence the results. Simply in terms of improvement agoraphobics improve more than animal phobics with desensitisation, but tend to improve slowly without treatment, unlike animal phobics which remain unchanged when left untreated in adults. However, despite such improvement agoraphobics tend to retain more disability than animal phobics after desensitisation. The longer the follow-up, the more the improvement which can be expected in some agoraphobics. Finally, how much improvement is reported depends upon whether the criterion is slight fluctuation or major change.

Phobias which begin as part of a depressive illness usually improve considerably as the depression clears, though a minority of patients are left with residual chronic phobias after such a depressive episode. Such phobias will be aggravated by subsequent depressive episodes and subside to their previous level as the depression clears once more.

Many patients have transient episodes of acute phobia, commonly of the agoraphobic variety, which last a few weeks or months and then clear completely and permanently. After road accidents or other traumas, short-lived fear of the situation concerned is frequent, but this disappears in most people unless the fear is reinforced by repeated trauma or if there is prolonged avoidance of the feared situation without opportunities for extinction of the fear by re-entry into the situation without dire consequences.

Once phobias have persisted continuously for a year or more then "spontaneous" recovery is much less likely to occur. Most series of phobic states in the literature are of this kind. Bearing in mind the difficulties in their interpretation, some of the results will be described.

Terhune (1949) described the outcome of 86 phobic outpatients, mainly of the agoraphobic variety. "Permanent relief from phobias" occurred in 67%, and "great improvement, working and living efficiently" in another 24%. It is not clear whether these figures refer to results at the end of treatment or an unspecified period of follow-up.

Friedman (1950) studied "travel phobics" in his private practice. Description of the patients makes it clear that they were similar to the outpatient agoraphobics of Gelder et al. (1967), but included patients with phobias of duration varying from 3 days to 32 years. At the end of treatment "recovery" was noted in 46% and "improvement" in a further 30%; males had a better prognosis and patients who were housebound had a worse outcome. Tucker (1956) reported "recovery" in 28% and "improvement" in a further 53% of 100 phobic outpatients, mainly of the agoraphobic type.

Roberts (1964) followed up 38 housewives (severe agoraphobics) for 1 to 16 years after they had been treated. At follow-up 24% were recovered without phobias (2 patients still needed treatment for depression and depersonalisation), 52% were improved in that they were able to leave their homes unaccompanied but still had their phobias, and 24% remained housebound. In this series the improvement was greater at discharge and decreased slightly over follow-up: 84% were improved at the time of discharge, 66% by 3-year follow-up and 53% at 5–16 year follow-up.

Sim and Houghton (1966) reported the outcome of treatment in 191 outpatients and inpatients, mostly of the agoraphobic kind. 45% of the patients had symptoms of less than 12 months duration. Six months after treatment 85% were improved, of whom 70% were much improved. Two to ten years later general practitioners reported 89% of them to be improved.

The outcome of desensitisation in several series of phobic patients was reported from the Maudsley Hospital (Marks and Gelder, 1965, Gelder and Marks, 1966; and Gelder et al. 1967). At the end of treatment in 2 series of severely agoraphobic outpatients about 45% were much improved while in 2 series of outpatients with less severe mixed phobias the percentage much improved was about 55% at the end of treatment. At the end of a year's follow-up the figures were not dissimilar. "Much improved" implied that patients were able to face phobic situations but still retained some fear and might still have a slight tendency to avoid them.

The prognosis of phobias might be summarised as follows: Acute phobias commonly remit completely after a short time. Once phobias have persisted for more than a year complete remission without treatment is less likely. In adults without treatment very circumscribed phobias such as phobias of animals, wind, darkness or examinations usually persist continuously and unchanged for many years. Such phobias are intensified by contact with the phobic situation, but most can improve markedly with desensitisation. With and without treatment the agoraphobic syndrome (phobic anxiety state) tends to run a fluctuating course over years and even decades. Periods of complete remission are rare once it has begun, but more than half of patients with less severe varieties will show useful improvement with treatment to the extent that they can lead reasonably active lives despite the persistence of residual symptoms. As long as panic attacks and anxiety at rest are continuing the phobias are unlikely to remit to any great extent.

Summary of Treatment of Phobias

Phobias are probably less likely to develop in children who grow in a milieu in which they are taught readiness to face difficulties and frightening situations. After sudden trauma it is probably wisest to return immediately into the situation connected with that trauma to prevent development of a phobia through cognitive rehearsal and repeated avoidance.

Once a phobia has developed and is causing persistent avoidance of the phobic situation more specific treatment is needed. Treatments for phobias abound, but few have been studied systematically. Desensitisation has been investigated the most thoroughly and is the commonest technique employed at present.

The procedure involves graduated exposure of the patient to phobic stimuli along a hierarchy of increasing intensity. First he visualises a series of images of phobic situations and later also goes out to meet those situations in practice. The idea of desensitisation was suggested independently by several workers since the beginning of this century, but the technique is now regarded as one of the behavioural psychotherapies.

Difficulties during desensitisation include problems in obtaining deep relaxation, problems in producing adequate visual imagery of the phobia, irrelevant or fluctuating hierarchies, and relapse of phobias which have already been desensitised. Lack of motivation may retard progress, and life situational problems can intrude into treatment.

At least 18 controlled studies of desensitisation have been completed in phobic subjects and patients, and more are in progress. Most of the studies were in volunteers with focal fears such as fears of snakes or spiders, stage fright or examination anxiety. An impressive uniformity of results has shown desensitisation to produce more change in the treated fear than did the corresponding control procedures, which included relaxation, suggestion and hypnosis, insight psychotherapy, drug placebo and no treatment or a period on a waiting list.

Desensitisation is an assembly of procedures which includes suggestions of improvement, praise of reports of progress, relaxation and exposure to phobic stimuli. Controlled studies suggest that all of these play a part and need to be combined together to produce the maximum effect. Most of the change can be thought of in terms of counterconditioning (pairing of the phobic stimulus with an opposing stimulus such as relaxation), operant conditioning (praise of the patient each time he makes small improvements) and cognitive rehearsal.

The more that psychiatric patients with phobias resemble phobic volunteers, the closer are the results of desensitisation in them to those in volunteers. Controlled clinical studies showed that in two separate groups of patients with more focal phobias, desensitisation produced significantly more improvement than did control procedures, but in 2 separate groups of severe agoraphobics desensitisation conferred no significant advantage over more traditional forms of hospital care. The type of patient being treated was a crucial variable, patients with circumscribed phobias and few other symptoms improving most with desensitisation. Predictors of poor response to desensitisation were the presence of agoraphobia, severe obsessions and other neurotic symptoms, high overt ("free floating") anxiety and physiological correlates of anxiety. Patients with severe agoraphobia improved significantly more once their free floating anxiety was relieved by modified leucotomy.

During follow-up after desensitisation most patients retain their improvement but are left with some residual disability. Desensitisation can be learned easily by clinicians, but it is time-consuming and boring, and is only applicable to a limited number of psychiatric patients. The cost effectiveness of the treatment is an important factor in determining whether to give it to a particular patient. In patients desensitisation is simply one tool in the total context of psychiatric management.

Desensitisation can be facilitated by administration in groups and by automated procedures, but these approaches are more applicable to volunteers than to patients. Controlled studies of intravenous short-acting barbiturates during desensitisation have not yet shown these to be particularly helpful adjuvants. Desensitisation produces rather better results with spaced than with massed practice, but it is not clear what the optimum rate should be. Desensitisation is most effective when given both in imagination and in practice, but this is not always feasible. Transfer of improvement from imagined to real situations is imperfect. A particularly powerful technique in volunteers is desensitisation in practice together with observation of live models gradually entering the phobic situation.

Processes other than relaxation which inhibit fear are eating, the presence of a trusted companion, self-assertion and sexual arousal. Each of these can be an aid to desensitisation in particular subjects. Subjects may give insightful statements about the origin of their phobias as they improve during desensitisation i.e. symptom alleviation can cause insight as well as result from it. Desensitisation can eliminate nightmares in which the content is the same as a phobia in the waking state.

Many processes other than desensitisation improve phobias, but most have not been tested thoroughly both in the laboratory and clinic. Modelling procedures are especially useful in eliminating fears in volunteers when combined with desensitisation, and can produce superior results to those of desensitisation alone. The uses of modelling in patients have not yet been explored properly. Flooding or implosion therapy is another promising technique which reduces fear in volunteers, but has not yet been tried adequately in patients. Paradoxical intention shares certain features with the method of flooding. Cognitive manipulation and rehearsal can also diminish fears in volunteers. Aversion relief has improved phobias in patients, but it is not yet acceptable clinically until further study shows it to be superior to less unpleasant treatments.

Relaxation techniques are helpful for patients mainly as an adjunct to desensitisation. Hypnosis can produce improvement by several mechanisms but is not a definitive treatment for phobias. Psychotherapy does not reduce phobias particularly well but is probably helpful for certain personality problems which occur with phobic disorders i.e. when a patient presents with a phobic disorder but is found to have troublesome personality difficulties, when improvement of a phobia by desensitisation discloses secondary gains from the phobia which prevent further progress, and when improvement of a phobia upsets a dynamic equilibrium in the patient's interpersonal relationships.

Certain drugs are good palliatives but not curatives for various features of phobic disorders. Both the phobic anxiety itself and background anxiety at rest away from the phobic situation can be relieved by sedative drugs, of which benzodiazepine derivatives such as chlordiazepoxide and diazepam are most commended at present. Panic attacks and depressive episodes are alleviated by anti-depressant drugs, the most suitable being iminodibenzyl derivatives such as imipramine or amitriptyline.

The psychiatric management of phobic patients requires full clinical assessment of the main problems and use of a variety of techniques appropriate to the patient's particular disorder. When phobias are part of another psychiatric disorder, that disorder requires treatment in its own right e.g. treatment of depression alone often alleviates secondary phobias as well. Where a phobic state is the dominant problem it requires definitive treatment. Where the phobia is a focal circumscribed problem it should respond well to desensitisation without much residual fear. Patients with less circumscribed fears will improve less with desensitisation alone, and where appropriate may also require sedative and antidepressant drugs. In the severest agoraphobics desensitisation is only useful for very limited aims of practical consequence to the patient, more support and drugs may be necessary, and the risk of addiction is greater. Hospitalisation for short periods may be necessary to tide patients over crises. Rarely, in the severest cases with chronic tension modified leucotomy is helpful.

Psychotherapy is indicated in any phobic disorders complicated by disabling interpersonal problems. Many supportive measures are useful for different patients e.g., provision of a telephone and car, a tape recording or record of relaxation instructions to take home, adjustment of their travel routine and daily activities to suit their individual needs.

BIBLIOGRAPHY

ABRAHAM, Karl (1913a): On the psychogenesis of agoraphobia in children. In Clinical Papers and Essays on Psychoanalysis, p. 42–3. New York, Basic Books 1955 (The Hogarth Press).

— (1913b): A constitutional basis of locomotor anxiety. In: Selected papers, London, Hogarth, 1948 (cited by Edward Weiss, 1964).

AGRAS, Stewart (1965): An investigation of the decrement of anxiety responses during systematic desensitisation therapy. Behav. Res. Ther. **2,** 267–260.

— (1966): Stimulus-response relationships in phobia. Paper to IV World Psychiatry Congress, Madrid, September, 1966.

— (1967): Transfer during systematic desensitisation therapy. Behav. Res. & Ther., **5,** 193–199.

— Sylwester, D. & Oliveau, D. (1969): The epidemiology of common fears and phobias. Awaiting publication.

AMBROSE, J. A. (1961): The development of the smiling response in early infancy. In: Determinants of Infant Behaviour. Ed. B. M. Foss, Methuen, London, p. 181.

— (1963): The concept of a critical period for the development of social responsiveness in early human infancy. In: Determinants of Infant Behaviour, Vol. II. p. 208–9. Ed. B. M. Foss, Methuen, London.

ANDREWS, J. D. W. (1966): Psychotherapy of phobias. Psychol. Bull., **66,** 455–480

ANGELINO, H., DOLLINS, J. & MECH, E. V. (1956): Trends in the "fears and worries" of school children. J. Genet. Psychol., **89,** 263–267.

(ANON.) F. H. (Mrs.) (1952): Recovery from a long neurosis. Psychiatry, **15,** 161–177.

(ANON.) Vincent (1919): Confessions of an agoraphobic victim. Am. J. Psychol., **30,** 295–299.

ARGYLE, M., & KENDON, A. (1967): The Experimental Analysis of Social Performance In: Advances in Experimental Social Psychology. Vol. 3. Ed. L. Berkowitz. New York and London, Academic Press.

ARIETI, S. (1961): A re-examination of the phobic symptom and of symbolism in psychopathology. Amer. J. Psychiat., **118,** 106–110.

ASHEM, B. (1963): The treatment of disaster phobia by systematic desensitisation. Behav. Res. Ther., **1,** 81–84.

AX, A. F. (1953): The physiological differentiation between fear and anger. Psychosom. Med. **15,** 433–442.

BAGBY, E. (1922–3): The etiology of phobias. J. abnorm. Psychol., **17,** 16–18.

BANCROFT, J. H. J. (1966): Aversion Therapy. Dissertation for Academic D.P.M., University of London.

— & MARKS, I. M. (1968): Electric aversion therapy of sexual deviations. Proc. Roy. Soc. Med., **61,** 796–798.

BANDURA, A. (1965): Vicarious processes. A case of no-trial learning. In: L. Berkowitz (Ed.) Advances in Experimental Social Psychology. Vol. II. New York, Academic Press, p. 1–55.

— (1967): Behavioural Psychotherapy. Scientific American, **216,** 78–86.

— (1968): Modelling approaches to the modification of phobic disorders. In Ciba Symposium on "The Role of Learning in Psychotherapy". Churchill, London.

— & MENLOVE, F. L. (1968): Factors determining vicarious extinction of avoidance behaviour through symbolic modelling. J. Pers. Soc. Psychol. In Press.

— & ROSENTHAL, T. L. (1966): Vicarious classical conditioning as a function of arousal level. J. Personal and Soc. Psychol., **3,** 54–62.

271

BANDURA, A., GRUSEC, J. E. & MENLOVE, F. L. (1967): Vicarious extinction of avoidance behaviour. J. Personal & Soc. Psychol., **5**, 16–23.

— ; BLANCHARD, E. D. & RITTER, B. J. (1968): The relative efficacy of desensitisation and modelling therapeutic approaches for inducing behavioural, affective and attitudinal changes. In preparation.

BARBER, T. X. (1962): Experimental controls and the phenomena of hypnosis: a critique of hypnosis: a critique of hypnotic research methodology. J. Nerv. Ment. Dis., **134**, 493–503.

— & HAHN, K. W. (1963): Hypnotic induction and "relaxation". Arch. Gen. Psychiat., **8**, 295–300.

BARLOW, D. H., AGRAS, S. & LEITENBERG, H. (1967): Control of classic neurotic "symptoms" through reinforcement and non-reinforcement. Paper to Association for Advancement of the Behavioural Therapies. Washington, D.C., September.

BAUM, M. (1966): Rapid extinction of an avoidance response following a period of response prevention in the avoidance apparatus. Psychol. Reports. **18**, 59–64.

BEARD, G. M. (1879): Morbid fear as a symptom of nervous disease. Hosp. Gaz., **6**, 305–308 (New York).

BEAUCHÊNE, E. P. C. De (1783): De l'Influence des Affections de l'Ame dans les Maladies Nerveuses des Femmes. (Cited by Errera, 1962). Méquignon, Amsterdam.

BENEDIKT, M. (1870): Uber Platschwindel. Allg. Wien. Med. Ztg. **15**, 488.

BERGER, S. M. (1962): Conditioning through vicarious instigation. Psychol. Review, **69**, 450–466.

BERLYNE, D. E. (1960): Conflict, Arousal and Curiosity. p. 122–127. McGraw-Hill, London.

BIGNOLD, B. C. (1960): Agoraphobia: A review of 10 cases. Med. J. of Australia, **2**, 332–333.

BORNSTEIN, B. (1931): Phobia in a 2½ year old child. Psychoan. Quart. **4**, 93–119.

BRADY, J. P. (1966): Brevital-Relaxation Treatment of neurosis. Paper to Symposium on Higher Nervous Activity, IV World Congress of Psychiatry, Madrid (Sept.).

BRADY, J. V. (1966): Autonomic and endocrine correlates of emotional conditioning in rhesus monkeys: In: Abstracts of XVIII Internat. Congress of Psychology, Moscow. Vol. I, p. 244.

— KELLY, D. & PLUMLEE, L. (1968): Autonomic and Behaviour responses of the rhesus monkey to emotional conditioning. Annals of N.Y. Acad. Sciences, —— In Press.

BROADHURST, P. L. & BIGNAMI, G. (1965): Correlative effects of psychogenetic selection: A study of the Roman High and Low Avoidance strains. Behav. Res. & Ther. **2**, 273–280.

BRODMAN, K. ERDMANN, A. J., LORGE, I., WOLFF, H. G. & BROADBENT, T. H. (1949): The Cornell Medical Index—an adjunct to medical interview. J. Amer. Med. Assoc., **140**, 530.

BRONSON, W. G. (1968): The fear of novelty. Psychol. Bull., **69**, 350–358.

BRU (1789): In Chambard, E. (1886): Ann. Med. Psychol., 7th ser. **4**, 198–207. Un cas de syphilophobie. (cited by Errera, 1962).

BUNNELL, B.N. (1966): Lesions of the amygdala and septal nuclei: effects upon aggressiveness and social dominance in rodents. Paper to XVIII Internat. Congr. of Psychol., Moscow, August. Abstracts Vol. I. p. 314–5.

BURTON, R. (1621): The Anatomy of Melancholy. 11th Ed. 1813, Vol. 1. London.

BUSS, A. H. (1961): The Psychology of Aggression (p. 102). John Wiley and Sons, New York.

CANNON, W. B. (1929): Bodily changes in pain, hunger, fear and rage. An account of researches into the function of emotional excitement. Harper and Row.

CARLSON, K. (1966): Aspects of avoidance learning stored subcortically. Paper presented to Eastern Psychological Association, New York, April.

CAUDILL, W. & DOI, L. T. (1963): Interrelations of psychiatry, culture and emotion in Japan. In: Galdston, I (Ed.) Man's Image in Medicine and Anthropology. Internat. Univ. Press. New York.

— & SCHOOLER, C. (1969): Symptom patterns and background characteristics of Japanese psychiatric patients. In: W. Caudill and Lin, T. (eds.) Mental Health Research in Asia and the Pacific. Honolulu, East-West Center Press.

CAUTELA, J. H. (1965): Desensitisation and insight. Behav. Res. & Ther., 3, 59–64.

— (1966): Desensitisation factors in the hypnotic treatment of phobias. J. Psychol., 64, 277–288.

CHARON, J. (1967): In Programme Notes to "A Flea in Her Ear", produced by The National Theatre, London.

CHAZAN, M. (1962): School phobia. Brit. J. Educ. Psychol., 32, 209–217.

CHURCH, R. M. (1959): Emotional reactions of rats to the pain of others. J. Compar. & Physiol. Psychol., 52, 132.

CLAPHAM, H. I., FREEMAN, T. & SCLARE, A. B. (1956): Some clinical observations on phobic states. Scottish Medical Journal, 1. (May) 165–172.

CLARK, D. F. (1963): The treatment of monosymptomatic phobia by systematic desensitisation. Behav. Res. Ther., 1, 63–68.

CLEVENGER, S. W. (1890). Heart disease in insanity and a case of panphobia. Alienist and Neurologist, VII, 535–543.

COHEN, S. I. & REED, J. (1968): The treatment of "nervous diarrhoea" and other conditioned autonomic disorders by desensitisation. Brit. J. Psychiat., 114, 1275–1280.

COHEN, M, E. & WHITE, P. D. (1950): Life situations, emotions and neurocirculatory asthemia (anxiety neurosis, neurasthenia, effort syndrome). Tr. Assoc. Res. Nerv. Ment. Dis., 29, 832–869.

CONNOLLY, J. (1830): An Inquiry concerning the Indications of Insanity. John Taylor.

COOK. S. W. (1939): A survey of methods used to produce "experimental neurosis". Amer. J. Psychiat., 95, 1259–1276.

COOKE, G. (1966): The efficacy of 2 desensitisation procedures. An analogue study Behav. Res. Ther., 4, 17–24.

COOLIDGE, J. E., WILLEN, M., TISSMAN, E., WALDFOGEL, S. (1960): School phobias in adolescence: a manifestation of severe character disturbance. Amer. J. Orthopsychiat., 30, 599.

COOPER, J. E., GELDER, M. G. & MARKS, I. M. (1965): Results of behaviour therapy in 77 psychiatric patients. Brit. Med. J., 1, 1222–1225.

COTT, H. B. (1940): Adaptive Coloration in Animals, pp. 387–9, p. 82. Methuen and Co.

COWDEN, R. C. & FORD, L. I. (1962): Systematic desensitisation with phobic schizophrenics. Amer. J. Psychiat., 119, 241–245.

CUMMINGS, J. D. (1944): The incidence of emotional symptoms in school children. Brit. J. Educ. Psychol., 14, 151–161 .

— (1946): A follow-up study of emotional symptoms in school children. Brit. J. Educ. Psychol., 16, 163–177.

CURRAN, D. & PARTRIDGE, M. (1963): Psychological Medicine. Livingstone, Edinburgh.

DALBIEZ, R. (1941): Psychoanalytical method and the doctrine of Freud. Longmans, London.

DARWIN, C. (1872): On the Expression of Emotions in Man and Animals. John Murray, London.

DAVISON, G. C. (1968): Systematic desensitisation as a counter-conditioning process. J. abn. Psychol., 73, 91–99.

DESCARTES, R. (1650): The Passions of the Soule, pp. 107–108. Martin and Ridley, London.

DEUTSCH, H. (1929): The genesis of agoraphobia. Internat. J. Psychoan. **10**, 51–69.

DIETHELM, O. (1936): Investigations with distributive analysis and synthesis. Arch. Neur. Psychiat., **35**, 484.

— (1936): Treatment in Psychiatry. The MacMillan Co., New York, p. 99.

DIGBY, K. (1644): In: Hunter, R. & MacAlpine, J. Three Hundred Years of British Psychiatry, 1963, p. 125. Oxford Univ. Press, London.

DIMOND, S. (1966): Imprinting and fear—a system governed by visual experience during the development of the embryo. Bull. Brit. Psychol. Soc. **19**, 63–4.

DIXON, J. J., de MONCHAUX, C. & SANDLER, J. (1957a): Patterns of anxiety: an analysis of social anxieties. Brit. J. Med. Psychol., **30**, 107.

— — — (1957b): Patterns of anxiety: the phobias. Brit. J. Med. Psychol., **30**, 34–40.

DOLLARD, J. & MILLER, N. E. (1950): Personality and Psychotherapy, pp. 157–158. McGraw-Hill.

DONNER, L. (1968): Effectiveness of a pre-programmed group desensitisation treatment for test anxiety with and without a therapist present. Ph.D. thesis, Rutgers State Univ. New Brunswick, N.J.

DUNSWORTH, F. A. (1961): Phobias in Children. Canad. Psychiat. Assoc. Journal, **6**, 291–294.

du SAULLE, Legrand (1895): De L'agoraphobie. Practicien, 8, 208–210. (Cited by Weiss, 1964).

— (1878): Étude clinique sur la peur des espaces (Agoraphobie des Alemands). Cited by Weiss, E. (1964), p. 2.

EDWARDS, J. G. (1965): Quantitative aspects of post-hypnotic effect. D.M. thesis. Univ. of Oxford.

EISENBERG, L. (1958): School phobia: a study in the communication of anxiety. Amer. J. Psychiat., **114**, 712–718.

EMERY, J. R. & KRUMBOLTZ, J. D. (1968): Standard vs. individualised hierarchies in desensitisation to reduce test anxiety. J. Counsel., Psychol. In Press.

ENGLISH, H. B. (1929): Three cases of the "conditioned fear response". J. abn. Soc., Psychol., **34**, 221–225.

ERNST, K. (1959): Die prognose der neurosen. Monogrm. Gesamtgeb. Neurol. Psychiat. **85**, Berlin, Springer Verlag.

ERRERA, P. (1962): Some historical aspects of the concept of phobia. The Psychiatric Quarterly, **36** (April), 325–336.

— & COLEMAN, J. V. (1963): A long-term follow-up study of neurotic phobic patients in a psychiatric clinic. J. nerv. ment. Dis., **136**, 267–271.

ERWIN, W. J. (1963): Confinement in the production of human neuroses: The barber's chair syndrome. Behav. Res. & Ther., **1**, 175–183.

EYSENCK, H. J. (1952): The effects of psychotherapy: An evaluation. J. consult. Psychol., **16**, 319–324.

— (1960): Behaviour Therapy and the Neuroses. Oxford: Pergamon Press.

— (1965): Letter to Editor. Brit. J. Psychiat., **111**, 1009.

— & EYSENCK, S. B. J. (1964): Manual of the Eysenck Personality Inventory. London.

— & RACHMAN, S. (1955): The application of learning theory to child psychology. In: Modern Perspectives in Child Psychiatry. (Ed. Howells, N. G.). Oliver & Boyd, Edinburgh.

FALCONER, M. A. & SCHURR, P. H. (1959): Surgical treatment of mental illness. In: Recent Progress in Psychiatry (Ed. Fleming, A. and Walk). London, Churchill, pp. 352–367.

FANTZ, R. L. (1958): Pattern vision in young infants. Psychol. Rec. **8.**
— (1961): The origins of form perception. Sci. American, 205 (May).
FENICHEL, O. (1944): Remarks on the common phobias. Psychoanal. Quart. **13,** 313–326.
— (1946): The Psychoanalytic Theory of Neurosis, p. 215. London, Routledge and Kegan.
FENZ, W. D. & EPSTEIN, S. (1966): Physiological reactions of experienced and novice parachutists as a function of the sequence of events leading up to and following a jump. Paper in Abstracts, Vol. II, p. 475, of XVIII Internat. Congr. of Psychol., Moscow.
FOLKINS, C. H., LAWSON, K. D., OPTON, E. M. & LAZARUS, R. S. (1968): Desensitisation and the experimental reduction of threat. J. abn. Psychol., **73,** 100–113.
FONBERG, E. (1963): Emotional reactions evoked by cerebral stimulation in dogs, pp. 47–49. In Bulletin de l'Academie Polonaise des Sciences Cl. II, Vol. XI, No. 1. Série des sciences biologiques.
— (1966): Emotional reactions evoked by electrical stimulation of subcortical structures and their role in the conditioning of alimentary and defensive reactions. Pages 125–129 in Symposium No. 3. Integrative forms of conditioned reflexes. Presented to XVIII Internat. Congr. of Psychol., Moscow, August.
FRANKL, V. E. (1960): Paradoxical Intention: A logotherapeutic technique. Amer. J. Psychother., **14,** 520–535.
FRANKS, C. M. & FRANKS, V. (1966): "Conditionability" as a general factor of man's performance in different conditioning situations. Paper in Abstracts Vol. I, p. 331 of XVIII Internat. Congr. of Psychol., Moscow.
FRAZIER, S. H. & CARR, A. C. (1967): Phobic Reaction. In: Freedman, A. M. & Kaplan, H. I. (Eds.). Comprehensive Textbook of Psychiatry. Williams and Wilkins, Baltimore.
FREEDMAN, D. (1965): Hereditary control of early social behaviour, pp. 149–155. In: B. M. Foss (Ed.): Determinants of Infant Behaviour III. Methuen.
FREEMAN, H. L. & KENDRICK, D. C. (1960): A case of cat phobia. Brit. Med. J. ii, 497–502.
FREUD, S. (1892): On the psychical mechanism of hysterical phenomena, pp. 24–6. In: Collected Works, Vol. I. Hogarth Press and Institute of Psychoanalysis.
— (1894): The justification for detaching from neurasthenia a particular syndrome: The anxiety neurosis, pp. 78–106. In: Collected Works, Vol. I. Hogarth Press and Institute of Psychoanalysis.
— (1895): A reply to criticisms on the anxiety neurosis, pp. 107–127. Collected Works, Vol. I, Hogarth Press and Institute of Psychoanalysis.
— (1909): A phobia in a 5-year old boy, p. 281. In: Collected Works, Vol. III, pp. 149–289. Hogarth Press and Institute of Psychoanalysis, London.
— (1913): Totem and Taboo, p. 127. Hogarth Press, London, 1955.
— (1919): Turnings in the world of psychoanalytic therapy. In: Collected Papers, **2,** 399–400. London, Hogarth Press and Institute of Psychoanalysis.
— (1950): From the history of an infantile neurosis. Collected papers, 3. London, Hogarth, p. 473–605.
FRIEDMAN, D. (1966a): A new technique for the systematic desensitisation of phobic symptoms. Behav. Res. & Therapy, **4,** 139–140.
— (1966b): Treatment of a case of dog phobia in a deaf mute by behaviour therapy. Behav. Res. & Ther. **4,** 141.
— & SILVERSTONE, J. T. (1967): Treatment of phobic patients by systematic desensitisation. Lancet, I, 470–2.
FRIEDMAN, J. H. (1950): Short term psychotherapy of "Phobia of Travel". Amer. J. Psychother., **4,** 259–278.

FRIEDMAN, P. (1959): The Phobias, chapter 15, pp. 292–306 in: American Handbook of Psychiatry, Vol. I. Ed. S. Arieti, Basic Books. New York.

GALE, D. S., STRUMFELS, G. & GALE, E. N. (1966): A comparison of reciprocal inhibition and experimental extinction in the psychotherapeutic process. Behav. Res. Ther. **4,** 149–156.

GALIBERT, J. (1963): Anxiety and conditioned reflex in agoraphobia. Evolut. Psychiat., **28,** 139–148.

GANTT, W. H. (1944): The Experimental Basis for Neurotic Behaviour. Psychosomatic Med. Monographs, **3,** Nos. 3 and 4.

— (1962): Factors involved in the development of pathological behaviour: Schizokinesis and autokinesis. In: Perspectives in Biology and Medicine, **5** (No. 4), pp. 473–482. Univ. of Chicago.

GARFIELD, Z. H., DARWIN, P. L., SINGER, B. A. & MCBREARTY, J. F. (1967): Effect of "in vivo" training on experimental desensitisation of a phobia. Psychol. Rep. **20,** 515–519.

GEER, J. H. (1965): The development of a scale to measure fear. Behav. Res. ; Ther., **3,** 45–53.

— (1966): Fear and autonomic arousal. J. abn., Psychol., **71,** 253–255.

— & SILVERMAN, I. (1967): Treatment of a recurrent nightmare by behaviour modification procedures. J. abn. Psychol., **72,** 188–190.

— & TURTELTAUB, A. (1967): Fear reduction following observation of a model. J. Person & Social Psychol., **6,** 327–331.

GELDER, M. G. & MARKS, I. M. (1966): Severe agoraphobia: A controlled prospective trial of behaviour therapy. Brit. J. Psychiat., **112,** 309–319.

— — (1968): Desensitisation and phobias: a crossover study. Brit. J. Psychiat. **114,** 323–328.

— — & WOLFF, H. H. (1967): Desensitisation and psychotherapy in the treatment of phobic states: A controlled enquiry. Brit. J. Psychiat., **113,** 53–73.

— & MATHEWS, A. M. (1968): Forearm blood flow and phobic anxiety. Brit. J. Psychiat., **114,** 1371–6.

GERZ, H. O. (1962): The treatment of the phobic and the obsessive-compulsive patient using paradoxical intention sec. Victor E. Frankl. J. Neuropyschiat. **3,** 375–387.

GEWIRTZ, J. L. (1961): A learning analysis of the effects of normal stimulation, privation and deprivation on the acquisition of social motivation and attachment. In: Determinants of infant behaviour, pp. 213–289. Ed. B. M. Foss. Methuen.

— & H. B. (1965): Stimulus conditions, infant behaviour and social learning in 4 Israeli child-rearing behaviours, pp. 161–179. In: B. M. Foss (Ed.): Determinants of infant behaviour III. Methuen.

GIBSON, E. J. & WALK, R. D. (1960): The "Visual Cliff". Scientific American, April.

GILL, M. M. & BRENMAN, M. (1943): Treatment of a case of anxiety hysteria by an hypnotic technique employing psychoanalytic principles. Bullet. Menninger Clinic., **7,** 163–171.

GLASER, K. (1959): Paediatrics, **23,** 371.

GLOOR, P. (1960): Amygdala. Chapter LVIII in Handbook of Physiology. Section I: Neurophysiology. Vol. II. Ed. John Field, Amer. Physiol. Soc.

GRAHAM, P. (1964): Controlled trial of behaviour therapy vs. conventional therapy: a pilot study. Unpublished D.P.M. dissertation: Univ. of London.

GRANT, Q. A. F. R. (1958): Age and sex trends in the symptomatology of disturbed children. D.P.M. dissertation, Univ. of London.

GROSSBERG, J. M. & WILSON, H. K. (1965): A correlational comparison of the Wolpe-Lang F. S. S. & Taylor M. A. S. Behav. Res. Ther., **3,** 125–128.

HAGMAN, E. (1932): A study of fears of children of pre-school age. J. Exp. Educ., **1**, 110–130.

HALL, G. S. (1897): A study of fears. Amer. J. Psychol., **8**, 147–249.

HANNAH, F., STORM, T. & CAIRD, W. K. (1965): Sex differences and relationships among neuroticism, extraversion and expressed fears. Perceptual and Motor Skills, **20**, 1214–1216.

HARE, E. H. (1965): Triennial Statistical Report, 1961–3. Bethlem Royal and Maudsley Hospital.

HARLOW, H. F. (1961): The development of affectional patterns in infant monkeys. In: Determinants of infant behaviour, p. 76. Ed. B. M. Foss Methuen.

— (1965): The affectional systems. In: Behaviour of Human Primates. Ed. by Schrier, A. M., Harlow & Stollnitz, Vol. II. Academic Press, N.Y.

HARPER, M. & ROTH, M. (1962): Temporal lobe epilepsy and the phobia-anxiety-depersonalisation syndrome. Compr. Psychiat., **3**, 129–151.

HASLERUD, G. M. (1938): The effect of movement of stimulus objects upon avoidance reactions in chimpanzees. J. comp. Psychol., **25**, 507-528.

HART, J. D. (1966): Fear reduction as a function of the assumption and success of a therapeutic role. Unpublished Master's thesis, Univ. of Wisconsin.

HEBB, D. O. & THOMPSON, W. R. (1954): The social significance of animal studies. In Handbook of Social Psychology, Vol. I, p. 554 (Ed. Gardner Lindzey). Addison-Wesley, Cambridge, Mass.

HENDERSON, D. & BATCHELOR, I. R. C. (1962): Henderson and Gillespie's Textbook of Psychiatry, 9th Edition. Oxford Univ. Press.

HERSOV, L. (1960a): Persistent non-attendance at school. J. Child Psychol. Psychiatry, **1**, 130–136.

— (1960b): Refusal to go to school. J. Child Psychol. Psychiat., **1**, 137–142.

HERZBERG, A. (1941): Short treatment of neuroses by graduated tasks. Brit. J. Med. Psychol., **19**, 19–36.

HILL, J. H., LIEBERT, R. M. & MOTT, D. E. W. (1968): Vicarious extinction of avoidance behaviour through films: An initial test. Psychol. Reports, **22**, 192.

HINGSTON, R. W. G. (1933): The meaning of animal colour and adornment, pp. 54–59, 142–145. Edward Arnold and Co., London.

HINKLE, L. E. & WOLFF, H. G. (1957): Health and the Social Environment. In: Explorations in Social Psychiatry, p. 131. (Eds.), Leighton, A. H., Clausen, J. A. & Wilson, J. N. Tavistock, London.

HIPPOCRATES: On Epidemics, V, Section LXXXII.

HITSCHMANN, E. (1913): Bemerkungen über Platzangst un andere neurotische Angstzustände. Int. Ztschr. f. Psa., **23**. (Cited by Fenichel, 1944).

HOENIG, J. & REED, G. F. (1966): The objective assessment of desensitisation. Brit. J. Psychiat., **112**, 1279–1283.

HOGAN, R. A. & KIRCHNER, J. H. (1967): Preliminary report of the extinction of learned fears via short term implosive therapy. J. abn. Psychol., **72**, 106–109.

— — (1968): Implosive, eclectic, verbal and bibliotherapy in the treatment of fears and snakes. Behav. Res. & Ther., **6**, 167–171.

HOLMES, F. B. (1936): An experimental investigation of a method of overcoming children's fears. Child Development, **7**, 6–30.

HUDSON, B. B. (1950): One trial learning in the domestic rat. Genet. Psychol. Monogr., **41**, 99–145.

INGRAM, I. M. (1961): Obsessional illness in mental hospital patients. J. Ment. Sci., **107**, 401.

IVEY, E. P. (1959): Recent advances in the psychiatric diagnosis and treatment of phobias. Amer. J. Psychother., **13**, 35–50.

JACKSON, J. H. (1879): In selected writings of John Hughling's Jackson Vol. I. On Epilepsy and Epileptiform Convulsions. Ed. J. Taylor, London. Hodder and Stoughton, 1937.

JASPERS, K. (1923): General Psychopathology, Springer Verlag, Berlin. Translated from German 7th ed. 1963, pp. 136–137. Manchester Univ. Press.

JERSILD, A. T. (1950): Child Psychology: 3rd Ed. Staple Press, London, pp. 260–284.

— & HOLMES, F. B. (1935): Children's Fears: Child Development. Monogr. No. 20.

— MARKEY, F. U. & JERSILD, C. L. (1933): Children's fears, dreams, wishes, daydreams, likes, dislikes, pleasant and unpleasant memories. Child Development Monogr. No. 12.

JOHN, E. (1941): A study of the effects of evacuation and air raids on pre-school children. Brit. J. Educ. Psychol. 11, 173–182.

JOHNSON, A., FALSTEIN, E., SZUREK, S. & SVENDSON, M. (1941): School phobia. Amer. J. Orthospychiat., 11, 702–711.

JONES, E. (1953): Sigmund Freud: Life and Work. Vol. I. Hogarth Press, London.

JONES, M. C. (1924a): The elimination of children's fears. J. exp. Psychol., 7, 382–390.

— (1924b): A laboratory study of fear: the case of Peter. Ped. Sem., 31, 308–315.

JONES, H. E. & M.C. (1928): Motivation and emotion: fear of snakes. Childhood Education, 5, 136–143.

JULIER, D. (1967): Agoraphobia in Men. D.P.M. Dissertation, Univ. of London.

KAHN, J. H. (1958): School refusal: some clinical and cultural aspects. Med. Officer, C, 337.

KARDINER, A. & SPIEGEL, H. (1941): War Stress and Neurotic Illness. Paul B. Hoeber, New York.

KATAN, A. (1937): The role of "displacement" in agoraphobia. Internat. J. Psychoan., (1951) 32, 41–50.

KELLOGG, R. (1959): What Children Scribble and Why. National Press Publications. Palo Alto.

KELLY, D. H. W. (1966): Measurement of anxiety by forearm blood flow. Brit. J. Psychiat., 112, 789–798.

— & WALTER, C. J. S. (1968): The relationship between clinical diagnosis and anxiety assessed by forearm blood flow and other measurements. Brit. J. Psychiat., 114, 611–626.

— WALTER, C. J. S. & SARGANT, W. (1966): Modified leucotomy assessed by forearm blood flow and other measurements. Brit. J. Psychiat. 112, 871–881.

KENDON, A. (1965): Some functions of gaze-direction in social interaction. (Unpublished). Institute of Exper. Psychol., Oxford.

KENNEDY, A. (1960): The general indications for psychological treatment. Lancet, 1, 1257.

KERRY, R. J. (1960): Phobia of outer space. J. Ment. Sci., 106, 1383–1387.

KIMBLE, G. A. (1961). Hilgard & Marquis' Conditioning and Learning. Methuen.

— (1966): Classical and instrumental conditioning: One process or two? Pages 55–62 in Symposium No. 4. Classical and instrumental conditioning. Presented to XVIII Int. Congr. Psychol., Moscow, August.

KING, A. (1962): Phenelzine treatment of Roth's calamity syndrome. Med. J. Aust., 1, 879–883.

— & LITTLE, J. C. (1959): Thiopentone treatment of the phobic-anxiety-depersonalisation syndrome. Proc. Roy. Soc. Med., 52, 595–596.

KIRCHNER, J. H. & HOGAN, R. A. (1966): The therapist variable in the implosion of phobias. Psychotherapy: Theory, research and practice, 3, 102–104

KLAUSNER, S. Z. (1966): The transformation of fear: A study of parachuting. Paper in Abstracts, Vol. II, p. 29 of XVIII Internat. Congr. of Psychol., Moscow.

KLEIN, D. F. (1964): Delineation of two drug-responsive anxiety syndromes. Psychopharmacologia, 5, 397–408.

KLEIN, E. (1945): The reluctance to go to school. Psychoanal. Study Child., 1, 263–292.

KOHLER, W. (1925): The Mentality of Apes. Routledge and Kegan Paul, London.

KOLANSKY, H. (1960): Treatment of a three-year old girl's severe infantile neurosis. Stammering and insect phobia. Psychoanal. Study Child., 15, 261–285.

KONDAS, O. (1967): Reduction of examination anxiety and "stage-fright" by group desensitisation and relaxation. Behav. Res. & Ther., 5, 275–281.

KRAEPELIN, E. (1913): Lectures on Clinical Psychiatry. Translation from 2nd ed., pp. 270–273.

KRAFT, T. & AL-ISSA, I. (1965): The application of learning theory to the treatment of traffic phobia. Brit. J. Psychiat., 111, 272–279.

KRAL, V. A. (1952): Psychiatric observations under severe chronic stress. Amer. J. Psychiat., 108, 105.

KRAUPL TAYLOR, F. (1966): Psychopathology: Its Causes and Symptoms, pp. 156–159. Butterworths, London.

KRIECKHAUS, E. E. (1966): The role of the mammillothalamic tract in conditioned avoidance behaviour. Paper in Abstracts, Vol. I, p. 312 of XVIII Internat. Congr. of Psychol., Moscow.

KRUSHINSKII, L. V. (1962): Animal Behaviour. Its normal and abnormal development. Consultants Bureau, N.Y. 1962. (Cited by Peters et al. 1966).

KUSHNER, (M.1965): Desensitisation of a post-traumatic phobia. In: Ullman, L. P. & Krasner, L. (1965): Case Studies in Behaviour Modification, pp. 193–196. Holt, Rinehart and Winston, New York.

LADEE, G. H. (1966): Hypochondriacal Syndromes. Elsevier, Amsterdam.

LADER, M. H. (1966): Predictive value of autonomic measures in patients with phobic states. D.P.M. Dissertation, Univ. of London.

— (1964): Effect of sedative drugs on autonomic measures in patients with anxiety. M.D. thesis, Univ. of Liverpool.

— & WING, L. (1966): Physiological Measures, Sedative Drugs and Morbid Anxiety. Maudsley Monograph No. 14. Oxford Univ. Press, London.

— GELDER, M. G. & MARKS, I. M. (1967): Palmar skin-conductance measures as predictors of response to desensitisation. J. Psychosom. Res. 11, 283–290.

LANCET (1952): Disabilities. Section entitled "Anxiety Neurosis", pp. 79–83.

LANDIS, C. (1964): Varieties of psychopathological experience. Ed. by F. A. Mettler, New York, Holt, Rinehart and Winston.

LANG, P. J. (1966): Fear reduction and fear behaviour. Problems in treating a construct. In 3rd Conference in Research in Psychotherapy, Chicago, Ill. June, 1966.

— (1968): The mechanics of desensitisation and the laboratory study of human fear. In: C. M. Franks, ed. Assessment and Status of the Behaviour Therapies. New York, McGraw-Hill.

— & LAZOVIK, A. D. (1963): Experimental desensitisation of a phobia. J. abn. soc. Psychol., 66, 519–525.

— LAZOVICK, A. D. & REYNOLDS, D. J. (1965): Desensitisation, suggestibility and pseudotherapy. J. abn. Psychol., 70, 395–402.

LANYON, R. I. & MANOSEVITZ, M. (1966): Validity of self-reported fear. Behav. Res. & Ther., 4, 17–24.

280   FEARS AND PHOBIAS

LAPOUSE, R. & MONK, M. A. (1959): Fears and worries in a representative sample of children. Amer. J. Orthopsychiat., **29**, 803–818.

LARSEN, S. R. (1965): Strategies for reducing phobic behaviour. Ph.D. Thesis. Stanford Univ., Calif.

LAUGHLIN, H. P. (1954): Fears and Phobias. Med. Annals of District of Columbia, **23**, 379–389, 441–448.

— (1956): The Neuroses in Clinical Practice. W. B. Saunders Co., London. Chapter on "The Phobic Reactions" (incl. p. 172).

— (1967): The Neuroses. Butterworths, Washington.

LAZARUS, A. A. (1961): Group therapy of phobic disorders by systematic desensitisation. J. abn. soc. Psychol., **63**, 504–510.

— (1963): The results of behaviour therapy in 126 cases of severe neurosis. Behav. Res. Ther., **1**, 66–79.

— (1966): Broad-spectrum behaviour therapy and the treatment of agoraphobia. Behav. Res. & Ther., **2**, 95–98.

— & ABRAMOVITZ (1962): The use of "emotive imagery" in the treatment of children's phobias. J. Ment. Sci., **108**, 191–5.

LE CAMUS, A. (1769): Medicine de l'Esprit. New Edition, Vol. I, pp. 259–265. Paris.

LEITENBERG, H., AGRAS, W. S., BARLOW, D. H. & OLIVEAU, D. C. (1968a): The contribution of selected positive reinforcement and therapeutic instructions to systematic desensitisation therapy. J. abn. Psychol., **73**,

— —, AGRAS, S., THOMSON, L. E. & WRIGHT, D. E. (1968b): Feedback in behaviour modification: an experimental analysis in two phobic cases. J. Applied Behav. Analysis, **1**, In Press.

LEONARD, W. E. (1928): The Locomotive God. Chapman and Hall.

LEONHARD, K. (1963): Individual therapie der Neurosen. Jena: Gustav Fischer Verlag.

LEVENSON, E. A. (1961): The treatment of school phobias in the young adult. Amer. J. Psychother., **15**, 539–552.

LEVINE, M. (1942): Psychotherapy in Medical Practice. New York, MacMillan, Co.

LEWIN, B. D. (1952): Phobic symptoms and dream interpretation. Psychoan. Quart., **21**, 295–321.

— (1935): Claustrophobia. Psychoan. Quart., **4**, 227–233.

LEWIS, A. J. (1938): Diagnosis and treatment of obsessional states. Practitioner, **141**, 21–30.

LIEF, H. A. (1955): Sensory association in the selection of phobic objects. Psychiatry, **18**, 331–338.

LITTLE, J. C. & JAMES, B. (1964): Abreaction of conditioned fear reaction after 18 years. Behav. Res. Ther., **2**, 59–63.

LOCKE, J. (1700): An essay concerning human understanding. In: The Philosophical Works of John Locke. Ed. St. John, J. A. (1913). G. Bell, London.

LOMONT, J. F. & EDWARDS, J. E. (1967): The role of relaxation in systematic desensitisation. Behav. Res. Ther., **5**, 11–25.

LURIA, A. C. (1961): The Role of Speech in the Regulation of Abnormal Behaviour, London.

MACALPINE, I. (1957): Syphilophobia: A psychiatric study. Brit. J. Vener. Dis., **33**, 92–99.

MACFARLANE, J. W., ALLEN, L. & HONZIK, M. P. (1954): A developmental study of the behaviour problems of normal children between 21 months and 14 years. Univ. of Calif. Press, Berkeley and Los Angeles.

MACRAE, D. (1954): On the nature of fear with reference to its occurrence in epilepsy. J. Nerv. Ment. Dis., **120**, 385–393.

MALAN, D. H. (1963): A study of brief psychotherapy. London, Tavistock publications.

MALLESON, N. (1959): Panic and Phobia: possible method of treatment. Lancet, 1, 225–227.

MANOSEVITZ, M. & LANYON, R. L. (1965): Fear Survey Schedule—a normative study. Psychol. Reports, 17, 699–703.

MARCHAIS, P. & JASON, M. (1962): De las hipothymie et du conditionnement dans la constitution des neuroses phobiques. Annales Medico-Psychologiques, 120, 572–577.

— — (1962): Attitude therapeutique dans les états phobiques survenus après hipothymie. Annales Medico-Psychologiques, 120, 577–583.

MARKS, I. M. (1965): Patterns of meaning in psychiatric patients: semantic differential responses in obsessives and psychopaths. Maudsley Monograph No. 13. Oxford Univ. Press.

— (1967): Components and correlates of psychiatric questionnaires. Brit. J. Med. Psychol., 40, 261-272.

— & GELDER, M. G. (1965): A controlled retrospective study of behaviour therapy in phobic patients. Brit. J. Psychiat., 111, 571–573.

— — (1966): Different onset ages in varieties of phobia. Amer. J. Psychiat., 123, 218–221.

— & HERST, E. (1969): The Open Door: A survey of agoraphobics in Britain. Awaiting publication.

— BIRLEY, J. L. T. & GELDER, M. G. (1966): Modified leucotomy in severe agoraphobia: A controlled serial inquiry. Brit. J. Psychiat., 112, 757–769.

— GELDER, M. G. & EDWARDS, J. G. (1968): Hypnosis and desensitisation for phobias: a controlled prospective trial. Brit. J. Psychiat., 114, 1263–1274.

— CROWE, M., DREWE, E., YOUNG, J. & DEWHURST, W. G. (1969): Obsessive neurosis in identical twins. Brit. J. Psychiat., 115. In Press.

MARTIN, I., MARKS, I. M. & GELDER, M. G. (1969): Conditioned eyelid responses in phobic patients. Behav. Res. Ther., 7, In Press.

MASSERMAN, J. H. (1943): Behaviour and Neurosis. Chicago, Univ. of Chicago Press.

— & YUM, K. S. (1946): An analysis of the influence of alcohol on experimental neurosis in cats. Psychosom. Med., 8, 36–52.

MATHEWS, A. M. & GELDER, M. G. (1969): A psychophysiological investigation of brief relaxation training. J. Psychosom. Res. In Press.

MAUDSLEY, H. (1895): The Pathology of Mind. London.

MAUPIN, E. W. (1962): Zen Buddhism: A psychological review. J. Consult. Psychol., 26, 362–378.

MECHANIC, D. (1962): The concept of illness behaviour. J. chron. dis., 15, 189–194.

— (1964): The influence of mothers on their children's health, attitudes and behaviour. Paediatrics, 33, 444–453.

— & VOLKART, E. H. (1961): Stress, illness behaviour and the sick role Amer. Sociol. Review., 26, 51–58.

MELAMED, B. & LANG, P. J. (1967): Study of the automated desensitisation of fear. Paper presented at Midwestern Psychol. Assoc. Convention, Chicago, Ill.

MELZACK, R. (1952): Irrational fears in the dog. Canad. J. Psychol., 6, 141–147.

MEYER, V. (1957): The treatment of two phobic patients on the basis of learning principles. J. abn. soc. Psychol., 55, 261–266.

MIGLER, B. & WOLPE, J. (1967): Automated self-desensitisation: a case report. Behav. Res. & Ther., 5, 133–135.

MILLER, M. L. (1946): Psychotherapy of a phobia in a pilot. Bull. Menninger Clinic., 10, 145.

— (1953): On street fear. Internat. J. Psychoan., 34, 232–252.

MILLER, N. E. (1951): Learnable drives and rewards, p. 435–472 in Handbook of Experimental Psychology, Ed. S. S. Stevens. Wiley, London.

— (1966): Experiments relevant to learning theory and psychopathology. Lecture to XVIII Internat. Congr. of Psychol., Moscow, August.

— (1968): In Ciba Symposium on "The Role of Learning in Psychotherapy". Churchill, London.

MOLL, A. (1891): Hypnotism. Walter Scott, London. (English translation of Der Hypnotismus, 1st Ed. Berlin, 1889).

MOORE, N. (1965): Behaviour therapy in bronchial asthma: a controlled study. J. Psychosom. Res. **9**, 257–276.

MORGAN, G. A. & RICCIUTI, H. N. (1967): Infants' response to strangers during the first year. In: Determinants of Infants Behaviour. Ed. B. M. Foss. Methuen.

MORRIS, R. & MORRIS, D. (1965): Men and Snakes. Hutchinson. Chapter 9, pp. 200–215.

MOSS, C. S. (1960): Brief successful psychotherapy of a chronic phobic reaction. J. abn. soc. Psychol., **60**, 266–270.

MOWRER, O. H. (1939): A stimulus response analysis of anxiety and its role as a reinforcing agent. Psychol. Rev., **46**, 553–565.

— (1947): On the dual nature of learning—a reinterpretation of "Conditioning" and "problem solving". Harv. Educ. Rev., **17**, 102–148.

— (1956): Two-factor learning theory reconsidered with special reference to secondary reinforcement and the concept of habit. Psychol. Rev. **63**, 114–128.

— & VIEK, P. (1948): An experimental analogue of fear. J. abn. soc. Psychol., **43**, 193–200.

MURPHREE, O. D., DYKMAN, R. A. & PETERS, J. E. (1966): Objective measures of behaviour in two strains of the pointer dog. Paper to Symposium on Higher Nervous Activity, IV World Psychiatry Congress, Madrid. (Sept.).

MURPHY, J. V., MILLER, R. F. & MIRSKY, I. A. (1955): Inter-animal conditioning in the monkey. J. Compar. & Physiol. Psychol., **48**, 211–214.

NAPALKOV, A. V. (1963): Information processes of the brain, pp. 64–67. In: Progress in Brain Research. Ed. Wiener and Schade, Elsevier, Amsterdam.

NURSTEN, J. P. (1958): The background of children with school phobia: A study of 25 cases. Med. Officer, **C**, 337–340.

OLDS, J. (1966): Chemical stimulation in subcortical reinforcement centres. In Abstracts of XVIII Internat. Congress of Psychol., Moscow., Vol. I, p. 243.

OSGOOD, C. E. (1953): Method and Theory in Experimental Psychology. Oxford Univ. Press.

PASKIND, H. A. (1931): A study of phobias. J. Neurol Psychopathol., **12**, 40–46.

PAUL, G. L. (1964): Modifications of systematic desensitisation based on a case study. Paper to 44th Annual Meeting of Western Psychol. Assoc., Portland, Oregon. (April).

— (1966): Insight versus Desensitisation in Psychotherapy: An experiment in anxiety reduction. Stanford Univ. Press.

— (1967): Insight versus desensitisation in psychotherapy two years after termination. J. consult. Psychol., **31**, 333–348.

— (1968a): Outcome of systematic desensitisation. In: Frank, C. M., Ed., Assessment and Status of the Behaviour Therapies. New York, McGraw-Hill.

— (1968b): A two year follow-up of systematic desensitisation in therapy. J. abn. Psychol. In Press.

— & SHANNON, D. T. (1966): Treatment of anxiety through systematic desensitisation in therapy groups. J. abn. Psychol., **71**, 124–135.

PERMAN, J. M. (1966): Phobia as a determinant of single-room occupancy. Amer. J. Psychiat., **123**, 609–613.

PETERS, J. E., MURPHREE, O. D., DYKMAN, R. A. & REESE, W. G. (1966): Genetically determined abnormal behaviour in dogs. Paper to Symposium on Higher Nervous Activity. IV World Psychiatry Congress, Madrid. (September).

PIAGET, J. (1966): Psychology, interdisciplinary relations and the system of sciences. Lecture to XVIII Internat. Congress of Psychol., Moscow.

PITTS, F. M. & McCLURE, J. N. (1967): Lactate metabolism in anxiety neurosis. New England J. Med. 277, 1329.

POLLITT, J. D. (1960): Natural history studies in mental illness. A discussion based on a pilot study of obsessional states. J. ment. Sci., 106, 93–113.

POPE, C. (1911): A note on tubercular phobia. The Medical Fortnightly, 39, 205–6.

PRATT, K. C. (1945): A study of the "fears" of rural children. J. Genet. Psychol. 67, 179–194.

PRINCE, M. (1898): Fear neurosis. Boston Med. Surg. J., 139, 613–616.

— & PUTNAM, J. J. (1912): Clinical study of a case of phobia: a symposium. J. abn. soc. Psychol., 7, 259–303.

RACHMAN, S. (1959): The treatment of anxiety and phobic reactions by systematic desensitisation psychotherapy. J. abn. soc. Psychol. 58, 259–263.

— (1965): Studies in Desensitisation I: The separate effects of relaxation and desensitisation. Behav. Res. Ther., 3, 245–251.

— (1966a): Studies in Desensitisation, II: Flooding. Behav. Res. & Ther. 4, 1.

— (1966b): Studies in Desensitisation, III: Speed of generalisation. Behav. Res. & Ther., 4, 7.

— (1968): Phobias. Their Nature and Control. Charles C. Thomas, Springfield, Illinois, Publication No. 721, American Lecture series.

— & COSTELLO, C. G. (1961): The aetiology and treatment of children's fears: A review. Amer. J. Psychiat., 118, 97–105.

RAMSAY, R. W. & VAN DIS, W. H. (1967): The role of punishment in the aetiology and continuance of alcohol drinking in rats. Behav. Res. & Ther., 5, 229–235.

— BARENDS, J., BREUKER, J. & KRUSEMAN, A. (1966): Massed versus spaced desensitisation of fear. Behav. Res. & Ther., 4, 205–7.

RANGELL, L. (1952): The analysis of a doll phobia. Internat. J. Psychoan., 33, 43.

RIGAL, J., RAYMOND, J. & FOURNIER, A. (1962): On agoraphobia appearing after intestinal amebiasis. Mechanism of conditioning. Ann. Medicopsychol., 120, 262–7.

RITTER, B. (1968): The group desensitisation of children's snake phobias using vicarious and contact desensitisation procedures. Behav. Res. & Ther., 6, 1–6.

ROBERTS, A. H. (1964): Housebound housewives—a follow-up study of a phobic anxiety state. Brit. J. Psychiat., 110, 191–197.

RODRIGUEZ, A., RODRIGUEZ, M. & EISENBERG, L. (1959): The outcome of school phobia. Amer. J. Psychiat., 116, 540–544.

ROGERSON, H. L. (1951): Venereophobia in the male. Brit. J. Vener. Dis. 27, 158–159.

ROSS, T. A. (1937): The Common Neuroses, p. 145. Edward Arnold, London.

ROTH, M. (1959): The phobic-anxiety-depersonalisation syndrome. Proc. Roy. Soc. Med., 52, 8, 587.

— GARSIDE, R. S. & GURNEY, C. (1965): Clinical Statistical enquiries into the classification of anxiety states and depressive disorders. In: Proceedings of Leeds Symposium on Behavioural Disorders. May and Baker.

RUBIN, B., KATKIN, R. & WEISS, G. (1968): Factor analysis of a fear survey schedule. Behav. Res. & Ther., 6, 65–76.

RUDDICK, B. (1961): Agoraphobia. Internat. J. Psychoanal., 42, 537–543.

RUTTER, M., TIZARD, J., & WHITMORE, K. (1968): Chapter 12 in Education, Health and Behaviour. Longman's, London.

RYLE, J. A. (1948): Nosophobia. J. Ment. Sci., **94**, 1–17.

SACKETT, G. P. (1966): Monkeys reared in isolation with pictures as visual input. Evidence for an innate relearning mechanism. Science, **154**, 1468–1472.

SANDERSON, R. E., CAMPBELL, D. & LAVERTY, S. G. (1962): Traumatically conditioned responses acquired during respiratory paralysis. Nature, **196**, 1235.

SARGANT, W. & DALLY, P. (1962): Treatment of anxiety states by antidepressant drugs. Brit. Med. J., **1**, 6–9.

SAUVAGES, F. B. de (1770–1): Nosologie Methodique. Translated by J. Nicolas. Vol. II, pp. 606–617. Herissant, Paris. (Cited by Errera, 1962).

SCHACHTER, S. (1957): Pain, fear and anger in hypertensives and normotensives. A psychophysiologic study. Psychosom. Med., **19**, 17–29.

— (1964): The interaction of cognitive and physiological determinants of emotional state. In: Psychobiological Approaches to Social Behaviour, pp. 138–173. Ed. P. H. Leiderman and D. Shapiro, Stanford Univ. Press, Stanford.

SCHACHTER, S. & SINGER, J. (1962) Cognitive, social and physiological determinants of emotional state. Psychol. Rev. , **69**, 379–399.

SCHERER, M. W. & NAKAMURA, C. Y. (1968): A fear-survey schedule for children (F.S.S.-F.C): A factor analytic comparison with manifest anxiety (CMAS). Behav. Res. & Ther., **6**, 173–182.

SCHILDER, P. (1921): Uber das Wisen der Hypnose. Berlin, Springer.

SCHILLER, P. H. (1952): Innate constituents of complex responses in primates. Psychol. Rev. , **59**, 177–191.

SCHMIDEBERG, W. (1951): Agoraphobia as manifestation of schizophrenia: analysis of case. Psychoanal. Rev., **38**, 343–352.

SCHNECK, J. M. (1952): Hypnotherapy of a patient with an animal phobia. J. Nerv. Ment. Dis., **116**, 48–57.

— (1954): The hypnoanalysis of phobic reactions, p. 465–476. In: L. M. Le Cron (Ed.). Experimental Hypnosis. MacMillan, New York.

SCHNEIRLA, T. C. (1965): Aspects of stimulation and organisation. In: Approach/ withdrawal processes underlying vertebrate behavioural development. In: Lehrman, D. S. Hinde, R. A. & Shaw, E. (Eds.) Advances in the study of behaviour, Vol. I, pp. 2–75. Academic Press, London and New York.

SCHNURMANN, A. (1949): Observations of a phobia. Psychoan. Study of the Child, **3–4**, 253–270.

SCHUBOT, E. D. (1966): The influence of hypnotic and muscular relaxation in systematic desensitisation of phobias. Unpublished. Ph.D. Stanford Univ.

SCHULTZ, J. H. & LUTH, W. (1959): Autogenic Training: Grune and Stratton. New York, N.Y.

SCOTT, R. B. (1966): Price's Textbook of Medicine, 10th Edition. Oxford Univ. Press.

SERGEANT, H. G. S. (1965): Systematic desensitisation. Unpublished D.P.M. dissertation. Univ. of London.

SHAKESPEARE, W. (1598): The Complete Works, p. 209. Oxford Univ. Press, London, 1955.

SHAPIRO, M. B., MARKS, I. M. & FOX, B.: (1963): A therapeutic experiment on phobic and affective symptoms in an individual psychiatric patient. Br. J. Soc. Clin. Psychol., **2**, 81–93.

SHERMAN, A. R. (1967): Therapy of maladaptive fear-motivated behaviour in the rat by the systematic gradual withdrawal of a fear-reducing drug. Behav. Res. & Ther., **5**, 131–129.

SHERRINGTON, C. S. (1952): The Integrative Action of the Nervous System, p. 98. Univ. of Cambridge Press.

SHIELDS, J. (1962): Monozygotic Twins brought up apart and brought up together. Oxford University Press.

SIDMAN, M. (1953): Avoidance conditioning with brief shock and no exteroceptive warning signal. Science, **118**, 157–158.

— (1955) On the persistence of avoidance behaviour. J. abn. soc. Psychol., **50**, 217–220.

SILVERMAN, I. & GEER, J. H. (1968): The elimination of recurrent nightmare by desensitisation of a related phobia. Behav. Res. Ther., **6**, 109–112.

SIM, M. & HOUGHTON, H. (1966): Phobic anxiety and its treatment. J. nerv. ment. Dis., **143**, 484–491.

SIMON, M. (1858): Du vertige nerveux et de son traitement. Mem. Acad. Med. Paris, **22**, 1–151. (Cited by Errera, 1962).

SLATER, E. (1939): Responses to a nursery school situation of 40 children. Soc. Res. Child Develop. Monogr. No. 4, Vol. 11, p. 7.

SLUCKIN, W. (1964): Imprinting and early learning. Methuen.

SMIRNOV, V. M. (1966): Neurophysiological Study of Human Emotion, pp. 116–118, in Symposium No. 3: Integrative forms of conditioned reflexes. Presented to XVIII Internat. Congr. of Psychol., Moscow. August.

SNAITH, R. P. (1968): A clinical investigation of phobias. Brit. J. Psychiat., **114**, 673–698.

SNOWDON, T., HAINSWORTH, F. R. & OVERMIER, J. P. (1966): Specific and permanent deficits in avoidance learning following forebrain ablation in the gold fish. Paper to XVIII Internat. Congr. of Psychol., Moscow. August. Abstracts, Vol. 1, p. 320.

SOLOMON, R. L. & TURNER, L. H. (1962): Discriminative classical conditioning in dogs paralysed by curare can later control discriminative avoidance responses in the normal state. Psychol. Rev., **69**, 202–219.

— & WYNNE, L. C. (1950): Avoidance conditioning in normal dogs and in dogs deprived of normal autonomic functioning. Amer. Psychologist, **5**, 264.

— — (1953): Traumatic avoidance learning: acquisition in normal dogs. Psychol. Monogr., **67**, No. 4 (Whole No. 354).

— — (1954): Traumatic avoidance learning: the principles of anxiety conservation and partial irreversibility. Psychol. Rev., **61**, 353–383.

— KAMIN, L. J. & WYNNE, L. C. (1953): Traumatic avoidance learning; the outcomes of several extinction procedures with dogs. J. abn. soc. Psychol., **48**, 291.

SOLYOM, L. & MILLER, S. B. (1967): Reciprocal inhibition by aversion relief in the treatment of phobias. Behav. Res. & Ther., **5**, 313–324.

SPENCE, K. W. (1964): Anxiety (Drive) level and performance in eyelid conditioning. Psychol. Bull. 1964, **61**, 129–139.

SPIEGLER, M. D., LIEBERT, R. M., McMAINS, M. J. & FERNANDEZ, L. E. (1968): Vicarious extinction of avoidance behaviour through a single presentation of a modelling film. Paper to A. Psychol. A. meeting.

SPITZ, R. (1965): The First Year of Life, p. 94. A psychoanalytic study of normal and deviant development of object relations. Internat. Universities Press, New York.

— & WOLFF, K. M. (1946): The smiling response: a contribution to the ontogenesis of social relations. Genet. Psychol. Monogr., **34**, 57–125, p. 68 and p. 81.

STENGEL, E. (1959): Classification of Mental Disorders. Bull. World Health Organ, **21**, 601–663.

STERBA, E. (1935): Excerpt from the analysis of a dog phobia. Psychoanal. Quart, **4**, 135.

STRAKER, M. (1951): Sickness fears: a manifestation of anxiety. Treat. Serv. Bull., **6**, 197–199.

TALBOT, M. (1951): Panic in school phobia. Amer. J. Orthopsychiat., **27,** 286–295.

TAYLOR, J. A. (1953): A personality scale of manifest anxiety. J. abn. soc. Psychol., **48,** 285–290.

TERHUNE, W. (1949): The phobic syndrome: A study of 86 patients with phobic reactions. Arch. Neurol. Psychiat., **62,** 162–172.

— (1961): The phobic syndrome: Its nature and treatment. J. Arkan. Med. Soc., **58,** 230–236.

THOMPSON, G. G. (1962): Child Psychology: Growth trends in psychological adjustment. Houghton Mifflin Co., Boston. 2nd Ed.

THORNDIKE, E. L. (1935): The Psychology of Wants, Interests and Attitudes, pp. 195–196. Appleton Century, London.

THORPE, J. G., SCHMIDT, E., BROWN, P. T. & CASTELL, D. (1964): Aversion relief therapy: A new method for general application. Behav. Res. & Ther., **2,** 71–82.

THORPE, W. H. (1961a): Sensitive Periods in the learning of animals and men. In: Thorpe, W. H. & Zangwill, O. L. (Eds.). Current problems in animal behaviour. Oxford University Press.

— (1961b): Introduction p. XXIII to King Solomon's Ring, by Lorenz, K. Z., Methuen, London.

TIMPANO, P. (1904): Clinical observation on a rare case of "phobia". J. ment. Path., **7,** 21–26.

TINBERGEN, N. (1951): The Study of Instinct (p. 31). Oxford University Press.

TOMKINS, S. (1963): Affect, Imagery, Consciousness. Vol. II, p. 157. N.Y. Springer Publishing Co.

TUCKER, W. I. (1956): Diagnosis and treatment of the phobic reaction. Amer. J. Psychiat., **112,** 825–830.

VALENTINE, C. W. (1930): The innate bases of fear. J. genet. Psychol., **37,** 394–419.

VALINS, S. & RAY, A. A. (1968): Effects of cognitive desensitisation on avoidance behaviour. J. Person & Soc. Psychol. **7,** 345–350.

WADA, J. A. (1961): Modification of cortically induced responses in brain stem by shift of attention in monkeys. Science, **133,** 40–42.

WAGNER, M. K. & CAUTHEN, N. R. (1968). A comparison of reciprocal inhibition and operant conditioning in the systematic desensitisation cf a fear of snakes. Behav. Res. & Ther., **6,** 225–227.

WALDFOGEL, S., COOLIDGE, J. & HAHN, P. (1957): Development, meaning and management of school phobia. Amer. J. Orthopsychiat., **27,** 754–780.

— TESSMAN, E. & HAHN, P. (1959): Learning problems III: A programme for early intervention in school phobia. Amer. J. Orthopsychiat., **29,** 324–332.

WALK, R. D. (1956): Selfratings of fear in fear-evoking situation. J. abn. soc. Psychol., **52,** 171–178.

— (1965): The study of visual depth and distance perception in animals. In: Lehrman, D. S., Hinde, R. A. & Shaw, E. (Eds.). Advances in the Study of Behaviour. Vol. I, pp. 99–154. Academic Press.

WALLIS, R. S. (1954): The overt fears of Dakota Indian children. Child Devel., **25,** 185–192.

WARBURTON, J. W. (1963): Some observations on the aetiology of phobic anxiety. Unpublished.

WARREN, W. (1965): A study of adolescent psychiatric in-patients and the outcome six or more years later. II. The Follow-up study. J. Child Psychol. Psychiat., **6,** 141–160.

WATSON, J. B. & RAYNER, R. (1920): Conditioned emotional reactions. J. exp. Psychol., **3,** 1–14.

WEBSTER, A. S. (1953): The development of phobias in married women. Psychol. Monograph, **67**, whole No. 367.

WEIL, A. A. (1959): Ictal emotions occurring in temporal lobe dysfunction. Arch. Neur., **1**, 87–97.

WEINBERG, N. H. & ZASLOVE, M. (1963): "Resistance" to systematic desensitisation of phobia. J. Clin. Psychol., **19**, 179–181.

WEISS, E. (1964): Agoraphobia in the light of ego psychology. Grune and Stratton, London.

— (1957): Ego disturbances in agoraphobia and related phenomena in the light of Federn's ego psychology. Psycho. **11**, 286–307.

WESTPHAL, C. (1871–2): Die agoraphobie: eine neuropathische erscheinung. Arch. für Psychiatrie und Nervenkrankheiten, **3**, pp. 138–171, pp. 219–221.

— (1878): Zwangvorstellungen. Archiv. Psychiat. Nervenkr., **8**, 734–750.

WICKERT, F. (Ed.) (1947): Psychological Research on Problems of Redistribution. Army Air Forces Aviation Psychology Program, Research Report No. 14. Washington, D.C.

WILLIAMS, D. (1956): The structure of emotions reflected in epileptic experiences. Brain, **79**, 29–67.

WILLMUTH, R. & PETERS, J. E. (1964): Recovery from traumatic experience in rats: Specific "treatment" vs. passage of time. Behav. Res. Ther., **2**, 111–116.

WILSON. G. D. (1966): An electrodermal technique for the study of phobias. N. Z. Med. J., **65**, 696–698.

— (1967a): Social desirability and sex differences in expressed fear. Behav. Res. & Ther., **5**, 136–137.

— (1967b): G. S. R. responses to fear related stimuli. Percept. Motor Skills, **24**, 401–402.

WING, L. (1965): Instruction Manual for Camberwell Register. M. R. C. Social Psychiatry Research Unit, Institute of Psychiatry, London.

WINOKUR, G., GUZE, S. B. & PFEIFFER, E. (1959): Developmental and sexual factors in woman: A comparision between control, neurotic and psychotic groups. Amer. J. Psychiat., **115**, 1097–1100.

— & HOLEMAN, E. (1963): Chronic anxiety neurosis: clinical and sexual aspects. Acta Psychiat. Scandin, **39**, 384–412.

— & LEONARD, C. (1963): Sexual life in patients with hysteria. Dis. Nerv. System, **24**, 1–7.

WITTENBORN, J. R. (1966): The Clinical Psychopharmacology of Anxiety. Charles C. Thomas, Springfield.

WOLFF, S. & WOLFF, H. G. (1947): Human gastric function. Oxford Univ. Press.

WOLPE, J. (1954): Reciprocal inhibition as the main basis of psychotherapeutic effects. Arch. Gen. Psychiat., **72**, 205.

— (1958): Psychotherapy by Reciprocal Inhibition. Stanford Univ. Press

— (1962): Isolation of a conditioning procedure as the crucial psychotherapeutic factor: A case study. J. nerv. ment. Dis. **134**, 316–329.

— (1964): Behaviour therapy in complex neurotic states. Brit. J. Psychiat. **110**, 28–34.

— (1965): Letter to Editor. Brit. Med. J., **1**, 1610.

— & LANG, P. J. (1964): A fear survey schedule for use in behaviour therapy. Behav. Res. Ther., **2**, 27–30.

— & LAZARUS, A. (1966): Behaviour Therapy Techniques. Oxford, Pergamon.

— & RACHMAN, S. (1960): Psychoanalytic "evidence". A critique based on Freud's case of Little Hans. J. nerv. ment. Dis., **130**, 135–148.

WOLPIN, M. & PEARSALL, L. (1965): Rapid de-conditioning of a fear of snakes. Behav. Res. Ther., **2**, 107.

— & RAINES, J. (1966): Visual imagery, expected roles and extinction as possible factors in reducing fear and avoidance behaviour. Behav. Res. & Ther., **4**, 25–37.

WOODWARD, J. (1959): Emotional disturbances of burned children. Brit. Med. J. **1**, 1009–1013.

WYNNE, L. C. & SOLOMON, R. L. (1955): Traumatic avoidance learning: acquisition and extinction in dogs deprived of normal peripheral autonomic function. Genet. Psychol. Monogr. **52**, 241–84.

YERKES, R. M. (1948): Chimpanzees: a laboratory colony. New Haven. Yale University Press.

— & YERKES, A. W. (1936): Nature and conditions of avoidance (fear) response in chimpanzees. J. Compar. Psychol., **21**, 53–66.

YORKSTON, N., SERGEANT, H. & RACHMAN, S. (1968): Methohexitone relaxation for desensitising agoraphobic patients. Lancet, **2**, 651–3.

ZBOROWSKI, M. (1952): Cultural components in response to pain. J. Soc. Issues, **8**, 16–30.

HUNTER, J. (1786): Treatise on Venereal Disease, in Hunter, R. & MacAlpine, J. Three Hundred Years of British Psychiatry, 1963, Oxford University Press, London.

MAY, R. (1950): The Meaning of Anxiety. Ronald Press, N.Y.

APPENDIX

Relaxation instructions from Wolpe and Lazarus (1966). In a good subject relaxation may be induced much faster than the times indicated, and many of the instructions may be omitted.

Relaxation of Arms (time: 4–5 min)

Settle back as comfortably as you can. Let yourself relax to the best of your ability . . . Now, as you relax like that, clench your right fist, just clench your fist tighter and tighter, and study the tension as you do so. Keep it clenched and feel the tension in your right fist, hand, forearm . . . and now relax. Let the fingers of your right hand become loose, and observe the contrast in your feelings . . . Now, let yourself go and try to become more relaxed all over. . . . Once more, clench your right fist really tight . . . hold it, and notice the tension again . . . Now let go, relax; your fingers straighten out, and you notice the difference once more . . . Now repeat that with your left fist. Clench your left fist while the rest of your body relaxes; clench that fist tighter and feel the tension—relax and feel the difference. Continue relaxing like that for a while. . . . Clench both fists tighter and tighter, both fists tense, forearms tense, study the sensations . . . and relax: straighten out your fingers and feel that relaxation. Continue relaxing your hands and forearms more and more . . . Now bend your elbows and tense your biceps, tense them harder and study the tension feelings . . . all right, straighten out your arms, let them relax and feel that difference again. Let the relaxation develop. . . . Once more, tense your biceps; hold the tension and observe it carefully . . . Straighten the arms and relax; relax to the best of your ability. . . . Each time, pay close attention to your feelings when you tense up and when you relax. Now straighten your arms, straighten them so that you feel most tension in the triceps muscles along the back of your arms: stretch your arms and feel that tension. . . . And now relax. Get your arms back into a comfortable position. Let the relaxation proceed on its own. The arms should feel comfortably heavy as you allow them to relax. . . . Straighten the arms once more so that you feel the tension in the triceps muscles; straighten them. Feel that tension . . . and relax. Now let's concentrate on pure relaxation in the arms without any tension. Get your arms comfortable and let them relax further and further. Continue relaxing your arms ever further. Even when your arms seem fully relaxed, try to go that extra bit further; try to achieve deeper and deeper levels of relaxation.

Relaxation of Facial Area with Neck, Shoulders, and Upper Back (time: 4–5 min)

Let all your muscles go loose and heavy. Just settle back quietly and comfortably. Wrinkle up your forehead now: wrinkle it tighter. . . . And now stop wrinkling your forehead, relax and smooth it out.   Picture the entire forehead and scalp becoming smoother as the relaxation increases. . . . Now frown and crease your brows and study the tension. . . . Let go of the tension again. Smooth out the forehead once more. . . . Now, close your eyes tighter and tighter. . . . Feel the tension . . . and relax your eyes. Keep your eyes closed, gently, comfortably, and notice the relaxation. . . . Now clench your jaws, bite your teeth together; study the tension throughout the jaws. . . . Relax your jaws now. Let your lips part slightly. . . . Appreciate the relaxation. . . . Now press your tongue hard against the roof of your mouth. Look for the tension. All right, let your tongue return to a comfortable and relaxed position. . . . Now purse your lips, press your lips together tighter and tighter. . . . Relax the lips. Note the contrast between tension and relaxation. Feel the relaxation all over your face, all over your forehead and scalp, eyes, jaws, lips, tongue and throat. The relaxation progresses further and further . . . Now attend to your neck muscles. Press your head back as far as it can go and feel the tension in the neck: roll it to the right and feel the tension shift; now roll it to the left. Straighten your head and bring it forward, press your chin against your chest. Let your head return to a comfortable position, and study the relaxation. Let the relaxation develop. . . . Shrug your shoulders, right up. Hold the tension. Drop your shoulders and feel the relaxation. Neck and shoulders relaxed. . . . Shrug your shoulders again and move them around. Bring your shoulders up and forward and back. Feel the tension in your shoulders and in your upper back. . . . Drop your shoulders once more and relax. Let the relaxation spread deep into the shoulders, right into your back muscles: relax your neck and throat, and your jaws and other facial areas as the pure relaxation takes over then grows deeper, deeper . . . ever deeper.

Relaxation of Chest, Stomach and Lower Back (time: 4–5 min)
Relax your entire body to the best of your ability. Feel that comfortable heaviness that accompanies relaxation. Breathe easily and freely in and out. Notice how the relaxation increases as you exhale; as you breathe out just feel that relaxation. . . . Now breathe right in and fill your lungs; inhale deeply and hold your breath. Study the tension. Now exhale, let the walls of your chest grow loose and push the air out automatically. Continue relaxing and breathe freely and gently. Feel the relaxation and enjoy it. . . . With the rest of your body as relaxed as possible fill your lungs again. Breathe in deeply and hold it again. . . . That's fine, breathe out and appreciate the relief; just breathe normally. Continue relaxing your chest and let the relaxation spread to your back, shoulders, neck and arms. Merely let go . . . and enjoy the relaxation. Now let's pay attention to your abdominal muscles, your stomach area. Tighten your stomach muscles, make your abdomen hard. Notice the tension. . . . And relax. Let the muscles loosen and notice the contrast. . . . Once more, press and tighten your stomach muscles. Hold the tension and study it. And relax. Notice the general well-being that comes with relaxing your stomach. Now draw your stomach in, pull the muscles right in and feel the tension this way. . . . Now relax again. Let your stomach out. Continue breathing normally and easily and feel the gentle massaging action all over your chest and stomach. . . . Now pull your stomach in again and hold the tension. . . . Now push out and tense like that; hold the tension. . . . Once more pull in and feel the tension. . . . now relax your stomach fully. Let the tension dissolve as the relaxation grows deeper. Each time you breathe out, notice the rhythmic relaxation both in your lungs and in your stomach. Notice thereby how your chest and your stomach relax more and more. . . . Try and let go of all contractions anywhere in your body. . . . Now direct your attention to your lower back. Arch up your back, make your lower back quite hollow, and feel the tension along your spine . . . and settle down comfortably again relaxing the lower back . . . just arch your back up and feel the tensions as you do so. Try to keep the rest of your body as relaxed as possible. Try to localise the tension throughout your lower back area. . . . Relax once more, relaxing further and further. Relax your lower back, relax your upper back, spread the relaxation to your stomach, chest, shoulders, arms and facial area. These parts relaxing further and further and further and ever deeper.

Relaxation of Hips, Thighs and Calves followed by Complete Body Relaxation
Let go of all tensions and relax . . . Now flex your buttocks and thighs. Flex your thighs by pressing down your heels as hard as you can . . . Relax and note the difference . . . Straighten your knees and flex your thigh muscles again . . . Hold the tension . . . Relax your hips and thighs. Allow the relaxation to proceed on its own . . . Press your feet and toes downwards, away from your face, so that your calf muscles become tense. Study that tension . . . Relax your feet and calves . . . This time, bend your feet towards your face so that you feel tension along your shins. Bring your toes right up . . . Relax again . . . Keep relaxing for a while . . . Now let yourself relax further all over. Relax your feet, ankles, calves and shins, knees, thighs, buttocks and hips. Feel the heaviness of your lower body as you

relax still further ... Now spread the relaxation to your stomach, waist, lower back. Let go more and more. Feel that relaxation all over. Let it proceed to your upper back, chest, shoulders and arms and right to the tips of your fingers. Keep relaxing more and more deeply. Make sure that no tension has crept into your throat; relax your neck and your jaws and all your facial muscles. Keep relaxing your whole body like that for a while. Let yourself relax.

Now you can become twice as relaxed as you are merely by taking in a really deep breath and slowly exhaling. With your eyes closed so that you become less aware of objects and movements around you and thus prevent any surface tensions from developing, breathe in deeply and feel yourself becoming heavier. Take in a long, deep breath and let it out very slowly ... Feel how heavy and relaxed you have become.

In a state of perfect relaxation you should feel unwilling to move a single muscle in your body. Think about the effort that would be required to raise your right arm. As you *think* about raising your right arm, see if you can notice any tensions that might have crept into your shoulder and your arm ... Now you decide not to lift the arm but to continue relaxing. Observe the relief and the disappearance of the tension ...

Just carry on relaxing like that. When you wish to get up, count backwards from four to one. You should then feel fine and refreshed, wide awake and calm.

Author Index

Abraham, K., 95, 119
Abramowitz, A. 230, 256
Agras, S., 6, 42, 66, 75, 76, 81, 124, 161, 169, 227
Ahrens, 25, 30
Allen, L., 75
Ambrose, J. A., 25, 29, 30
Andrews, J. D. W., 184, 248
Angelino, H., 169, 170
Argyle, M., 29
Arieti, S., 95
Ashem, B., 81, 159
Ax, A. F., 37, 39, 40, 41

Bagby, E., 87, 159
Bancroft, J. H. J., 55, 59, 69
Bandura, A., 62, 65, 191, 201, 226–8, 234–6
Barber, T. X., 246
Barlow, D. H., 241–3
Batchelor, I. R. C., 102
Baum, M., 61
Beauchène, E. P. C. de, 10
Benedikt, M., 10
Berger, S. M., 65
Berlyne, D. E., 26, 27
Bignami, G. 16
Bignold, B. C., 125
Birley, J. L. T., 83, 92, 217–221
Blanchard, E., 226–7
Bornstein, B., 95
Brady, J. V., 44, 49, 228
Bregman, 68
Brenman, M., 246
Brever, 90, 92
Broadhurst, P. L., 16
Brodman, K., 205
Bronson, W. G., 26, 28
Bru, 10
Bunnell, B. N., 47
Burton, R., 1, 8, 81, 139, 152, 160

Cannon, W. B., 36–7
Carlson, K., 47
Carr, A. C., 7, 77, 105, 181
Caudill, W., 155
Cautela, J. H., 231–2, 246
Cauthern, N. R., 243
Celsus, 3, 7, 179–180
Chazan, M., 173, 176
Chalmers Mitchell, 28
Church, R. M., 65
Clapham, H. I., 77
Clark, D. F., 147
Clevenger, S. W., 12, 73
Cohen, M. E., 84
Cohen, S. I., 166

Coleman, J. V., 77, 105, 125, 135
Connolly, J., 10
Cook, S. W., 135
Cooke, G., 225
Coolidge, J. E., 177
Cooper, J. E., 189, 203–5, 218, 265
Cott, H. B., 30
Cowden, R. C., 260
Cummings, J. D., 167
Curran, D., 102

Dalbiez, R., 95
Dally, P., 252
Darwin, C., 11
Davison, G. C., 93, 191, 194, 200, 201, 228
Denker, 265
Descartes, R., 90
Deutsch, H., 95, 140
Diethelm, O., 80
Digby, K., 8, 183,
Dimond, S. 20
Dixon, J. J., 130, 203
Doi, L. T., 155
Dollard, J., 59, 90
Donner, L. 191, 199–201, 223
Dunsworth, F. A., 169, 171, 176
du Saulle, L., 12, 134

Edwards, J. E., 191, 200, 228
Edwards, J. G., 214–216, 246
Eisenberg, L., 176, 257
Emery, J. R., 225
English, H. B., 62, 67–9
Epstein, S., 2
Ernst, K., 189
Errera, P., 3, 11, 77, 105, 125, 135
Erwin, W. J., 135
Eysenck, H. J., 67, 91, 184, 203, 207, 265

Falconer, M. A., 218
Fantz, R. L., 14, 21
Fenichel, O., 95
Fenz, W. D., 2
Folkins, C. H., 239
Fonberg, E., 45–47, 49, 57
Ford, L. I., 260
Frankl, V. E., 239–240
Franks, C. M., 64, 68
Frazier, S. H., 7, 77, 105, 181
Freedman, D., 17, 25
Freeman, H. L., 147
Freind, 10
Freud, S., 12, 90–2, 94–5, 99, 102, 119, 147, 149, 183, 233, 256
Friedman, D., 85, 147, 224
Friedman, J. H., 125, 128, 266

Friedman, P., 94, 263

Gale, D. S., 63
Galen, 9
Galibert, J., 88
Gantt, W. H., 62, 92
Garfield, Z. H., 225
Geer, J. H., 41 76–8, 232–3, 235
Gelder, M. G., 42, 74–5, 80, 83, 92, 107, 109, 125–8, 140, 143, 147, 156, 169, 199–223, 234, 245, 247, 249, 266–7
Gerz, H. O., 239
Gewirtz, J. L., 25
Gibson, E. J., 20
Gill, M. M., 246
Glaser, K., 257–8
Gloor, P., 47, 49
Graham, P., 168, 173
Grant, Q.A.F.R., 168
Grossberg, J. M., 76, 77, 78

Hagman, E., 81, 169–71, 255–6
Hall, G. S., 11, 18, 73, 77, 168
Hannah, F., 76–8
Hare, E. H., 77, 105, 112, 125–6
Harlow, H. F., 17, 19, 24, 26
Harper, M., 80, 127, 138
Haslerud, G. M., 29, 31
Hart, J. D., 235, 241
Hebb, D. O., 26
Henderson, D., 102
Hersov, L., 174–76
Herst, E. R., 81, 98, 124, 126, 247
Herzberg, A., 183
Hill, J. H., 235
Hingston, R. W. G., 30
Hinkle, L. E., 86
Hippocrates, 3, 7, 81, 102, 152
Hitschmann, E., 95
Hogan, R. A., 235, 237–9
Hohmann, G. W., 37–8
Holeman, E., 128
Holmes, F. B., 168, 170
Honzik, M. P., 75
Houghton, H., 124–5, 253, 267
Hudson, B. B., 91
Hunter, J., 10, 230–1, 240

Il-Issa, I., 85
Ingram, I. M., 165
Ivey, E. P., 89–90, 94

Jackson, J. H., 47
James, B., 88
James, W., 36
Jamieson, 30
Jason, M., 91
Jaspers, K., 3
Jersild, A. T., 32, 168–80, 181, 183, 255–6
John, E., 81, 171
Johnson, A., 257
Jones, E., 12, 89, 95, 126, 233

Jones, M. C., 29, 67, 89, 171, 183
Jones, H. E., 29
Julier, D., 76–7

Kahn, J. H., 257
Kardiner, A., 85, 181
Katan, A., 95
Kellogg, R., 30
Kelly, D. H. W., 42–3, 82, 107, 109
Kendon, A., 29
Kendrick, D. C., 147
Kennedy, A., 98
Kerry, R. J., 81, 159
Kimble, G. A., 55, 57–8, 69
King, A., 252–4
Kirchner, J. H., 235, 237–9
Klausner, S. Z., 2
Klein, D. F., 80, 120, 125–6, 138, 252
Kohler, W., 26
Kolansky, H., 147
Kondas, O., 191, 200–1, 223
Kora, 155, 240
Kraepelin, E., 12, 102
Kraft, T., 85
Kral, V. A., 5
Kraupl Taylor, F., 4, 5, 7, 153
Krieckhaus, E. E., 47
Krumboltz, J. D., 225
Krushinskii, L. V., 17
Kushner, M., 85

Ladee, G. H., 160
Lader, M. H., 41, 82–3, 93, 107, 109–10, 114, 138–9, 216–7, 245
Landis, C., 1, 133
Lang, P. J., 5, 49, 76–8, 105, 191–4, 199, 200–1, 215, 228–9, 234
Lange, 36
Lanyon, R. I., 76–8
Lapouse, R., 167–8, 170–1
Larsen, S. R., 235, 239, 246
Laughlin, H. P., 3, 6, 7, 81, 88, 90, 102, 140, 147
Lawlor, M., 30
Lazarus, A. A., 185–6, 189, 191, 199, 200, 207–8, 214, 216, 223, 229, 247, 249, 256, 289
Lazovick, A. D., 76–78, 191
Le Camus, A., 9
Leitenberg, H., 191, 198, 201–2, 241, 243
Leonard, C., 128
Leonard, W. E., 122
Leonhard, K., 184
Levenson, E. A., 177
Levine, M., 183
Lewin, B. D., 95
Lewis, A. J., 165
Lief, H. A., 89–90, 92, 247
Little, J. C., 88, 246, 253–4
Locke, J., 9, 90–1
Lomont, J. F., 191, 200, 228
Lorenz, K., 20
Luria, A. C., 66

Luth, W., 246

MacAlpine, I., 10, 162–3
Macfarlane, J. W., 75, 107, 167, 169, 171
MacLure, J. N., 84
Macrae, D., 48
Malan, D. H., 147
Malleson, N., 237, 240
Manosevitz, M., 76–8
Maranon, 39
Marchais, P., 91
Marks, I. M., 69, 74–5, 79–81, 83, 92, 98,
    107, 111, 116, 124–8, 130, 140, 143,
    147, 156, 165, 169, 119–223, 246–7,
    249, 254, 267
Martin, I., 82, 107, 109, 110, 114
Masserman, J. H., 60–1
Mathews, A. M., 42, 245
Maudsley, H., 12, 102
Maupin, E. W., 241
Mawson, A., 224
May, R. 170
Mechanic, D., 149, 248
Melamed, B., 191, 194, 199–201, 223,
    228
Melzack, R., 29
Menlove, F. L., 234–5
Meyer, V., 184
Migler, B., 223
Miller, M. L., 1, 15, 95, 119
Miller, N. E., 45, 55, 57–9, 61, 90, 203,
    260
Miller, R. F., 65
Miller, S. B., 244–5
Mirsky, I. A., 65
Moll, A., 246
Monk, M. A., 167–8, 171
Moore, N., 166
Morgan, G. A., 25
Morris, R. & D., 13, 28
Moss, C. S., 88, 147, 247
Mowrer, O. H., 57–9
Murphree, O. D., 16
Murphy, J. V., 65

Nakamura, C. Y., 77, 169
Napalkov, A. V., 61, 91
Nursten, J. P., 175

Olds, J., 45
Osgood, C. E., 66, 93

Partridge, M., 102
Paskind, H. A., 77, 124, 147
Paul, G. L., 66, 93, 191, 194–8, 199,
    200–1, 212–3, 223
Pavlov, I. P., 65
Pearsall, L., 147
Perman, J. M., 5
Peters, J. E., 16, 85, 181
Piaget, J., 14
Pitts, F. M., 84

Pollitt, J. D., 165
Pope, C., 161
Pratt, K. C., 168–70
Prince, M., 12, 80, 120, 127, 130, 182

Rachman, S., 67, 91, 95, 184–6, 191,
    200–1, 227, 230, 235, 237
Raines, J., 235, 239
Ramsay, R. W., 60, 224
Rangell, L., 4, 159, 250
Ray, A. A., 241
Rayner, R., 62, 67, 89, 91, 173
Reed, J., 166
Reynolds, D. J., 191
Ricciuti, H. N., 25
Rigal, J., 91
Ritter, B., 191, 201, 223, 225–8, 235–6
Roberts, A. H., 125, 127–8, 267
Rodriguez, A., 175, 257–8
Rogerson, H. L., 162
Rosenthal, T. L., 65
Ross, T. A., 3
Roth, M., 80, 111, 119, 125, 127–8,
    137–8, 253
Rubin, B., 77
Ruddick, B., 250
Rutter, M., 74, 126, 148, 156, 168, 173,
    255
Ryle, J. A., 80, 160–1

Sackett, G. P., 22, 172
Sanderson, R. E., 61
Sargant, W., 252
Sauvages, F. B. de, 10
Schachter, S., 36–41, 49, 241
Scherer, M. W., 77, 169
Schilder, P., 246
Schiller, P. H., 62
Schmideberg, W., 250
Scheck, J. M., 246
Schneirla, T. C., 18–21, 171
Schooler, C., 155
Schnurman, A., 256
Schubot, E. D., 191, 199–200, 228
Schultz, J. H., 185, 246
Schurr, P., 218
Scott, R. B., 102
Sergeant, H. G. S., 224
Shakespeare, W., 8
Shannon, D. T., 191, 194–6, 200–1, 223
Shapiro, M. B., 136
Sherman, A. R., 61, 251
Sherrington, C. S., 63
Shields, J., 17, 79
Sidman, M., 56, 60
Silverman, I., 232–3
Silverstone, T., 224
Sim, M., 124–5, 251, 253, 267
Simon, M., 10
Singer, J., 36, 241
Slater, E., 172, 174
Sluckin, W., 21
Smirnov, V. M., 45

Snaith, R. P., 111, 120, 125
Snowdon, T., 47, 59
Solomon, R. L., 37, 57–8, 61–2, 91, 245
Solyom, L., 244–5
Spence, K. W., 64
Spiegel, H., 85, 181
Spiegler, M. D., 235
Spitz, R., 25, 30
Spitzer, R., 77
Stekel, W., 94
Stengel, E., 102
Sterba, E., 95, 147, 250, 256
Straker, M., 80, 161

Talbot, M., 258
Taylor, J. A., 64
Terhune, W., 3, 77, 80, 125, 127, 128, 251, 266
Thompson, G. G., 169, 171
Thompson, W. R., 26
Thorndike, E. L., 68, 171, 173
Thorpe, J. G., 244
Thorpe, W. H., 14, 20
Timpano, P., 159
Tinbergen, N., 20
Tomkins, S., 30
Tucker, W. I., 80, 125, 127, 266
Turner, L. H., 58, 245
Turteltaub, A., 235

Valentine, C. W., 14, 17, 27, 31, 33–4, 69, 73
Valins, S., 235, 241
Van Dis, W. H., 60
Viek, P., 58
Vincent, 73, 122–3, 135
Volkart, E. H., 248

Wada, J. A., 30

Wagner, M. K., 243
Waldfogel, S., 174, 176, 257–8
Walk, R. D., 2, 3, 14, 20–1
Wallis, R. S., 170
Walter, C. J., 42
Warburton, J. W., 125
Warren, W., 258
Watson, J. B., 33–4, 62, 67, 89, 91, 173
Webster, A. S., 90, 127–8
Weil, A. A., 48–52
Weinberg, N. H., 186, 188–9
Weiss, E., 8, 11, 73, 80, 120, 134–5
Westphal, C., 11–2, 73, 102, 116, 133, 135
White, P. D., 84
Wickert, F., 2
Williams, D., 47–51
Willmuth, R., 85, 181
Wilson, G. D., 41, 43, 76–8
Wilson, H. K., 76–8
Wing, L., 41, 82–3, 103, 107, 217
Winokur, G., 128
Wittenborn, J. R., 250
Wolff, H. G., 39, 86
Wolff, H. H., 80, 140, 143, 208–12, 221
Wolff, K. M., 25, 30
Wolff, S., 39
Wolpe, J., 62–3, 77, 85, 91, 95, 147, 159, 184–86, 189, 207–8, 223, 230, 289
Wolpin, M., 147, 235, 239
Woodward, J., 173
Wynne, L. C., 37, 57, 62, 91

Yerkes, R. M., 17, 29, 31
Yorkston, N., 224
Yum, K. S., 60

Zaslove, M., 186, 188–9
Zborowski, M., 81
Zimmerman, 26

Subject Index

Abreaction, 88–9, 93, 98, 101, 239, 246

Acetylcholine, 253

Acquisition of fear, 57–60

Age incidence of phobias, 74–5, 100, 108–116

Agoraphobia, 5, 8, 10–12, 75, 80–3, 86, 89, 92–100, 106, 117–8
  in animals, 30–1

Agoraphobic factor, 111, 135

Agoraphobic syndrome, 108–114, 118–146
  acute phase, 141–4
  age of onset, 86, 125–6
  aggravating factors, 133–44
  anxiety in, 137–8
  autobiographical accounts, 121–4
  childhood background ,126–7
  clinical features in, 111–2, 129–44
  confinement, effect of, 135
  depersonalisation in, 138
  depression in, 136, 139, 218–9, 260–2, 266
  employment problems, 145–6
  family, effect on, 136
  leucotomy in, 143
  motivation, role of, 136, 140–4
  natural history of, 124–6
  non-phobic symptoms, 137–40
  obsessions in, 139–40
  onset of, 130–1
  organic disorders in, 140
  panic attacks in, 131–2, 137, 141
  personality background, 126–7, 143
  physiological features, 108–12, 130, 138
  precipitating factors, 128
  prevalence, 76, 124–6
  prognosis, 216–7, 220, 266–7
  reasons for treatment, 145–6
  relieving factors, 123, 133–44, 263–5
  response to desensitisation, 109–14, 143
  sex incidence, 124–6
  sexual function in, 127–8
  treatment of, 203–70
  willpower in, 123, 136, 140–4

Alcohol, for fear, 59–61, 70
  in phobias, 136

Alcoholism, 251, 262

Amitriptyline, 252–4, 262, 270

Androgens, 75–6, 78

Anger
  compared to fear, 39–41

Animals
  fear in, 16–47

Animals—(contd.)
  fear of, 33–4, 67, 74, 81–3
  phobias of, 86–9, 91, 94, 106–14, 118, 147–52
    age of onset, 147–8
    background in, 150
    clinical picture in, 150–2
    onset, 149
    reasons for treatment, 148–9
    sex incidence, 148

Antidepressant drugs, 252–4, 260, 262, 270

Antipathies, 9

Anxiety, 6, 86, 92, 99
  and conditioning, 64
  autonomic correlates of
    forearm blood flow, 42–3
    skin conductance, 41–2, 216–7
  free floating, diffuse, general, 83, 93, 116–7, 123, 194, 216–20, 251–2, 262, 269

Anxiety hysteria, 94, 119

Anxiety neurosis
  see "Anxiety state"

Anxiety state, 75, 80–5, 94, 105, 109, 112, 116, 120, 124, 132, 138

Approach-withdrawal
  alternation of, 21–7
  conflict, 27, 59–60
  stimuli producing, 18–25, 45–7

Assertion, as anxiety reducer, 230

Asthma, 166

Autogenic training, 185, 246

Autokinesis, 92

Autonomic equivalents to phobias, 165–6

Autonomic responses, operant conditioning of, 57
  Also see "Fear, autonomic components"

Aversion relief, 244–5, 269

Barbiturates, 59–60, 224, 250–4, 269

Behavioural psychotherapy, 182

Behavioural rehearsal, 230

Benzodiazepine drugs, 250–4, 261, 269

Biochemistry of fear, 43–5, 70, 84–5

Birds
  embryonic experience in, 20
  fear in, 19–22, 35
  fear of novelty, 27

Brain mechanisms subserving fear, 45–54, 57, 70

Burnt out habits, 99, 142, 262

Caesar, Augustus, 8

Calamity syndrome, 86

Catharsis, role of, 98–9
Children's fears and phobias, 66–9, 116, 166–77
  age incidence, 169–70
  associated disturbances, 171
  cultural influences, 170, 173
  family influences, 170
  incidence, 167–8
  modelling in, 34, 171
  of particular situations
    animals, 33–4, 67, 169, 170, 234–7
    dark, 33–4, 169, 170
    school, 172–7
    sea, 33, 35
    snakes, 29
    sudden movement, 31
    uncanniness, 27, 33–4
  sex incidence, 168
  treatment of, 183, 234–7, 255–9
Chimpanzees
  fear of novelty, 26
  fear of snakes, 28–9, 62–3
  fearfulness in twins, 17
Chlordiazepoxide, 250–4, 261, 270
Classification of phobias, 102–118
Claustrophobia, 75, 120
Cognitive manipulation, 235, 241, 269
Companionship relieving fear, 33, 62, 70, 98, 230, 256, 264, 269
Concentration camp, fear in, 5
Conditionability, 63–4, 68, 70, 82–3
Conditioned avoidance responses, 16–17, 45–7, 56, 70, 184, 245
  acquisition during curarisation, 58
  effect of sympathectomy, 62
  extinction of, 60–3, 70, 184
Conditioned emotional response, 57–9
Conditioned fear as drive, 58–60, 70
Conditioning of fear, avoidance, classical, escape instrumental, operant, 56–71, 90–4
  higher order responses, 58, 65, 93
  summation of responses, 58
Confinement, effect on fear, 31, 58
Contiguity learning, 58, 70, 91
Counterconditioning, 63, 93, 101, 184, 202–3, 268
Counterphobic behaviour, 6–7, 233
Cultural influences on phobias, 80–1, 99, 170, 173

Damocles, 8
Darkness, fear of, 33, 53, 75, 169, 170
Deconditioning, 184
Demosthenes, 8
Depersonalisation, 77, 93, 97, 99, 138
Depression, 86, 93, 98, 105, 115, 119, 121, 152, 218–9, 253, 260–2, 266, 270
Depressive illness, phobias in, 105, 260
Desensitisation, 8, 62–3, 82–3, 93, 101, 109, 182–233, 260–3, 268–70

Desensitisation—(contd.)
  anxiety during, 187
  automated, 194, 199, 223
  components of, 199–203
  cost effectiveness of, 222, 262, 269
  depression during, 187
  difficulties during, 186–9, 268
  dissociation during, 187–8, 228
  expectation of improvement in, 198–9
  facilitation of, 223–5
  hierarchies, construction of, 185, 188
      ,,   , standard vs. individually tailored, 225
  history of, 183–4
  imagery during, 187–8
  in autonomic disorders, 166
    groups, 223
    imagination vs. in practice, 225–7
    obsessive phobias, 164–5, 208
  indications for, 212, 220–1, 260–1, 269–70
  insight during, 231–2
  massed vs. spaced practice in, 224–5, 269
  motivation during, 187
  of nightmares, 232–3
  operant conditioning in, 202–3, 268
  positive reinforcement in, 194
  prognostic factors, 211–2, 216–7, 220–2, 268–70
  results of
    in patients, 203–223, 256, 268–70
    in volunteers, 189–203, 268
  speed of change during, 228
  technique, 184–6
  therapist, effect of, 194, 199, 223
  transfer of improvement, 227–8, 269
Diazepam, 250–4, 261, 270
Displacement of anxiety, 94–101
Dissociation, 228
Dogs, genetics of fearfulness in, 16–17
Dogs, as fear reducers, 59–61, 70
  in obsessions, 164
  in phobias, 224, 250–4, 260, 269–70
Drug dependence, 251, 262

ECT, 262
EEG during fear, 51–3
Emotions
  physiological and cognitive elements, 36–9, 69
Emotive imagery, 230, 256
Epilepsy and fear, 47–54, 70
Experimental paradigms of fear, 55–8, 70, 91
Extinction of fear, 60–3
Extroversion, 109
Eye spots, 30
Eyelid conditioning, 64, 108–117

Eyes
  as innate releasers, 25
  fear of, 29–30

Families, phobias in, 81
Fear (also see "Phobias")
  acquisition of, 57–60, 67–70
  adrenalin-produced, 39
  age influences, 74–5
  alternation to approach behaviour, 21–6
  as a trait, 16
  autonomic components, 36–45, 228–9
    compared with anger, 39–41
    forearm blood flow, 42–3, 69
    skin conductance, 41–2, 69, 78
  behavioural effects of, 1
  biochemistry of, 2, 43–5, 70, 84–5
  brain mechanisms in, 45–54, 70
  chronic effects of, 2
  cognitive components, 36–9, 49–51, 69
  components of, 5, 36–9, 46–51, 70, 77–8, 228–9
  disturbances associated with, 79–80
  EEG during, 51–3
  effect of confinement, 31, 58, 70, 91
  effect of social interaction, 22–6
  embryonic experience, 20
  enthusiasm and, 2
  epileptic fear, 47–54, 70
  evolution and, 11, 12
  experimental paradigms, 55–8, 70, 91
  extinction of, 60–3, 67–70
  genetics of, 16–18, 33, 35, 79, 100
  innate factors, 13–35
  learning of, 36–71
    physiological mechanisms, 36–54, 69–70
    psychological mechanisms, 55–71
  maintenance of, 58–60, 69
  maturational factors, 15–35
  modelling in, 34, 64–5, 69–70
  phylogenetic influences, 18
  physiological aspects, 2, 11, 36–54, 69
  postictally, 51, 53–4
  relieving factors
    antagonistic responses, 62–4, 229–30
    assertion, 230, 269
    companionship, 33, 62, 70, 98, 230, 256, 264, 269
    drugs, 59–61
    feeding, 62–3, 70, 229, 256, 269
    sexual stimuli, 62, 70, 230, 269
  sex incidence of, 75–8
  species specifity of, 16
  species variability of, 17
  superstitions, 6, 9
  symbolic aspects, 65–7, 71, 81
  temporal lobe and, 48–54
Fear of particular situations, 18–35
  animals, 33–4, 67, 74, 99, 169, 170, 225, 234–7
  dark, 33–4, 53, 75, 169, 170

Fear of particular situations—(contd.)
  fear, 4
  gaze, 29–30, 74
  heights, 20–1, 30, 32, 35, 73
  illness, 74–5, 94
  light, 30–2, 35
  noise, 32, 35, 74, 99, 170, 183
  novelty, 26–8, 33–5
  parachuting, 2–3
  snakes, 5, 28–9, 35, 62–3, 76, 105, 169, 200–1, 225–8, 235
  space, 31–2, 99
  spiders, 42
  strangers, 25–6, 32, 73–4, 99
  sudden movement, 29, 31, 33, 35, 73–4
  threat displays, 22–3, 35, 172
  thunder, 75
  uncanny. See "novelty"
  unfamiliar. See "novelty"
Fear Survey Schedules, 76–9, 192
Feydeau, 12
Flooding, 60–2, 200, 235–240, 269
Forearm blood flow, 42–3, 69, 108–118
Freud, fears of, 89, 94–5, 126
Frigidity, 93, 99

Gaze, fear of, 30, 74, 85, 152–6
Generalisation gradient, 66–7
Genetics of fearfulness, 16–18, 33, 79, 100
Germanicus, 9
Guilt in phobias, 91, 99

Habituation, 184, 245
  of galvanic skin response, 41, 83, 216–7
Hawk effect, 16, 19–20
Heights, fear of, 20–1, 30, 32, 35, 55, 73, 75, 92, 158, 233
Henry III of France, 10
Hydrophobia, 3, 7, 179
Hyerhydrosis, 166
Hypochondriasis, 115, 160
Hysteria, 91–2
  conversion, 80

Illness phobias, 74–6, 115, 159–63
Iminodibenzyl derivatives, 252–4, 270
Imipramine, 252–4, 262, 270
Imitative learning, 64, 67
Implosion. See "Flooding"
Impotence, 159, 230–1, 240
Imprinting, 21–2, 25, 83, 172
Infants
  experience, role of, 14
  fear of heights, 21, 32, 35, 73
    movement, 32
    noise, 32, 35
    strangers, 25–6, 32, 35, 55
    uncanny, 27
  innate responses in, 14, 25–6
  maturation in, 14

Infants—(*contd.*)
  smiling response, 25, 30
  visual perception in, 20
Innate fear responses, 13–34, 55, 69,
  73–4, 171
  as unconditioned response, 20
  effect of social interaction, 23
  interaction with learning, 33, 35, 55,
    69, 73
Innate releasing mechanism, 20, 22–4, 30
  as unconditioned stimulus, 20
Insight and improvement, 88–9, 231–2

James I of England, 9
James–Lange theory of emotions, 36–9

Kenophobia, 110, 120

Lactate as anxiety producer, 84–5
Lag phase in development of phobias,
  85, 92, 101, 181
Latent fear, 15
Learning of fear, 14, 36–71, 89–93
  acquisition, 57–60, 70
  different kinds of learning, 56–7
  facilitatory periods for, 83
  in single trial, 61, 91–2
  interaction with innate elements, 34,
    69
Learning theory, 90–4, 101
Leucotomy, 92, 117–8, 143, 217–20,
  254–5, 263, 270
Light, fear of, 30–2, 35
Light deprivation, 20, 21
Locomotor anxiety, 110, 119
Logotherapy, 239

Maintenance of fear, 58–60
Manzoni, 10
Maturation of fear, 13–35, 74, 167, 171
Meditation, 241, 246
Meprobamate, 251
Methohexitone, 224, 254
Modelling, 34, 64–5, 171, 173, 225–7,
  234–7
Monkeys (Also see "Chimpanzees")
  approach behaviour, 24–6
  biochemical changes during fear, 44–5
  different components of emotion, 228
  fear of particular situations
    gaze, 30
    heights, 21
    novelty, 26–7, 35
    snakes, 28–9, 35
    strangers, 55
    threat displays, 22–3, 35, 172
  modelling of fear in, 65
Monoamine oxidase inhibitors, 252
Montaigne, 9
Montanus, 8
Morel, 11
Morita therapy, 240
Mother, as relief stimulus, 27–8

Motion parallax, 21
Movement, fear of, 29, 31, 33, 35, 73–4

Neuroticism, 109
Nicanor, 7
Nightmares, as expression of phobias,
  232–3
Noise, fear of, 32, 35, 74, 99, 170, 183
Normal fear, 8, 11, 13–69, 106–7
Nosophobia, 160
No-trial learning, 64
Novelty, fear of, 26–8, 33, 35

Obsessions, 6, 8, 79, 93, 98–9, 102, 105,
  112, 119, 124, 269
Obsessive phobias, 106, 115, 163–5
Open Door, The, 124, 144–6, 265
Operant conditioning, 56–71, 90–4, 202,
  241–4

Panic, 6, 90
Panic attacks, 83, 86, 92–3, 119, 131–2,
  207, 220, 252, 262, 267, 270
Parachuting, fear during, 2–3
Paradoxical intention, 239–41, 269
Paranoid delusions, 6
Pascal, 8
Personality disorders, phobias in, 105,
  260
Personality of phobic patients, 80, 99,
  219–20
Phenothiazine drugs, 250–4, 260
Phobias (also see "Fear")
  acute phase, 85–6, 181
  aetiology, 72–101, 116–7
  associated symptoms, 79–80, 93, 99
  autonomic changes in, 82–3
    eyeblink conditioning, 82–3, 99,
      108–118
    forearm blood flow, 42–3, 82–3, 99,
      108–118
    skin conductance, 41–2, 53–4, 66–7,
      69, 78 82–3, 108–118, 164–5,
      216–7, 227
  autonomic equivalents to, 165–6
  classification of, 102–118
  components of, 5, 36–9, 46–51, 70,
    77–8, 228–9
  concealment of, 4
  definition, 3
  difficulties in recognising, 5
  discrimination from allergy, 8
  effect of expressing emotion, 98–9
  effect of psychological pressure, 5
  exposure, influence of, 74
  external situations, 105–115, 118
  extinction of, 93
  family influences on, 80–1, 89
  genetics of, 79
  historical aspects, 7–12

Phobias—(*contd.*)
incidence, 74–7, 107
  age, 74–5, 99, 108–115
  sex, 75–8, 99
internal situations, 105–6, 115–6, 118
marital problems and, 99–100
maturational influences on, 74
modelling of, 79, 89
  (also see "Modelling")
obsessive, 106, 115, 163–5
onset age of, 108
onset of, 85–9, 93
personality background in, 80, 143, 180–1
phylogenetic influences, 11, 72–4, 100
physiological aspects, 2, 36–54, 69, 93, 99
postictal, 51, 53–4
prevention of, 180–1
prognosis, 211–2, 216–7, 220–2, 234, 258–9, 265–7
reasons for treatment, 48–9, 145–6, 248–9
relieving factors, 11, 73, 98 (also see "Fear")
secondary gain from, 99
selective attention in, 4, 151
symbolic aspects, 65–7, 71, 81, 90–101, 247
treatment of, 178–270
trauma, role of, 85–9, 91–3, 99–100, 122, 173, 181–2, 266, 268
will power in, 9, 123, 136, 140–4
Phobias of particular situations, 4, 72
(also see "Fear")
animals, 74, 79, 81, 86, 88, 94, 106
being grasped from behind, 87–8
darkness, 158
dental treatment, 159
falling, 158
heat, 89
heights, 73, 92, 158, 233
illness and death, 66–7, 74–6, 80–1, 106, 115, 159–63
injections, 159
insanity, 81, 97
open spaces, 72, 79, 81 (also see "Agoraphobia")
school, 74, 173–7, 257–9
sharp instruments, 81
snakes, 76, 105, 191–4, 200–1, 243
social situations, 75, 82–3, 106, 118, 152–7
spiders, 95–6, 147, 151, 200, 235
texture, 159
thunderstorms, 92, 158
travel, 72, 79, 97, 140, 159
vomiting, 154
water, 87
wind, 159
Phobic-anxiety-depersonalisation syndrome, 80, 86, 110, 119, 121, 139
Phobic anxiety state, 110, 119, 121, 155

Phobic clubs, 124, 144–6, 265
Phobic disorders vs. phobic symptoms, 105, 118, 124, 260–1
Phobic patients, psychiatric management of, 222–3, 260–1, 269–70
Phobic state, 105, 118
Phobos, 3
Platzangst, 110, 120
Platzschwindel, 10
Postictal phobias, 51, 53–4
Preoccupations, 6
Prevention of phobias, 180–1
Pseudoconditioning, 15
Pseudoneurotic schizophrenia, 120
Psychiatric management of phobic patients, 222–3, 260–1, 269–70
Psychoanalysis, 249–50, 256
Psychotherapy, indications for, 249
  (also see "Treatment of phobias")
Punishment training, 56, 70

Rats
  extinction of conditioned responses, 61, 63
  fear of light, 30–1
  genetics of fearfulness, 16
  modelling of fear, 65
Recall of forgotten traumas
  effect on phobias, 86–9, 101
Reciprocal inhibition, 63, 184
Relaxation, 185–7, 199–200, 202, 215, 245, 263, 268–9
  instructions for, 289–91
Representational mediation process, 66–7, 101
Repression, 87, 94, 98
Responses antagonistic to fear, 229–30

Schizophrenia, phobias in, 105
Schonberg, Duke of, 10
School refusal, 74, 173–7, 257–9
  distinction from separation anxiety, 176
Second signalling system, 65, 93
Secondary gain, 99
Selective attention in phobias, 4, 151
Sensitive ideas of reference, 6
Sensory association, 89–90, 101
Separation anxiety, 80, 97–8, 176
Sex incidence of phobias, 75–8, 99
Sexual deviations, 69
Sexual fears, 96, 159
Sexual role, influence on phobias, 75–8
Shinkeishitsu, 155
Sidman avoidance schedule, 56
Single trial learning, 61, 91–2
Skin conductance (also see "Phobias, autonomic changes")
  after relaxation, 245
  as prognostic variable, 216–7, 220
  during anxiety and fear, 41–2, 53–4, 66–7, 69, 78, 93

Skin conductance (*contd.*)
  habituation of, 41, 101–118, 216–7, 220
  in phobic disorders, 108–118, 164–5, 216–7, 220
Smiling response in infants, 25, 30
Snakes. See "Fear of particular situations".
Social fears, 29–30, 152, 182
Social learning, 64
Social phobias, 75, 82–3, 99, 106, 109, 113–4, 118, 152–7, 166
  clinical features, 108–9, 113–4, 153–6
  onset, 156–7
  physiological features, 109, 113
  reasons for treatment, 156
Social reinforcement, 242
Soterias, 7
Space, fear of, 31–2, 72–4
Spiders, fear of, 42, 95–6, 147, 151, 200, 235
Spinal cord lesions, emotions after, 37–9
Stage fright, 182, 194–8
Stimulus generalisation, 89–90, 92, 101
Stimulus prepotency, 18–9, 22, 34–5, 69, 72–4, 100, 116
Strangers, fear of, 25–6, 32, 55, 73–4
Street fear, 119
Superstitious fear, 6, 107
Symbolism of fear, 65–7, 81, 90–101, 247
Syphiliphobia, 10, 162–3
Symptom substitution, 220

Taboos, 6
Tavistock phobic inventory, 111
Temporal lobe and fear, 48–54
Temporal pacing, 56, 70
Test anxiety, 200–1, 225, 237
Theresienstadt, 5
Timidity, 16–18, 33, 35, 64, 99
  twin studies of, 17, 79
Thiopentone, 253–4
Topophobia, 110
Trauma in origin of phobias, 74, 85–9, 91–3, 266
Treatment of phobias, 63, 97–8, 178–270
  (also see "Desensitisation")
  abreaction, 88–9, 93, 239, 246
  acetylcholine, 253
  after trauma, 181–2
  amitriptyline, 252–4, 262, 270
  autogenic training, 185, 246
  automated, 194, 199, 223, 238–9

Treatment of phobias—(*contd.*)
  aversion relief, 244–5, 269
  chlordiazepoxide, 250–4, 261, 270
  cognitive manipulation, 235, 241
  community services, 264–5
  desensitisation, 182–233
  diazepam, 250–4, 261, 270
  drugs, 224, 250–4, 263, 269–70
  ECT, 262
  expectation of improvement, 198, 201–2
  exposure, 181–3, 199–202, 227, 238, 248, 255–7, 268
  faith healing, 247
  flooding, 200, 235–40, 269
  hypnosis, 88–9, 185, 191–4, 199–202, 214–6, 239, 245–6, 268–9
  imipramine, 252–4, 262, 270
  leucotomy, 92, 217–220, 254, 263, 270
  limited goals in, 261, 270
  methohexitone, 224, 254
  modelling, 180–1, 201–2, 225–7, 234–7, 255–6, 269
  Morita therapy, 240
  operant conditioning, 202, 241–4
  positive reinforcement, 198, 202
  psychoanalysis, 249–50, 256
  psychotherapy, 97–9, 183–4, 195–7, 199, 202, 208–15, 232, 239, 247–9, 260, 268–70
  relaxation, 185–7, 199–200, 202, 215, 245, 263, 268–70
  social reinforcement, 241–4
  supportive measures, 263–5, 270
  therapeutic relationship, 202
  therapist, effect of, 194, 199, 200, 223, 238–9
  thiopentone, 253–4
  transfer of improvement, 227–8
Truancy, 174
Tully, 8
Two-factor theory, 57–9

Uncanniness, fear of. See "Novelty"

Vertigo hypocondriaque, 10
Vertigo hysterique, 10
Vicarious learning, 64–5
  Also see "Modelling"
Visual cliff, 20–1, 30
Visual perception, 14, 21

War neuroses, 85, 88, 181–2
Writer's cramp, 126